Hormone Receptors in Breast Cancer

Cancer Treatment and Research
Steven T. Rosen, M.D., *Series Editor*

Burt, R.K., Brush, M.M. (eds): *Advances in Allogeneic Hematopoietic Stem Cell Transplantation.* 1999. ISBN 0-7923-7714-1.
Angelos, P. (ed.): *Ethical Issues in Cancer Patient Care* 2000. ISBN 0-7923-7726-5.
Gradishar, W.J., Wood, W.C. (eds): *Advances in Breast Cancer Management.* 2000. ISBN 0-7923-7890-3.
Sparano, J. A. (ed.): *HIV & HTLV-I Associated Malignancies.* 2001. ISBN 0-7923-7220-4.
Ettinger, D. S. (ed.): *Thoracic Oncology.* 2001. ISBN 0-7923-7248-4.
Bergan, R. C. (ed.): *Cancer Chemoprevention.* 2001. ISBN 0-7923-7259-X.
Raza, A., Mundle, S.D. (eds): *Myelodysplastic Syndromes & Secondary Acute Myelogenous Leukemia* 2001. ISBN: 0-7923-7396.
Talamonti, M. S. (ed.): *Liver Directed Therapy for Primary and Metastatic Liver Tumors.* 2001. ISBN 0-7923-7523-8.
Stack, M.S., Fishman, D.A. (eds): *Ovarian Cancer.* 2001. ISBN 0-7923-7530-0.
Bashey, A., Ball, E.D. (eds): *Non-Myeloablative Allogeneic Transplantation.* 2002. ISBN 0-7923-7646-3.
Leong, S. P.L. (ed.): *Atlas of Selective Sentinel Lymphadenectomy for Melanoma, Breast Cancer and Colon Cancer.* 2002. ISBN 1-4020-7013-6.
Andersson, B., Murray D. (eds): *Clinically Relevant Resistance in Cancer Chemotherapy.* 2002. ISBN 1-4020-7200-7.
Beam, C. (ed.): *Biostatistical Applications in Cancer Research.* 2002. ISBN 1-4020-7226-0.
Brockstein, B., Masters, G. (eds): *Head and Neck Cancer.* 2003. ISBN 1-4020-7336-4.
Frank, D.A. (ed.): *Signal Transduction in Cancer.* 2003. ISBN 1-4020-7340-2.
Figlin, R. A. (ed.): *Kidney Cancer.* 2003. ISBN 1-4020-7457-3.
Kirsch, M.; Black, P. McL. (ed.): *Angiogenesis in Brain Tumors.* 2003. ISBN 1-4020-7704-1.
Keller, E.T., Chung, L.W.K. (eds): *The Biology of Skeletal Metastases.* 2004. ISBN 1-4020-7749-1.
Kumar, R. (ed.): *Molecular Targeting and Signal Transduction.* 2004. ISBN 1-4020-7822-6.
Verweij, J., Pinedo, H.M. (eds): *Targeting Treatment of Soft Tissue Sarcomas.* 2004. ISBN 1-4020-7808-0.
Finn, W.G., Peterson, L.C. (eds.): *Hematopathology in Oncology.* 2004. ISBN 1-4020-7919-2.
Farid, N. (ed.): *Molecular Basis of Thyroid Cancer.* 2004. ISBN 1-4020-8106-5.
Khleif, S. (ed.): *Tumor Immunology and Cancer* Vaccines. 2004. ISBN 1-4020-8119-7.
Balducci, L., Extermann, M. (eds): *Biological Basis of Geriatric Oncology.* 2004. ISBN
Abrey, L.E., Chamberlain, M.C., Engelhard, H.H. (eds): *Leptomeningeal Metastases.* 2005. ISBN 0-387-24198-1
Platanias, L.C. (ed.): *Cytokines and Cancer.* 2005. ISBN 0-387-24360-7.
Leong, S.P.L., Kitagawa, Y., Kitajima, M. (eds): *Selective Sentinel Lymphadenectomy for Human Solid Cancer.* 2005. ISBN 0-387-23603-1.
Small, Jr. W., Woloschak, G. (eds): *Radiation Toxicity: A Practical Guide.* 2005. ISBN 1-4020-8053-0.
Haefner, B., Dalgleish, A. (eds): *The Link Between Inflammation and Cancer.* 2006. ISBN 0-387-26282-2.
Leonard, J.P., Coleman, M. (eds): *Hodgkin s and Non-Hodgkin s Lymphoma.* 2006. ISBN 0-387-29345.
Leong, S.P.L. (ed): *Cancer Clinical Trials: Proactive Strategies.* 2006. ISBN 0-387-33224-3.
Meyers, C. (ed): *Aids-Associated Viral Oncogenesis.* 2007. ISBN 978-0-387-46804-4.
Ceelen, W.P. (ed): *Peritoneal Carcinomatosis: A Multidisciplinary Approach.* 2007. ISBN 978-0-387-48991-9.
Leong, S.P.L. (ed): *Cancer Metastasis and the Lymphovascular System: Basis for rational therapy.* 2007. ISBN 978-0-387-69218-0.
Raizer, J., Abrey, L.E. (eds): *Brain Metastases.* 2007. ISBN 978-0-387-69221-0.
Woodruff, T., Snyder, K.A. (eds): *Oncofertility.* 2007. ISBN 978-0-387-72292-4.
Angelos, P. (ed): *Ethical Issues in Cancer Patient Care, Second Edition.* 2008. ISBN 978-0-387-73638-9.
Ansell, S. (ed): *Rare Hematological Malignancies.* 2008. ISBN 978-0-387-73743-0.
Gradishar, W.J., Wood, W.C. (eds): *Advances in Breast Care Management, Second Edition.* 2008. 978-0-387-73160-5.
Blake, M., Kalra, M. (eds): *Imaging in Oncology.* 2008. ISBN 978-0-387-75586-1.
Bishop, M. R. (ed): *Hematopoietic Stem Cell Transplantation.* 2008. ISBN 978-0-387-78579-0.
Stockfleth, E., Ulrich, C. (eds): *Skin Cancer after Organ Transplantation.* 2008. ISBN 978-0-387-78573-8.
Fuqua, S.A.W. (ed): *Hormone Receptors in Breast Cancer,* 2009. ISBN: 978-0-387-09462-5.

Suzanne A.W. Fuqua
Editor

Hormone Receptors in Breast Cancer

Springer

Editor
Suzanne A.W. Fuqua
Baylor College of Medicine
Houston, TX
USA
sfuqua@bcm.tmc.edu

ISBN 978-1-4899-9680-0 ISBN 978-0-387-09463-2 (eBook)
DOI 10.1007/978-0-387-09463-2

Printed on acid-free paper

springer.com

Preface

Since radiolabeled estrogens were first observed in the early 1960s to be preferentially concentrated in estrogen target organs — observations that gave rise to the concept of an "estrogen receptor (ER)," it has become clear that many human breast cancers are dependent on estrogen for their growth. Estrogens' mitogenic effects are mediated through ERs α and β, which is the therapeutic target for hormonal therapies. The purpose of the book is to provide an up-to-date resource on the role of hormone receptors in breast cancer. Since approximately 1 of 8 women in the United States and 1 of 12 women in European countries are affected by breast cancer, there has been a massive effort to understand the mechanisms of hormone action. This explosion of information has led to exciting new areas of gene-specific targeting of the disease and breast cancer prevention. Paradigm shifts in treatment options and sequencing of hormonal therapies have recently occurred in breast cancer management, necessitating close cooperation and communication between translational scientists and physicians. This book is focused on providing this communication.

The 11 chapters of this book examine many aspects of hormone receptors, including basic and translational information on the molecular biology of the ERs, the utility of the ERs for the clinical management of breast cancer as it relates to assessing clinical outcome and selecting appropriate therapy, a review on the biology of ER and its role in the diagnosis and treatment of breast cancer, the importance of non-nuclear ER expression in breast cancer and other endocrine target tissues, the importance of ERs α and β inaggressive breast tumors of African-American women, cross-talk between BRCA1 and ER, and a detailed discussion of the role of ER in metastasis of breast cancer. We have included the latest clinical information on sequencing of hormonal therapies in breast cancer, the use of biomarkers in presurgical neoadjuvant trials, the problem of clinical hormone resistance, strategies to utilize hormonal prevention in high-risk patients, and the elucidation of hormone-responsive phenotypes as defined by state-of-the-art molecular expression profiling.

I would like to express my deep thanks to all the authors for their valuable contribution to the chapters and the successful completion of this book, as well as Ms. Laura Walsh and Maureen Tobin at Springer US.

Houston, TX Suzanne A.W. Fuqua

Contents

Contributors

Kathy S. Albain Loyola University Chicago Stritch School of Medicine, Department of Medicine, Division of Hematology/Oncology, Cardinal Bernardin Cancer Center, Maywood, IL, USA

Powel H. Brown Lester and Sue Smith Breast Center, Baylor College of Medicine, Houston, TX, USA, pbrown@bcm.tmc.edu

Yukun Cui Breast Center, Baylor College of Medicine, Houston, TX, USA

Regina M. Fearmonti Department of Surgical Oncology, The University of Texas M. D. Anderson Cancer Center, Houston, TX, USA, gfearmo@aol.com

Suzanne A.W. Fuqua Breast Center, Baylor College of Medicine, Houston, TX, USA, sfuqua@bcm.tmc.edu

Matthew H. Herynk Breast Center, Baylor College of Medicine, Houston, TX, USA

Kelly K. Hunt Department of Surgical Oncology, The University of Texas M. D. Anderson Cancer Center, Houston, TX, USA, khunt@mdanderson.org

Stephen R.D. Johnston Department of Medicine, Royal Marsden NHS Foundation Trust, Chelsea, London, UK, Stephen.Johnston@rmh.nhs.uk

Khandan Keyomarsi Department of Experimental Radiation Oncology, The University of Texas M. D. Anderson Cancer Center, Houston, TE, USA

Marleen Kok The Netherlands Cancer Institute, Amsterdam, The Netherlands

Sabine Linn The Netherlands Cancer Institute, Amsterdam, The Netherlands, m.kok@nki.nl

Ellis R. Levin Division of Endocrinology and Metabolism, University of California, Irvine and the Long Beach VA Medical Center, Long Beach, CA, USA, ellis.levin@va.gov

Yuxin Li Lester and Sue Smith Breast Center, Baylor College of Medicine, Houston, TX, USA

Shelly S. Lo Loyola University Chicago Stritch School of Medicine, Department of Medicine, Division of Hematology/Oncology, Cardinal Bernardin Cancer Center, Maywood, IL, USA, shlo@lumc.edu

Indira Poola Department of Surgery and Breast Center, Howard University College of Medicine, Washington, DC, USA, ipoola@howard.edu

Kathleen I. Pritchard Sunnybrook Research Institute, Sunnybrook Odette Cancer Centre, Faculty of Medicine, University of Toronto, Toronto, ONT, Canada

Monica M. Richert Department of Pathology, Division of Molecular and Cellular Pathology, University of Alabama at Birmingham, Birmingham, Alabama, USA, mrichert@PATH.UAB.EDU

Eliot M. Rosen Department of Oncology, Lombardi Comprehensive Cancer Center, Georgetown University, Washington, DC, USA, emr36@georgetown.edu

Patricia Robinson Loyola University Chicago Stritch School of Medicine, Department of Medicine, Division of Hematology/Oncology, Cardinal Bernardin Cancer Center, Maywood, IL, USA

Jennifer Selever Breast Center, Baylor College of Medicine, Houston, TX, USA

Valerie Speirs Section of Pathology and Tumor Biology, Leeds Institute of Molecular Medicine, University of Leeds, St James's University Hospital, Leeds, UK, V.Speirs@leeds.ac.uk

Abeer M. Shaaban Section of Pathology and Tumor Biology, Leeds Institute of Molecular Medicine, University of Leeds, St James's University Hospital, Leeds, UK

Janagi Thirugnanasampanthan Breast Center, Baylor College of Medicine, Houston, TX, USA

Marc van de Vijver Academic Medical Center, Amsterdam, The Netherlands, mj.vandevijver@amc.uva.nl

Danny R. Welch Department of Pathology, Division of Molecular and Cellular Pathology, University of Alabama at Birmingham, Birmingham, AL, USA, danwelch@uab.edu

Hormone Action and Clinical Significance of the Estrogen Receptor α

Matthew H. Herynk, Jennifer Selever, Janagi Thirugnanasampanthan, Yukun Cui, and Suzanne A.W. Fuqua

Clinical Relevance of ERα

ERα expression in breast cancer has many functions, including tumor growth enhancement, serving as an efficacious therapeutic target, and being a prognostic and predictive factor. Thus, a great deal of research has attempted to delineate the roles of ERα in human breast cancer. It has long been known that approximately two-thirds of human breast cancers express ERα and that estrogen drives tumor growth through its receptor. Because of its role in tumor growth, the ERα signaling pathway is a highly useful axis for hormonal manipulation. Several types of drugs have been developed for this purpose, including SERMs (selective estrogen receptor modulators), aromatase inhibitors, and pure antagonists. These agents will be discussed in greater detail in subsequent chapters.

Several assays have been developed for the detection of ERα in breast cancer patients. The dextran-coated charcoal (DCC) assay utilizes radiolabeled steroid ligand to detect ERα (reviewed in [1]). Since cutoff values for defining ERα status vary among different laboratories using this assay, there can be ambiguity in the definition of certain tumors. However, using this assay can be advantageous in that it can provide reproducible quantitation of ERα under proper conditions. Another method that detects ERα is the use of antibodies directed against specific epitopes of the receptor [2, 3]. This method also has a disadvantage in that there are procedural variations among different laboratories [4]. However, if this assay can be standardized, then the subjective nature of the assay will not pose a significant problem. The detection of ERα in patients can be carried out in different ways with assays that have problematic disadvantages but still serve important roles in the treatment of these patients.

S.A.W. Fuqua (✉)
Breast Center, Baylor College of Medicine, One Baylor Plaza, Houston, TX 77030, USA
e-mail: sfuqua@bcm.tmc.edu

S.A.W. Fuqua (ed.), *Hormone Receptors in Breast Cancer*,
Cancer Treatment and Research 312, DOI 10.1007/978-0-387-09463-2_1,

ERα has utility as both a prognostic and a predictive factor. The former indicates the inherent biologic aggressiveness of the disease if left untreated, whereas the latter indicates the likelihood of a response to treatment. In terms of prognostic factors, positive ERα expression correlates with a better outcome [5]. However, prognostic evaluations can change at the time of first relapse, and this is partly based on ERα status at the time of diagnosis as well as the time interval between primary treatment and relapse [6]. ERα expression also correlates with other factors indicative of better prognosis such as greater differentiation, diploidy, lower number of dividing cells, and lower mutation rates of breast cancer-associated genes.

As a predictive factor, ERα expression generally reflects that the patient is likely to respond to hormonal therapy, including second-line therapies [7]. On the other hand, lack of ERα expression predicts that the patient may not respond to hormone-based therapies [8]. The intensity of ERα expression also directly correlates with the degree of responsiveness to hormonal manipulation. While the ERα status of metastases may not always be consistent with that of the primary tumor, the ERα status of metastases is more predictive of response to hormonal therapy [9]. Thus, the ERα status of a patient is useful in determining the most appropriate method of treatment.

ERα Activation Domains

Transcription of estrogen-responsive genes is stimulated predominantly via two transactivation domains, activation function 1 (AF-1) at the amino terminus and activation function 2 (AF-2) at the carboxyl terminus of ERα (Fig. 1). These two domains span large areas of the receptor, and both are necessary for maximal ERα transcriptional activity. AF-1 and AF-2 bind various receptor co-regulatory proteins leading to different transcriptional outcomes (for a

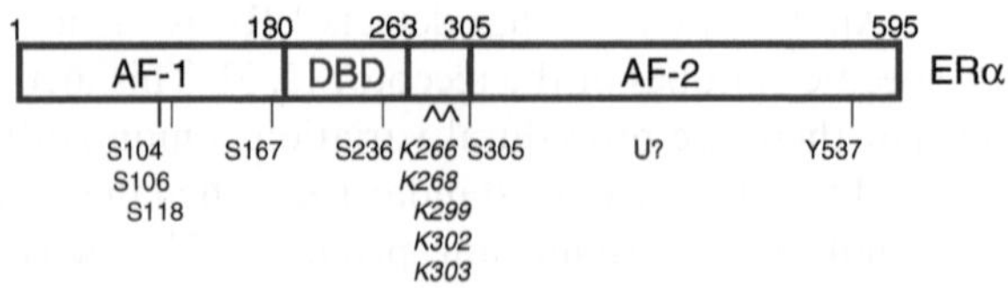

Fig. 1 ERα is divided into four important functional domains: the amino-terminal transactivation domain containing the AF-1 motif spanning amino acids 1–180, the DNA-binding domain spanning amino acids 181–263, the hinge domain spanning amino acids 264–305, and the ligand-binding domain containing the AF-2 motif spanning amino acids 306–595. AF-2a is located between amino acids 282 and 351 (not shown). The post-translational modified residues are depicted in the figure: phosphorylated residues are marked with a vertical line, ^^ indicates the region containing the known acetylation and/or sumoylation sites. Ubiquitination is depicted as a black U? because the exact residue within the ligand-binding domain is not known

complete review, see Hall and McDonnell [10]). Transcription can also be stimulated to a lesser extent by a less-described transactivation domain referred to as AF-2a [11], and the significance of this domain is less understood.

AF-1 and AF-2 each function in distinct ways, and depending on the nature of the cell and the promoter type, one or both can affect signaling. AF-1 functions in a ligand-independent manner to exert transcriptional activity [12]. AF-1 can be differentially phosphorylated by a number of important signaling molecules, such as AKT2 (also known as protein kinase B or PKB) and Erk1/2 (extracellular regulated kinase 1/2), resulting in diverse responses to SERMs. For example, phosphorylation of serine 167 by AKT2 leads to insensitivity to tamoxifen, whereas phosphorylation of serine 118 by Erk1/2 leads to sensitivity to tamoxifen [12]. AF-2, on the other hand, stimulates transcription in a ligand-dependent manner [13]. Thus, transcription of ERα-regulated genes depends on these two main transactivation domains which function in a highly regulated manner.

Crystal Structure of ERα

To date, the three-dimensional structure of full-length ERα has not yet been solved. However, due to ERα's similarity with other nuclear hormone receptors and molecular modeling, we can infer a broad model of ERα structure. Crystallization efforts have focused on the DNA-binding and the ligand-binding domains, which have revealed the mechanism of action for several ERα agonists as well as antagonists. Estradiol binds ERα within a carboxy-terminal hydrophobic pocket, and upon ligand binding, helix 12 repositions itself over this pocket [14]. This new confirmation stabilizes helix 12 in the receptor, allowing it to recruit transcriptional receptor coactivators [15]. The large side chains of the antagonists tamoxifen, faslodex, or raloxifene prevent helix 12 from adopting an agonist-bound confirmation, thus antagonizing coactivator binding to the receptor. In contrast, compounds without large side chains, such as genistein or 5,11-*cis*-diethyl-5,6,11,12-tetrahydrochrysene-2,8-diol (THC), inhibit ER activation by stabilizing nonproductive conformations of the ligand-binding pocket [16, 17]. Recently, a number of groups have utilized the crystal structure and molecular modeling in an attempt to identify better, more specific drugs for disrupting estrogen receptor signaling [18, 19], an effort which is currently underway.

Formation of the Transcriptome

Stimulation of transcription by ERα occurs via a number of distinct molecular events in the nucleus. ERα homo- or heterodimerizes with other nuclear receptors such as estrogen receptor β (ERβ) or androgen receptor (AR) and binds, via the DNA-binding domain (DBD), to estrogen response elements (EREs) located on the promoters of estrogen-responsive genes [20]. This allows interaction with other components of the transcription factor complex, including receptor co-regulatory proteins which will be discussed in the following sections of this chapter and the basal transcription machinery (for a complete review, see Klein and Hitpass [21]). ERα also has the ability to dimerize with proteins such as stimulating protein 1 (Sp1) and activating protein 1 (AP1) and affects transcription through the binding of these proteins to non-ERE-containing sites [22, 23]. Thus, the regulation of ERα transcriptional activity is complex and involves a myriad of proteins from those specific to nuclear hormone receptors to components of the basal transcription machinery.

Estrogen Receptor Cofactors

It was well known that ER's function is tissue specific and ligand dependent, indicating that ERα alone could not account for its diversified functions, thus requiring additional signaling factors [24]. This concept led to the discovery of the first ER cofactors in 1995 [25]. Using techniques such as yeast two-hybrid and protein library screening, a growing body of proteins and RNAs affecting ERα transcriptional activity, either directly and/or indirectly, have been identified [26]. To date, the Nuclear Receptor Signaling Atlas (NURSA) website (www.nursa.org) lists over 170 known nuclear cofactors. These factors are generally categorized as coactivators (enhance ER transcriptional activity) or corepressors (reduce ER transcriptional activity). In general, these cofactors do not bind to DNA directly but rather through association with sequence-specific DNA-binding proteins, including but not limited to nuclear receptors. Upon recruitment to the promoter complex, these factors may affect transcription directly or via recruiting additional cofactors. In this section, we will focus on the fundamentals of ER cofactors and some of the latest findings in this field.

Coactivators

The first subcloned steroid receptor coactivator, SRC-1 or NcoA1, enhanced the transcriptional activity of ERα when cells were treated with estrogen [25]. Additionally, SRC-1 also has been shown to be involved in ligand-independent activation of ERα. The second member of this coactivator family, SRC-2, also known as GRIP1 in mice or TIF2 in human tissues, can only activate ERα transcriptional activity in the presence of estrogen [27, 28]. Like SRC-1, SRC-3 (also called RAC3, p/CIP, AIB1, or ACTR) activated both ligand-dependent and ligand-independent ERα transcriptional activity [29, 30]. Sequence analysis of these family members elucidated an LxxLL nuclear receptor-binding motif (the so-called NR box, L = leucine, isoleucine, or other large hydrophobic amino acid residues) that is conserved among other coactivators such as CBP/p300 and TRAP220 [31]. While the coactivators mentioned above act in a ligand-dependent manner, additional coactivators directly interact with the ligand-independent AF1 domain (e. g., p68 RNA helicase) [32], hinge domain (e.g., PGC-1α) [33], or the DBD (e.g., Ciz1) [34]. In addition to the coactivators that directly interact with ERα, additional cofactors such as protein arginine methyl transferase, CARM1, and PRMT2 [35] affect ER transcriptional activity through indirect association with ERα mediated by the SRC family of coactivators. Coactivator regulation of ERα is a complex process that leads to enhanced transcriptional activity in both a ligand-dependent and -independent manner.

Corepressors

Compared with coactivators, there are far fewer corepressors identified so far. Corepressors inhibit transcription of ERα target genes through directly or indirectly interacting with steroid receptors. Sequence analysis between nuclear corepressors, including NcoR1 and SMRT, identified an LxxxI/HIxxxI/L conserved nuclear corepressor-binding motif (the so-called CoNR box), which has been demonstrated to mediate either ligand-independent or anti-estrogen-stimulated association with the AF2 domain of ERα [36]. Similar to coactivators, corepressors have been shown to interact with other domains of ERα, including the AF1 (HDAC4) [37] and hinge domains (SAFB and MTA2) [38, 39]. It has been reported that overexpression of the nuclear corepressors NCoR and SMRT enhances tamoxifen antagonist activity without interfering with estrogen-stimulated gene expression [40]. This is consistent with a later discovery that reduced levels of NCoR correlate with hormone resistance in breast cancer cells [41]. Furthermore, we have recently shown that overexpression of the MTA2 corepressor resulted in hormone-independent and anti-estrogen-resistant cell growth [39]. These findings, in combination with many additional corepressor studies, suggest that corepressors may be involved in the processes of anti-estrogen function and the development of resistance as well.

Transcriptional Cofactor or Transcriptional Factor?

Some ERα cofactors also contain specific DNA-binding domains (e.g., NcoR, MTA1/2, or Ciz1), raising the possibility that they may affect gene transcription directly. One study demonstrated that MTA1, an ERα corepressor, could activate breast cancer amplified sequence 3 (BCAS3) promoter activity, probably through direct interaction and recruitment of the p300 coactivator [42]. To date, the majority of studies have analyzed the ability of these proteins to alter transcriptional activity as cofactors, however, it is clear that some may directly effect the transcriptional activity of their target genes.

Chromatin Remodeling and the Cyclical Occupancy of ERα Cofactors

Acetylation and/or methylation of histones promote decondensation of chromatin structure, thereby favoring gene transcription. In contrast, deacetylation and/or demethylation lead to chromatin condensation, thus abrogating transcription. A large number of steroid receptor cofactors are implicated in these chromatin remodeling processes by either directly modifying histones (e.g., CBP/p300, P/CAF, SRC-1, CARM1, and HDAC1) or indirectly deacetylating histones through interaction with histone deacetylases (e.g., MTA1 and 2 or SIN3; for a review, see [26]). The importance of these co-regulatory proteins in controlling gene activity is further emphasized by the findings that these cofactors or cofactor complexes are recruited to estrogen-responsive promoters in an ordered, cyclical manner. There is some evidence suggesting that histone premodification is essential to direct the recruitment of individual cofactors. For example, the recruitment of histone methyl transferase PRMT1 to the pS2 promoter requires the SET (patient SE translocation) protein [43], which demethylates histone H4 arginine 3 and provides a target for the histone methyl transferase activity of PRMT1. In addition, ERα and cofactors are also modified during transcriptional activation. These modifications may represent a signal to release these cofactors from the promoter. For example, acetylation of ERα results from agonist-induced interactions with certain coactivators that leads to decreased transcriptional activity [44]. SRC-3, an ERα coactivator with intrinsic histone acetyl transferase activity, loses its coactivator ability upon acetylation by p300 [45]. In addition, the presence of SRC-3 enhances ERα recruitment to the promoter, however, SRC-3 also helps to direct agonist-induced ERα degradation [46]. Collectively, these studies suggest that a common physiologic network exists controlling both the "ON" and "OFF" signals for ERα action.

Alternative Exons in the 5′UTR

One mechanism of regulating ERα protein expression is through differential usage of upstream untranslated exons. As many as eight exons have been identified, and this review will use the nomenclature suggested by Flouriot et al. [47], as modified by Kos et al. [48]. ERα exon 1 contains an acceptor splice site at +163 permitting the splicing of several different exons encoding various 5′UTRs. At least seven different promoters have been described that show relative tissue specificity (for a complete review, see Kos et al. [48]). Promoter A in exon 1 is the most common promoter expressed in tissues and cell lines. Promoter C was first described in 1991 [49], but a longer version of promoter C was described in subsequent years [50]. Additional exons A–E have been described and have also been shown to affect reporter gene expression levels [51]. One hypothesis is that the numerous AUG start codons found in the ERα 5′UTRs inhibit scanning ribosomes from reaching the start codon, thereby reducing ERα protein expression [51]. Promoters within 2 kilobase pairs of the acceptor splice site (generally A, B, and C) are utilized in cell lines and tissues that express high levels of ERα. The more distal promoters, E and F, are found in tissues where ERα expression is less abundant, such as the liver and human osteoblasts [52]. Additionally, promoters T1 and T2 are expressed predominately in the testis and epididymis [53]. While these alternative promoters can account for the tissue-specific expression of ERα, they may also play a role in the regulation of ERα levels. In vitro studies analyzing promoter usage have demonstrated increased use of promoter A in breast cancer cells when compared with normal mammary epithelium [54]. Additionally, in breast tumor cell lines, Weigel et al. have shown activation of promoters not normally activated in breast epithelium [55].

Epigenetic and Post-translational Regulation of ERα

Epigenetic information on the genome provides directions on when, where, and how the genetic information should be used. Post-translational regulation of nuclear steroid receptors is an exciting field of study, which is comprised of events encompassing methylation, phosphorylation, acetylation, ubiquitination, and most recently protein sumoylation [56]. Post-translational regulation of the nuclear receptor family is dynamic, with member proteins being differentially affected by modifications either singly or in combination, thereby influencing receptor conformation, ligand binding, DNA binding, and coactivator interactions [57]. It has been postulated that post-translational modifications of ERα play a key role in the regulation of its functions.

Methylation

DNA methylation is one of the most important forms of post-translational modifications in which a methyl group is covalently bonded to the 5-carbon on the cytosine base by DNA methyltransferases [58]. Methylation of the estrogen receptor occurs on cytosine within the CpG islands associated with the promoter [59]. CpG islands are regions close to the promoter of genes that contain cytosine (C) and guanine (G) residues at a greater than 50% frequency. Hypermethylation of the ERα promoter silences the gene by repressing transcription and in some cases is associated with malignant transformation of cells, whereas hypomethylation of ERα is associated with gene activation indicating an inverse relationship between promoter methylation and transcriptional activity [60].

Acetylation

ERα is known to be acetylated on lysines, and the conserved acetylated amino acids in ERα are lysines (K) 266, K268, K299, K302, and K303 (Fig. 1). The acetylation of K266 and K268 has opposite effects compared to the acetylation of K302 and K303. K266 and K268 induce DNA-binding and ligand-dependent activation, whereas K302 and K303 inhibit ERα ligand-dependent activation [61]. Our recent experiments using ERα deletion constructs suggest that the phosphorylation status of S305 within the hinge domain of ERα coordinately regulates the acetylation of lysines 302 and 303 [44]. Although mass spectrometry has previously identified these same two lysines as sites of acetylations [62], Kim et al. have recently shown that these two lysine residues may not be acetylated in the full-length protein, although these results need to be validated [63]. Thus, the hinge domain of the receptor is replete with post-translational modifications having the potential for important functional consequences.

Phosphorylation

ERα is phosphorylated on multiple residues and a complete list of phosphorylation sites and their respective kinases is found in Table 1. The diversity of kinases and responses to phosphorylation illustrate the range of effector pathways that are utilized in the complex regulation of ERα or amplification of its signal. For instance, phosphorylation of S305 ERα can be mediated by both the protein kinase A (PKA) and p21-activated kinase 1 (PAK-1) signaling networks [44, 64, 65]. PKA-mediated phosphorylation of ERα does not alter its DNA-binding abilities but instead enhances ligand-binding affinity [64]. Additionally,

Table 1 ERα phosphorylation sites

Amino acid	Modification	Effect	References
S104	Phosphorylation by Cyclin A-CDK	Enhanced transcriptional activity	[86]
S106	Phosphorylation by Cyclin A-CDK	Enhanced transcriptional activity	[87]
S118	Phosphorylation by MAPK	Enhanced transcriptional activity	[88]
S167	Phosphorylation by Akt2	Enhanced transcriptional activity	[89]
S236	Phosphorylation by PKA	Enhanced ER dimerization and DNA binding	[64, 90]
S305	Phosphorylation by PKA or PAK1	Enhanced ligand-binding affinity, tamoxifen resistance	[64, 65]
Y537	Phosphorylation by Src kinase	Enhanced transcriptional activity	[74, 90, 91]

the PKA-mediated phosphorylation of S305 allows tamoxifen to act as an agonist of ERα, and PKA is known to be frequently overexpressed in breast tumors [44, 64, 66]. Clearly, ERα phosphorylation has a variety of effects in the physiologic actions of ERα and is an emerging area of study.

Ubiquitination

The tight regulation of ERα function is partially due to the ubiquitin–proteasome pathway regulating the levels of protein and the receptor's response to ligand [67]. Ubiquitination is the reversible covalent bonding of the highly conserved 76 amino acid ubiquitin to lysine residues on target proteins. Upon ligand binding to ERα, ubiquitin binds the receptor on lysine residues within the AD core region of the ligand-binding domain inducing the protein to undergo ubiquitin-mediated proteasomal degradation. This has been shown to be an important step in the transactivation of ERα, and transactivation can be inhibited by proteasome inhibitors [67–69]. While ubiquitination and proteasomal degradation are important mechanisms of regulating ERα protein levels, the ubiquitination of ERα may play an important role in the transactivation of ERα.

Sumoylation

SUMO-1, a small ubiquitin-like modifier, covalently and reversibly bonds to target proteins with the assistance of conjugating enzymes. Recent experiments by Sentis et al. reveal that ligand-dependent sumoylation occurs on lysine residues within the hinge domain of ERα and that sumoylation regulates transcriptional activity of this nuclear receptor [70]. The same lysine residues that are acetylated can also be sumoylated including K266, K268, K302, and K303 (Fig. 1), suggesting a tight regulatory pathway governing the occupation of these residues and subsequent downstream effects.

ERα Mutations

A number of mutations and polymorphisms have been identified in ERα from numerous diseases including psychiatric diseases, precocious puberty, and many cancers (for a complete review, see Herynk and Fuqua [2]). While over 20 different mutations have been identified, rarely has any independent mutation been found in more than one sample, in contrast are the A86V, K303R, and Y537S/N ERα mutations. The A86V mutation was found in 12% of the breast cancer specimens analyzed and has been associated with lower levels of ERα protein and spontaneous abortions [71, 72]. The tyrosine at 537 is the only site that has been found to be mutated to two different residues, serine and asparagine [73, 74]. This residue lies at the amino-cap of H12, therefore it is not surprising that mutations at this site would significantly affect the activity of ERα [74–76].

We originally identified the K303R ERα mutation in 34% of premalignant breast hyperplasias [77]. More recently, utilizing a sensitive primer extension sequencing technique, we have demonstrated that this mutation was present in invasive breast cancer specimens and the presence of the K303R ERα mutation correlated with older age, larger tumor size, and lymph node-positive disease [78]. In comparison, Conway et al. have identified this mutation in only 5.7% of breast cancers utilizing a different gel electrophoresis detection method [79]. Therefore, we propose that while the absolute frequency of this mutation remains to be validated, it is clearly present in a significant number of breast cancer samples.

Analysis of the K303R ERα mutation has shown that this mutated receptor exhibits hypersensitive growth to low concentrations of estrogen [77]. Additionally, the mutated ERα has increased binding to the coactivator TIF2, and the corepressor MTA2 was unable to repress the activity of the mutant receptor [39]. The presence of an arginine at the 303 position removes a key acetylation site and allows ERα to be more highly phosphorylated by PKA signaling [44]. Collectively, these data indicate that this residue plays a key role in ERα signaling, and whether or not this mutation will affect other epigenetic regulatory mechanisms of ERα remains to be determined. While identification of mutations has been rare, the role of mutations in breast cancer may be underappreciated, and is an underexplored field, which might effect future breast cancer therapeutic decisions with hormone-based therapies. The use of alternative sequencing strategies, employing accurate primer extension sequencing to replace standard dye terminator approaches, may be warranted in this regard.

Mouse Modeling of ERα

Mice lacking ERα expression are viable and demonstrate a wide range of phenotypes altering normal functions including effects on sexual organs and function, bone, brain, and cardiovascular, to name a few (for a complete review, see Couse and Korach [80]). Additionally, mice deficient in ERα exhibit normal early development of mammary glands, however, these glands never develop beyond the newborn stage [81]. In contrast, ERβ knockout (KO) mice develop normal ductal structures with reduced side branching [82], thereby demonstrating that ERα has a central role and is the predominant receptor involved in mammary gland development.

While ERα has a vital role in normal mammary gland development, aberrant ERα signaling has been shown to function in the development of preneoplastic mammary lesions and breast cancer development and progression.

Ninety-five percent of mice conditionally overexpressing wild-type ERα displayed abnormal ductal structures at 4 months of age [83]. While 52 and 36% of 4-month-old virgin mice had lobular and ductal hyperplasias, respectively, 21% of 4-month-old virgin mice displayed DCIS [84]. Earlier, the same group reported 37% of mice overexpressing T antigen – ERα had developed adenocarcinomas by 11 months of age [83]. While exogenous estrogen stimulation did not alter the incidence of hyperplasias or DCIS in the wild-type receptor system [84], aromatase overexpression was sufficient to cause preneoplastic changes within the mammary gland [85]. These data demonstrate that increased ERα can lead to preneoplastic changes contributing to mammary tumorigenesis.

Conclusions

The role of ERα in the human breast has been extensively studied over the past several decades. The development of transgenic mice overexpressing or lacking ERα expression has greatly aided in defining the roles of ERα in both normal mammary gland development and breast cancer development and progression. Laboratory studies have clearly shown that ERα is a highly regulated molecule demonstrating complex, multilayered regulation including organ-specific alternate promoters, epigenetics, cofactor levels and interactions, and a highly regulated degradation. Additionally, disruption of this complex regulation can drastically effect the physiologic regulation and homeostasis of the body leading to a variety of disease states. The presence of ERα in human breast cancer has proven to be clinically useful, both as a prognostic indicator to suggest the inherent biologic aggressiveness of the disease and as a predictive factor to guide therapies for the treatment of this widespread disease. Clearly, ERα has proven to be an important molecule in breast cancer and will further demonstrate its important roles in the future.

References

1. Elledge RM, Fuqua SAW. Estrogen and Progesterone Receptors. In: Harris JR, Lippman ME, Morrow M, Osborne CK, eds. Diseases of the Breast. Philadelphia: Lippincott, Williams & Wilkins; 2000:471–88.
2. Herynk MH, Fuqua SA. Estrogen receptor mutations in human disease. Endocr Rev 2004;25:869–98.
3. King WJ, Greene GL. Monoclonal antibodies localize oestrogen receptors in the nuclei of target cells. Nature 1984;307:745–7.
4. Biesterfeld S, Veuskens U, Schmitz FJ, Amo-Takyi B, Bocking A. Interobserver reproducibility of immunocytochemical estrogen- and progesterone receptor status assessment in breast cancer. Anticancer Res. 1996;16:2497–500.
5. Fuqua SAW. The role of estrogen receptors in breast cancer metastasis. J Mam Gland Bio Neoplasia. 2002;6:407–17.
6. Cocconi G. The natural history of operable breast cancer after primary treatment. Ann Oncol. 1995;6 Suppl 2:11–21.

7. Bundred NJ. Prognostic and predictive factors in breast cancer. Cancer Treat Rev. 2001;27:137–42.
8. Early_Breast_Cancer_Trialists'_Collaborative_Group. Tamoxifen for early breast cancer: an overview of the randomised trials. Lancet 1998;351:1451–67.
9. Lower EE, Glass EL, Bradley DA, Blau R, Heffelfinger S. Impact of metastatic estrogen receptor and progesterone receptor status on survival. Breast Cancer Res Treat 2005;90:65–70.
10. Hall JM, McDonnell DP. Coregulators in nuclear estrogen receptor action: from concept to therapeutic targeting. Mol Interv. 2005;5:343–57.
11. Norris JD, Fan D, Kerner SA, McDonnell DP. Identification of a third autonomous activation domain within the human estrogen receptor. Mole Endocrinol. 1997;11:747–54.
12. Glaros S, Atanaskova N, Zhao C, Skafar DF, Reddy KB. Activation function-1 domain of estrogen receptor regulates the agonistic and antagonistic actions of tamoxifen. Mol Endocrinol. 2006;20:996–1008.
13. Green S, Gronemeyer H, Chambon P. Structure and function of steroid hormone receptors. In: Sluyser M, ed. Growth factors and oncogenes in breast cancer. Chichester, England: Ellis Horwood Ltd; 1987. p. 7–28.
14. Brzozowski A, Pike ACW, Dauter A, et al. Molecular basis of agonism and antagonism in the oestrogen receptor. Nature 1997;389:753–8.
15. Shiau AK, Barstad D, Loria PM, et al. The structural basis of estrogen receptor/coactivator recognition and the antagonism of this interaction by tamoxifen. Cell 1998;95:927–37.
16. Shiau AK, Barstad D, Radek JT, et al. Structural characterization of a subtype-selective ligand reveals a novel mode of estrogen receptor antagonism. Nat Struct Biol. 2002;9:359–64.
17. Pike AC, Brzozowski AM, Hubbard RE, et al. Structure of the ligand-binding domain of oestrogen receptor β in the presence of a partial agonist and a full antagonist. Embo J. 1999;18:4608–18.
18. Vedani A, Dobler M, Lill MA. Combining protein modeling and 6D-QSAR. Simulating the binding of structurally diverse ligands to the estrogen receptor. J Med Chem. 2005;48:3700–3.
19. Wang CY, Ai N, Arora S, et al. Identification of previously unrecognized antiestrogenic chemicals using a novel virtual screening approach. Chem Res Toxicol. 2006;19:1595–601.
20. Panet-Raymond V, Gottlieb B, Beitel LK, Pinsky L, Trifiro MA. Interactions between androgen and estrogen receptors and the effects on their transactivational properties. Mol Cell Endocrinol. 2000;167:139–50.
21. Klein-Hitpass L, Ryffel GU, Heitlinger E, Cato ACB. A 13 bp palindrome is a functional estrogen responsive element and interacts specifically with estrogen receptor. Nucleic Acids Res. 1988;16:647–64.
22. Safe S. Transcriptional activation of genes by 17 beta-estradiol through estrogen receptor-Sp1 interactions. Vitam Horm. 2001;62:231–52.
23. Jakacka M, Ito M, Weiss J, Chien PY, Gehm BD, Jameson JL. Estrogen receptor binding to DNA is not required for its activity through the nonclassical AP1 pathway. J Biol. Chem. 2001;276:13615–21.
24. Halamachi S, Marden E, Martin G, MacKay H, Abbondanza C, Brown M. Estrogen receptor-associated proteins: possible mediators of hormone-induced transcription. Science 1994;264:1455–8.
25. Onate SA, Tsai SY, Tsai MJ, O'Malley BW. Sequence and characterization of a coactivator for the steroid hormone receptor superfamily. Science 1995;270.
26. McKenna NJ, Lanz RB, O'Malley BW. Nuclear receptor coregulators: cellular and molecular biology. Endocrine Rev. 1999;20:321–44.

27. Voegel JJ, Heine MJS, Tini M, Vivat V, Chambon P, Gronemeyer H. The coactivator TIF2 contains three nuclear receptor-binding motifs and mediates transactivation through CBP binding-dependent and -independent pathways. EMBO J. 1998;17:507–19.
28. Hong H, Kohli K, Trivedi A, Johnson DL, Stallcup MR. GRIP1, a novel mouse protein that serves as a transcriptional coactivator in yeast for the hormone binding domains of steroid receptors. Proc Natl Acad Sci USA. 1996;93:4948–52.
29. Anzick SL, Kononen J, Walker RL, et al. AIB1, a steroid receptor coactivator amplified in breast and ovarian cancer. Science 1997;277:965–8.
30. Li H, Gomes PJ, Chen JD. RAC3, a steroid/nuclear receptor-associated coactivator that is related to SRC-1 and TIF2. Proc Natl Acad Sci USA. 1997;94:8479–84.
31. Chang C-Y, Norris JD, Gron H, et al. Dissection of the LXXLL nuclear receptor-coactivator interaction motif using combinatorial peptide libraries: discovery of peptide antagonists of estrogen receptors α and β. Mol Cell Biol. 1999;19:8226–39.
32. Endoh HK, Maruyama Y, Masuhiro Y, et al. Purification and identification of p68 RNA helicase acting as a transcriptional coactivator specific for the activation function 1 of human estrogen receptor α. Mol Cell Biol. 1999;19:5363–72.
33. Tcherepanova I, Puigserver P, Norris JD, Spiegelman BM, McDonnell DP. Modulation of estrogen receptor-alpha transcriptional activity by the coactivator PGC-1. J Biol Chem. 2000;275:16302–8.
34. den Hollander P, Rayala SK, Coverley D, Kumar R. Ciz1, a Novel DNA-binding coactivator of the estrogen receptor alpha, confers hypersensitivity to estrogen action. Cancer Res. 2006;66:11021–9.
35. Chen D, Huang SM, Stallcup MR. Synergistic, p160 coactivator-dependent enhancement of estrogen receptor function by CARM1 and p300. J Biol Chem. 2000;275:40810–6.
36. Leers J, Treuter E, Gustafsson J-A. Mechanistic principles in NR box-dependent interaction between nuclear hormone receptors and coactivator TIF2. Mol Cell Biol. 1998;18:6001–13.
37. Leong H, Sloan JR, Nash PD, Greene GL. Recruitment of histone deacetylase 4 to the N-terminal region of estrogen receptor alpha. Mol Endocrinol. 2005;19:2930–42.
38. Oesterreich S, Zhang Q, Hopp T, et al. Tamoxifen-bound estrogen receptor (ER) strongly interacts with the nuclear matrix protein HET/SAF-B, a novel inhibitor of ER-mediated transactivation. Mol Endocrinol. 2000;14:369–81.
39. Cui Y, Niu A, Pestell R, et al. Metastasis-associated protein 2 is a repressor of estrogen receptor alpha whose overexpression leads to estrogen-independent growth of human breast cancer cells. Mol Endocrinol. 2006;20:2020–35.
40. Smith CL, Nawaz Z, O'Malley BW. Coactivator and corepressor regulation of the agonist/antagonist activity of the mixed antiestrogen, 4-Hydroxytamoxifen. Mol Endocrinol. 1997;11:657–66.
41. Scott DJ, Parkes AT, Ponchel F, Cummings M, Poola I, Speirs V. Changes in expression of steroid receptors, their downstream target genes and their associated co-regulators during the sequential acquisition of tamoxifen resistance in vitro. Int J Oncol. 2007;31:557–65.
42. Gururaj AE, Singh RR, Rayala SK, et al. MTA1, a transcriptional activator of breast cancer amplified sequence 3. Proc Natl Acad Sci USA. 2006;103:6670–5.
43. Wagner S, Weber S, Kleinschmidt MA, Nagata K, Bauer UM. SET-mediated promoter hypoacetylation is a prerequisite for coactivation of the estrogen-responsive pS2 gene by PRMT1. J Biol Chem. 2006;281:27242–50.
44. Cui Y, Zhang M, Pestell R, Curran EM, Welshons WV, Fuqua SAW. Phosphorylation of estrogen receptor α blocks its acetylation and regulates estrogen sensitivity. Cancer Res. 2004;64:9199–208.
45. Chen H, Lin RJ, Xie W, Wilpitz D, Evans RM. Regulation of hormone-induced histone hyperacetylation and gene activation via acetylation of an acetylase. Cell 1999;98:675–86.

46. Shao W, Keeton EK, McDonnell DP, Brown M. Coactivator AIB1 links estrogen receptor transcriptional activity and stability. Proc Natl Acad Sci USA. 2004;101:11599–604.
47. Flouriot G, Griffin C, Kenealy M, Sonntag-Buck V, Gannon F. Differentially expressed messenger RNA isoforms of the human estrogen receptor-alpha gene are generated by alternative splicing and promoter usage. Mol Endocrinol. 1998;12:1939–54.
48. Kos M, Reid G, Denger S, Gannon F. Minireview: genomic organization of the human ERalpha gene promoter region. Mol Endocrinol. 2001;15:2057–63.
49. Keaveney M, Klug J, Dawson MT, et al. Evidence for a previously unidentified upstream exon in the human oestrogen receptor gene. J Mol Endocrinol. 1991;6:111–5.
50. Piva R, Del Senno L. Analysis of a DNA sequence upstream of the human estrogen receptor gene. Ann N Y Acad Sci. 1993;684:235–8.
51. Kos M, Denger S, Reid G, Gannon F. Upstream open reading frames regulate the translation of the multiple mRNA variants of the estrogen receptor alpha. J Biol Chem. 2002;277:37131–8.
52. Reid G, Denger S, Kos M, Gannon F. Human estrogen receptor-alpha: regulation by synthesis, modification and degradation. Cell Mol Life Sci. 2002;59:821–31.
53. Brand H, Kos M, Denger S, et al. A novel promoter is involved in the expression of estrogen receptor alpha in human testis and epididymis. Endocrinology. 2002;143:3397–404.
54. Grandien K, Backdahl M, Ljunggren O, Gustafsson JA, Berkenstam A. Estrogen target tissue determines alternative promoter utilization of the human estrogen receptor gene in osteoblasts and tumor cell lines. Endocrinology. 1995;136:2223–9.
55. Weigel RJ, Crooks DL, Iglehart JD, deConinck EC. Quantitative analysis of the transcriptional start sites of estrogen receptor in breast carcinoma. Cell Growth Differ. 1995;6:707–11.
56. Selever J, Fuqua SAW. Sumoylation of estrogen receptor a: Are post-translational modification coordinated. Breast Cancer Online 2007.
57. Likhite VS, Stossi F, Kim K, Katzenellenbogen BS, Katzenellenbogen JA. Kinase-specific phosphorylation of the estrogen receptor changes receptor interactions with ligand, deoxyribonucleic acid, and coregulators associated with alterations in estrogen and tamoxifen activity. Mol Endocrinol. 2006;20:3120–32.
58. Wajed SA, Laird PW, DeMeester TR. DNA methylation: an alternative pathway to cancer. Ann Surg. 2001;234:10–20.
59. Giacinti L, Claudio PP, Lopez M, Giordano A. Epigenetic information and estrogen receptor alpha expression in breast cancer. Oncologist. 2006;11:1–8.
60. Fan M, Yan PS, Hartman-Frey C, et al. Diverse gene expression and DNA methylation profiles correlate with differential adaptation of breast cancer cells to the antiestrogens tamoxifen and fulvestrant. Cancer Res. 2006;66:11954–66.
61. Faus H, Haendler B. Post-translational modifications of steroid receptors. Biomed Pharmacother. 2006;60:520–8.
62. Wang C, Fu M, Angeletti RH, et al. Direct acetylation of the estrogen receptor alpha hinge region by p300 regulates transactivation and hormone sensitivity. J Biol Chem. 2001;276:18375–83.
63. Kim MY, Woo EM, Chong YT, Homenko DR, Kraus WL. Acetylation of estrogen receptor alpha by p300 at lysines 266 and 268 enhances the deoxyribonucleic acid binding and transactivation activities of the receptor. Mol Endocrinol. 2006;20:1479–93.
64. Michalides R, Griekspoor A, Balkenende A, et al. Tamoxifen resistance by a conformational arrest of the estrogen receptor alpha after PKA activation in breast cancer. Cancer Cell 2004;5:597–605.
65. Rayala SK, Talukder AH, Balasenthil S, et al. P21-activated kinase 1 regulation of estrogen receptor-alpha activation involves serine 305 activation linked with serine 118 phosphorylation. Cancer Res. 2006;66:1694–701.

66. Zwart W, Griekspoor A, Berno V, et al. PKA-induced resistance to tamoxifen is associated with an altered orientation of ERalpha towards co-activator SRC-1. EMBO J. 2007;26:3534–44.
67. Tateishi Y, Kawabe Y, Chiba T, et al. Ligand-dependent switching of ubiquitin-proteasome pathways for estrogen receptor. Embo J. 2004;23:4813–23.
68. Ohta T, Fukuda M. Ubiquitin and breast cancer. Oncogene 2004;23:2079–88.
69. Nawaz Z, Lonard DM, Dennis AP, Smith CL, O'Malley BW. Proteasome-dependent degradation of the human estrogen receptor. Biochemistry 1999;96:1858–62.
70. Sentis S, Le Romancer M, Bianchin C, Rostan MC, Corbo L. Sumoylation of the estrogen receptor alpha hinge region regulates its transcriptional activity. Mol Endocrinol. 2005;19:2671–84.
71. Garcia T, Lehrer S, Bloomer WD, Schachter B. A variant estrogen receptor messenger ribonucleic acid is associated with reduced levels of estrogen binding in human mammary tumors. Mol Endocrinol. 1988;2:785–91.
72. Lehrer S, Sanchez M, Song HK, et al. Oestrogen receptor B-region polymorphism and spontaneous abortion in women with breast cancer. Lancet 1990;335:622–4.
73. Kohler MF, Berkholz A, Risinger JI, Elbendary A, Boyd J, Berchuck A. Mutational analysis of the estrogen-receptor gene in endometrial carcinoma. Obstet Gynecol. 1995;86:33–7.
74. Zhang QX, Borg A, Wolf DM, Oesterreich S, Fuqua SA. An estrogen receptor mutant with strong hormone-independent activity from a metastatic breast cancer. Cancer Res. 1997;57:1244–9.
75. Carlson KE, Choi I, Gee A, Katzenellenbogen BS, Katzenellenbogen JA. Altered ligand binding properties and enhanced stability of a constitutively active estrogen receptor: evidence that an open pocket conformation is required for ligand interaction. Biochemistry 1997;36:14897–905.
76. Weis KE, Ekena K, Thomas JA, Lazennec G, Katzenellenbogen BS. Constitutively active human estrogen receptors containing amino acid substitutions for tyrosine 537 in the receptor protein. Mol Endocrinol. 1996;10:1388–98.
77. Fuqua SAW, Wiltschke C, Zhang QX, et al. A hypersensitive estrogen receptor-α mutation in premalignant breast lesions. Cancer Res. 2000;60:4026–9.
78. Herynk MH, Parra I, Cui Y, et al. Association between the estrogen receptor alpha A908G mutation and outcomes in invasive breast cancer. Clin Cancer Res. 2007;13:3235–43.
79. Conway K, Parrish E, Edmiston SN, et al. The estrogen receptor-alpha A908G (K303R) mutation occurs at a low frequency in invasive breast tumors: results from a population-based study. Breast Cancer Res. 2005;7:R871–80.
80. Couse JF, Korach KS. Estrogen receptor null mice: what have we learned and where will they lead us? Endocr Rev. 1999;20:358–417.
81. Bocchinfuso WP, Korach KS. Mammary gland development and tumorigenesis in estrogen receptor knockout mice. J Mammary Gland Biol Neoplasia. 1997;2:323–34.
82. Krege JH. Generation and reproductive phenotypes of mice lacking estrogen receptor beta. Nat Acad Sci. 1998;95:15677–82.
83. Tilli MT, Frech MS, Steed ME, et al. Introduction of estrogen receptor-alpha into the tTA/TAg conditional mouse model precipitates the development of estrogen-responsive mammary adenocarcinoma. Am J Pathol. 2003;163:1713–9.
84. Frech MS, Halama ED, Tilli MT, et al. Deregulated estrogen receptor alpha expression in mammary epithelial cells of transgenic mice results in the development of ductal carcinoma in situ. Cancer Res. 2005;65:681–5.
85. Tekmal RR, Kirma N, Gill K, Fowler K. Aromatase overexpression and breast hyperplasia, an in vivo model – continued overexpression of aromatase is sufficient to maintain hyperplasia without circulating estrogens, and aromatase inhibitors abrogate these preneoplastic changes in mammary glands. Endocr-Relat Cancer. 1999;6:307–14.

86. Rogatsky I, Trowbridge JM, Garabedian MJ. Potentiation of human estrogen receptor alpha transcriptional activation through phosphorylation of serines 104 and 106 by the cyclin A-CDK2 complex. J Biol Chem. 1999;274:22296–302.
87. Joel PB, Smith J, Sturgill TW, Fisher TL, Blenis J, Lannigan DA. pp90rsk1 regulates estrogen receptor-mediated transcription through phosphorylation of Ser-167. Mol Cell Biol. 1998;18:1978–84.
88. Joel PB, Traish AM, Lannigan DA. Estradiol and phorbol ester cause phosphorylation of serine 118 in the human estrogen receptor. Mol Endocrinol. 1995;9:1041–52.
89. Arnold SF, Obourn JD, Jaffe H, Notides AC. Serine 167 is the major estradiol-induced phosphorylation site on the human estrogen receptor. Mol Endocrinol. 1994;8:1208–14.
90. Feng W, Webb P, Nguyen P, et al. Potentiation of estrogen receptor activation function 1 (AF-1) by Src/JNK through a serine 118-independent pathway. Mol Endocrinol. 2001;15:32–45.
91. Herynk MH, Beyer AR, Cui Y, et al. Cooperative action of tamoxifen and c-Src inhibition in preventing the growth of estrogen receptor-positive human breast cancer cells. Mol Cancer Ther. 2006;5:3023–31.

Role of ERβ in Clinical Breast Cancer

Valerie Speirs and Abeer M. Shaaban

Introduction

A second estrogen receptor (ER), ERβ, was cloned from rat in 1996 by Jan-Ake Gustafsson [1] and soon afterward human and murine isoforms were identified [2, 3]. Although unexpected, the discovery of ERβ was not totally surprising as other members of the steroid receptor superfamily, to which ER belongs, had multiple family members, and up to this point ER was an exception in this regard. As shown in Fig. 1, ERβ is structurally and genetically distinct from its sib ERα: mature full-length ERα is 595 amino acids and located on chromosome 6q while ERβ comprises 530 amino acids and resides on chromosome 14q22-25 [4, 5]. Because of the recognized importance of ERα in the breast, it follows that ERβ may also fulfill an important role. In this chapter we review the current understanding of ERβ in clinical breast cancer and discuss the potential role it may play in the future management of this disease.

ERβ Isoforms and Their Function

ERβ exists as five distinct isoforms, termed ERβ1–5, each distinguished by a unique exon 8 sequence. Moreover, in breast cancer, these variants are usually found in greater abundance than wtERβ (ERβ1) at least in terms of RNA expression [6–8]. Ethnic differences in expression of ERβ isoforms have been reported with ERβ1 and in particular, ERβ5 expressed at significantly higher levels in African Americans compared to Caucasians [9]. Tumors from African

V. Speirs (✉)
Section of Pathology and Tumor Biology, Leeds Institute of Molecular Medicine, University of Leeds, Wellcome Trust Brenner Building, St James's University Hospital, Leeds, LS9 7TF, UK
e-mail: V.Speirs@leeds.ac.uk

S.A.W. Fuqua (ed.), *Hormone Receptors in Breast Cancer*,
Cancer Treatment and Research 312, DOI 10.1007/978-0-387-09463-2_2,

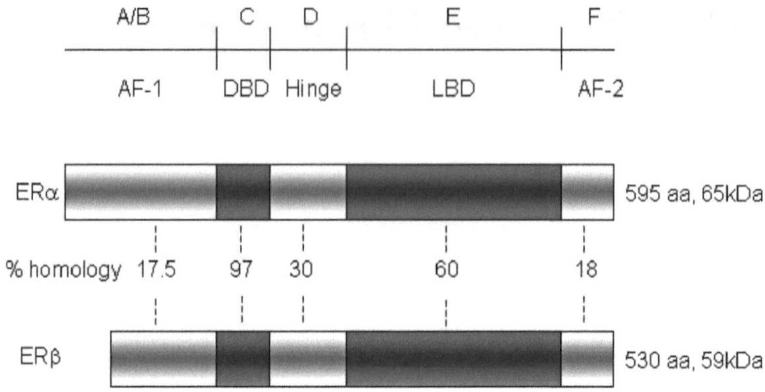

Fig. 1 Schematic illustration of human ERα and ERβ

Americans are often ERα negative with poorer survival [10]; so the high expression of ERβ isoforms suggests that these patients may well benefit from specific ERβ-targeted therapies (discussed later). These isoforms are schematically illustrated in Fig. 2 and described in detail below.

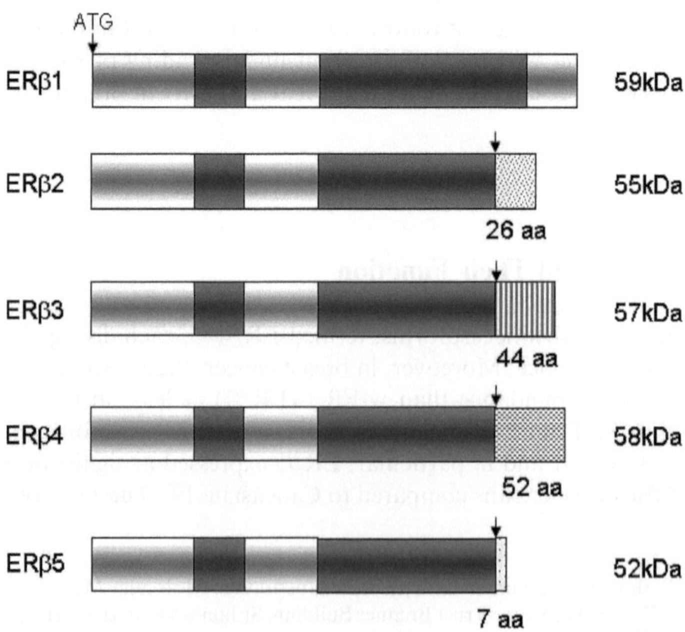

Fig. 2 Structure of ERβ1–5. All five isoforms are identical in structure through exons 1–7 but have a unique exon 8 sequence

ERβ1

The first published human ERβ1 cDNA was initially believed to encode a protein of ~53 kDa [2]. However, a longer version was subsequently identified, which is now accepted as full-length ERβ1 comprising 530 amino acids and encoding a protein of ~59 kDa [11]. A longer, functionally distinct 548 amino acid form of ERβ has also been described with an additional 18 amino acids at the N-terminus [12], but this is not commonly expressed, as evidenced from studies in three ethnically diverse populations (Caucasian, African or Asian; [13]).

ERβ1 binds estradiol with high affinity [4, 14] via a functional steroid-binding pocket [15], and the AF-2 domain recruits p160 co-activators necessary for transcriptional activation [16]. ERβ1 exhibits transcriptional activity on "classic" and "non-classic" EREs [17, 14] and can induce gene transcription in vitro [18, 19].

Introduction of ERβ1 into ER-negative cells has inhibitory effects on cell proliferation and invasion [20–22]. Coupled with the observation that ERβ1 expression is reduced in many clinical breast cancers (discussed in detail below), this has led to the conclusion that ERβ1 is a good prognostic factor in breast and other cancers [23, 24].

ERβ2/cx

Originally named ERβcx, ERβ2 is identical to *ERβ1* from exons 1 to 7 but has a unique 26 amino acid sequence in exon 8 [17, 11]. ERβ2 cannot bind estradiol and by itself does not exhibit any significant transcriptional activity on an ERE reporter gene [14, 25]. However, it can influence the action of other ERs, through heterodimerization with ERα and ERβ2 which subsequently inhibits DNA binding and ligand-dependent transactivation [17, 11, 14, 26].

ERβ3

Two independent studies failed to show ERβ3 expression in a panel of breast cancer cell lines [7, 17] and it is believed to be a testis-specific isoform. However, unpublished work from our laboratory has shown the presence of ERβ3 by RT-PCR in MCF-7 cells, with sporadic expression and low-level expression in other studies [27, 28].

ERβ4 and ERβ5

Originally believed to be truncated isoforms [17], ERβ4 and ERβ5 have subsequently been shown to represent full-length distinct isoforms that bind promoter sequences on DNA but do not bind estrogen. They translocate to the nucleus and exhibit three to four times higher estrogen-independent transcriptional activity than ERβ1.

In vitro band shift studies indicate that ERβ1–3 are able to form DNA-binding homodimers and heterodimers with each other with the ERα [17]. Similarly, ERβ4 and ERβ5 form heterodimers with ERα, negatively regulating its transcriptional activity [9, 29]. The ability of ER isoforms to influence the action of other ERs through heterodimerization is a very important finding with the potential implications of antagonizing the growth-promoting function of ERα.

ERβ Splice Variants

Many splice variants have been identified and comprise deletions, insertions and point mutations. These have been reviewed in detail elsewhere [30]; so only selected examples are given below. Their prognostic significance is still under debate as it is not clear whether or not they are translated into protein. No significant difference in expression of exon deletion variants ER$\beta\Delta$2 or Δ4 has been reported between tumor tissue and normal breast [31, 32]. Exon 5–6 deletions tend to be decreased in breast cancers while ER$\beta\Delta$5 expression was significantly increased in higher grade tumors and post-menopausal patients [32]. ER$\beta\Delta$5 lacks part of the ligand-binding domain and although cannot itself bind ligand it acts as a dominant-negative repressor of estrogen-induced ERα and ERβ transactivation [14, 33]. However, ER$\beta\Delta$5 is also common in normal mammary gland [34]. Deletion of ER$\beta\Delta$6 results in a truncated translation product which, although common, does not correlate with general clinico-pathological variables [31, 32].

Distribution of ERβ Isoforms in the Breast

ERβ is the principal ER in normal breast [35]. Unlike ERα which is localized to luminal epithelial cells (Fig. 3a), ERβ is expressed in luminal epithelium, myoepithelium, stromal cells and endothelium of blood vessels [35]. The protein is also expressed in the reactive lymphocyte population within normal breast.

Immunohistochemical studies showed that ERβ isoforms are differentially expressed in normal breast with ERβ wild type and ERβ1 staining the majority of nuclei of interlobular ducts and terminal duct lobular units [35, 36] (Fig. 3b). ERβ2 immunoreactivity was also reported in nerve tissue within normal breast [27]. Data from our laboratory also show an abundance of ERβ5 protein within the nuclei of luminal cells, myoepithelial cells and stromal cells (Fig. 3c). ERβ2, however, appears to be less expressed in normal mammary ducts [37]. This is illustrated in Fig. 3d.

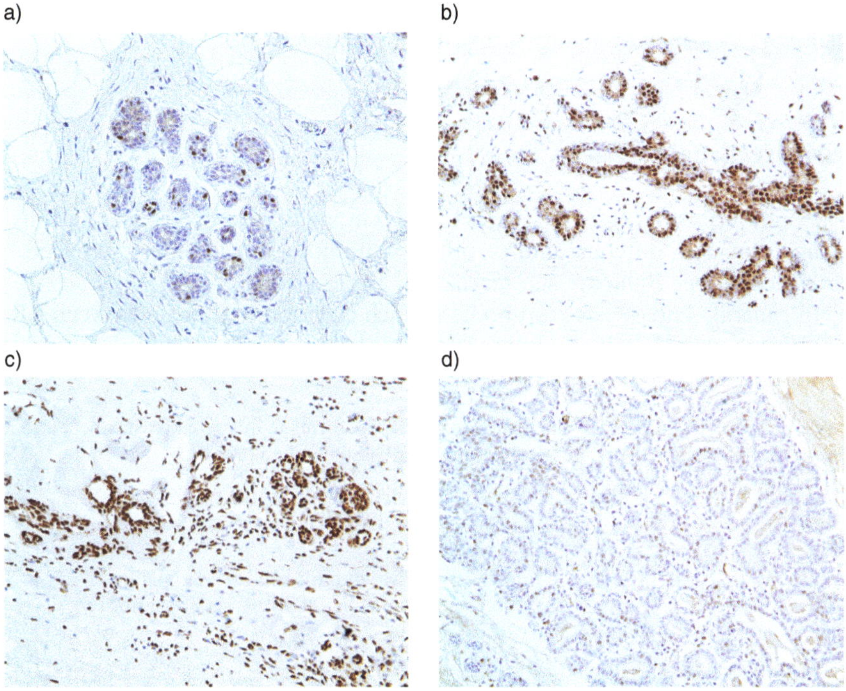

Fig. 3 (**a**) ERα immunohistochemistry in a normal mammary lobule showing scattered positive luminal epithelial cells. Myoepithelial cells and stromal cells do not express the protein, (**b**) Normal terminal duct lobular unit showing strong immunoreactivity for ERβ1 in luminal epithelium, myoepithelium and stromal cells, (**c**) Strong positive ERβ5 staining in the majority of luminal, myoepithelial and stromal cells within normal mammary lobules, (**d**) Expression of ERβ2 in epithelial cells of normal lobules. Both the proportion of positive cells and intensity of staining are less than ERβ1 (**c**)

Clinical Data

Prior to the availability of reliable antibodies for ERβ, the first studies addressing the significance of ERβ in clinical breast cancer were conducted at the mRNA level. Often these considered total mRNA, which did not take into account the potential role of individual isoforms. Additionally, many studies used mRNA extracted from non-microdissected tissue which potentially contains not only tumor cells but also adjacent normal tissue, adipose tissue, blood vessels and immune infiltrates, all known to express ERβ [38]. These early studies have been reviewed in detail elsewhere [23, 39]; so we will focus predominantly on antibody-based studies since these have greater clinical applicability. Following the development of antibodies against ERβ and its isoforms, in the last few years, studies have determined their efficacy to detect the protein in breast cancer [40–42]. These studies are important because if ERβ is to fulfill any future prognostic role, it will be necessary to have a simple and robust assay that can be easily adopted by histopathology laboratories.

Invasive Breast Cancer

The immunohistochemistry studies of ERβ in invasive breast cancer and their association with outcome and/or other pathobiological features published to date (September 2008) are summarized in Table 1.

In general, studies using antibodies, which do not discriminate between ERβ isoforms, have been mixed. However, it must be noted that study size is variable,

Table 1 Summary of protein-based studies of ERβ isoforms in invasive breast cancer and its association with clinico-pathological features (1999–September 2008)

ERβ isoform	Number	Clinical associations	Ref
Total	353	Increased OS and DFS in ERα-negative cases.	[104]
Total	319	ERα, PR	[57]
Total	305*	Improved survival in tamoxifen-treated patients. No correlation with ERα, PR, size, age, node status, ploidy	[47]
Total	234	Aneuploidy	[93]
Total	165	Increased DFS	[45]
Total	92	Node-negative patients, low S-phase fractions, pre-menopausal	[44]
Total	77	Improved response to endocrine therapy	[43]
Total	71	Inverse correlation with ERα, trend with node status. No correlation with Ki67	[94]
Total	65	ERα, PR and well-differentiated tumors	[46]
Total	59	No correlation with ERα, size, grade, node status or survival	[95]
Total	44	Ki67 and cyclin A	[96]
Total	41	No association with ERα, LN, size or differentiation state	[97]
Total	27	PR. High ERβ expression has improved outcome	[64]
Total	79	<2 cm, high grade	[98]
Total, β2	43	Both increased in invasive cancer	[51]
Total, β2	50	Total correlates with β2. β2 correlates with MIB1 in tamoxifen-resistant tumors. No correlation with ERα, PR, age, grade, tumor type or node status	[68]
β1	936	Better survival in triple negative and node negative cases but associated with more aggressive disease in node positive cases	[105]
β1	181	DFS, ERα, PR, increased topoisomerase IIa. Inverse correlation with c-erbB2 overexpression, no correlation with p53	[48]
β1	141	Reduced expression in malignant cells	[36]
β1	170	Correlation with PPARγ	[99]

Table 1 (continued)

ERβ isoform	Number	Clinical associations	Ref
β1	167	Ki67. No correlation with ERα, PR, grade or node status	[100]
β1	150	DFS. Inverse correlation with HER-2 and SRC-1	[49]
β1	88	Increased DFS	[50]
β1	52	Node-negative patients and those showing a positive response to endocrine treatment	[101]
β1	41	Not reported	[102]
β2	141	Better prognosis	[106]
β2	73	Favorable response to endocrine therapy	[67]
β1, β2	150	β1 with small tumor size, negative node status and low histological grade β2 with ERβ and low histological grade. β1 and β2 associated with better DFS and OS	[107]
ND	147	HER-2, cathepsin D, p53, pS2, Ki-67. No correlation with grade, ploidy or S-phase	[103]
βw	57	ERα, PR, low grade	[53]
βN		Low grade	
βC		ERα, PR, low grade, better prognosis	
β2		No correlation	
Total, β1, β2	225#	Total and β1 correlated with Ki67 and CK5/6, β2 with c-Jun and NFκBp65. No effects on survival	[108]
Total, β1, β2	442	Total and β1 associated with better survival, especially in triple negative cases. β2 uninformative	[109]
β1, β2, β5	757	β1 with ERα, PR, AR, BRCA1. β2 with ERα, PR, AR, BRCA1 and better OS and DFS and response to tamoxifen. β5 with better OS. Cytoplasmic β2 associated with poor OS and DFS	[110]
β1, β2, β3, β5	17	β3 and β5 with increased tumor size and increased proliferation. β3 with LN status	[27]

*Western blot study, #ERα negative cohort, ND = not defined, DFS = disease-free survival, OS = overall survival. Article dealing with specific histopathological subtypes have been excluded.

ranging from 27 to 319 cases. We believe that the most valid data will come from larger datasets (>50 cases), and of these some trends are beginning to emerge in terms of improved response to endocrine therapy, increased survival and association with well-differentiated tumor [43–46, 107] in ERβ-positive tumors. The positive association of ERβ with improved survival has also been independently confirmed in a Western blot study of 234 cases [47]. This association appears even stronger when the role of isoform-specific antibodies is examined, with ERβ1 correlating with improved disease-free survival [48–50, 105–107, 109].

The pathobiological role of ERβ2 in breast cancer is just starting to be defined and protein studies are inconsistent. A study of 26 DCIS, 43 invasive breast cancers and 39 adjacent normal tissues reported a significant increase of ERβ2 in DCIS and invasive breast cancer compared to normal gland [51]. This correlates with mRNA studies in which *ERβ2* mRNA was the most abundantly expressed *ERβ* isoform in breast tumors [6, 52, 53]. However, a significant decrease in ERβ2 mRNA was reported in 66 breast cancers compared to adjacent normal tissue from the same individuals, with the opposite trend observed with ERβ5 [54]. More recent studies focussing exclusively on protein expression and in large cohorts seem to indicate that ERβ2 is a good prognostic factor [106, 107, 110].

While there have been several mRNA studies comparing expression of ERβ isoforms, comparative immunohistochemical studies are rare. A small study of 17 invasive breast carcinomas showed that expression of both ERβ3 and ERβ5 was associated with larger tumor size and high proliferative activity whereas ERβ5 alone was associated with nodal metastasis [27]. The largest and most comprehensive study of ERβ isoforms conducted to date involved immunohistochemical analysis of ERß1, ERß2 and ERß5 in 757 invasive breast carcinomas with long term clinical follow up and made into tissue microarrays [110]. Nuclear expression of ERβ2 significantly correlated with tumor grade and size, Nottingham Prognostic Index, cumulative survival (CS), distant metastasis, death from breast cancer, and ERα, PR, AR and BRCA1 expression. Positive ERβ1 expression was not associated with any pathological parameter. ERβ5 was predominantly expressed in grade 3 carcinomas, showed a highly significant positive correlation with ERβ1 and a trend towards shorter survival associated with high Allred scores ($\geq$7). Notably, this study also highlighted the importance of cytoplasmic expression, a feature that had been consistently reported by different groups, but the significance of which had not been elucidated. In our study, cytoplasmic ERβ2 staining, whether alone or in combination with nuclear expression, was associated with a decrease in CS. The mechanism behind this remains unexplored.

A few studies have examined ERβ in ERα negative cohorts [reviewed in 111]. Interestingly, in these cohorts ERβ expression seems to be associated with more aggressive disease. Thus when expressed independently of ERα, the role of ERβ is markedly different. ERβ has also been examined in triple negative/basal phenotype breast cancers which are currently receiving much attention and its presence is predictive of better outcome and response to endocrine therapy [109], suggesting that any type of ER confers favorable outcome in breast cancer.

ERβ is also expressed in male breast cancer [55], but because of the rarity of the disease in men, it is not yet known if this contributes to prognosis.

Role in Neoplastic Progression

A handful of studies have examined ERβ expression in DCIS. Using antibodies which detect either total ERβ or ERβ1 widespread expression of ERβ was seen in DCIS [44, 56, 57]. The relationship between DCIS nuclear grade and ERβ expression has also been studied. Both the two largest studies on DCIS thus far have examined ERβ expression in 59 paraffin wax-embedded cases [56, 58]. An inverse correlation was seen with nuclear grade [56], however in the second series, this was not observed [58]. In another series of 35 DCIS examples, 28 cases were classified as positive, but no association was found between nuclear expression of ERβ and DCIS grade [36]. However, when stained for ERβ2 a different expression pattern was noted in DCIS (n = 26), with low expression in normal breast which was increased in DCIS and continued to increase further in invasive carcinoma [51]. The relationship with HER2 has also been studied where 50% of HER2-negative DCIS cases expressed ERβ, suggesting that these tumors might represent a distinct phenotypical subtype [58].

Comparative studies indicate that ERβ1 protein expression decreases progressively from normal breast, through intraductal proliferation, to in situ and invasive neoplasia [56, 36], although most breast carcinomas express at least some ERβ protein. Similar conclusions were drawn from RNA studies and therefore loss of ERβ appears to be a hallmark of mammary carcinogenesis. It has been hypothesized that ERβ acts as a dominant suppressor inhibiting the mitogenic effect of ERα [26]. Loss of ERβ1 is therefore implicated in the development of estrogen-dependent tumors [24]. There is experimental evidence that reduction of ERβ1 in invasive carcinomas might be the result of reversible promoter hypermethylation [59]. Indeed, more than two-thirds of invasive breast carcinomas showed increased methylation when compared with normal breast. Many pre-invasive lesions also showed increased methylation indicating that promoter methylation might be an early indication of malignancy [59]. Furthermore, in epithelial hyperplasia of usual type, higher ERα:ERβ protein ratio was found in patients who subsequently developed breast cancer [60]. Interestingly, ERβ2 seems to follow the reverse pattern where its protein expression increased progressively with neoplastic progression [51] and has also been borne out in mRNA studies [53].

Role in Tamoxifen Response/Resistance

Studies investigating the relationship between ERβ expression response/resistance and hormonal therapy have produced conflicting results. In a prospective study of 47 patients over 65 years, both ERα (protein) and ERβ (mRNA) were analyzed prior to and after neoadjuvant hormone therapy. The response rate was assessed by the degree of tumor shrinkage. In this cohort ERβ expression did not predict pre-operative response to hormone therapy whereas higher ERα levels correlated with better response [61]. However, tumors with positive ERβ mRNA expressed higher levels of the EGFR protein, a feature often associated with hormone resistance [62], which may have accounted for the lack of predictive response. In a series of 118 breast cancer patients treated with adjuvant tamoxifen, positive nuclear expression of total ERβ, using a 10% cutoff value for positivity, was associated with better survival in node-positive ($P = 0.007$) and -negative patients ($P = 0.0069$) [45]. High levels of ERβ were predictive of overall survival and disease-free survivals in patients treated with tamoxifen (n = 186 patients) [47]. ERβ1 has also been shown to correlate with a longer disease-free survival ($P = 0.008$) and a negative HER2 status ($P < 0.001$) [49].

An mRNA study in a cohort of 105 patients treated with adjuvant endocrine therapy showed that expression of *ERβ2* was significantly related to improved disease-free survival [63]. Conversely, others showed no correlation between *ERβ2* mRNA expression and tamoxifen response [64], also been borne out at the protein level [65]. A pilot study of 18 core needle biopsies revealed that ERβ2 expression correlated with poor response to endocrine therapy [66]. The same study showed that ERβ2 in ERα+ cells was associated with lack of PR expression [66]. This was contradicted in a combined immunohistochemistry and Western blotting study where ERβ2 expression correlated with a favorable response to endocrine therapy, with ERβ2-positive patients having increased survival [67]. A third study with a cohort of 50 breast tumors, including 34 tamoxifen sensitive and 16 cases of relapse failed to show any difference in ERβ2 expression, leading the authors to conclude that ERβ2 is not predictive of tamoxifen resistance [68].

ERβ2 but not ERβ1 was significantly associated with a good relapse-free survival ($P < 0.005$) and was predictive of overall survival in ERα-positive cases and in patients who received adjuvant tamoxifen therapy [63, 100, 106]. Conversely, ERβ1, but not ERβ2, appears to be predictive of response to tamoxifen therapy with low levels being associated with tamoxifen resistance [68, 109]. Tumors that responded to endocrine therapy were shown to contain lower ratios of ERβ2:ERβ1 protein when compared with non-responders [43].

Tamoxifen-resistant tumors were shown to have less-frequent methylation of the ERβ gene when compared with ERα, leading the authors to hypothesize that the ERβ methylation inversely correlated with tamoxifen resistance [69]. One of the obvious drawbacks of these studies is the small cohorts, and further validation on larger datasets with defined clinical outcome is now required as advocated in a recent review outlining retrospective clinical studies where ERβ expression was associated with increased likelihood of response to hormone therapy [70].

ERβ Polymorphisms and Breast Cancer Risk

In Africans, five novel ERβ polymorphisms have been described and one of these, a valine to glycine substitution at position 320 (V320G), was significantly less transcriptionally active in reporter gene assays than wtERβ [71]. A further novel variant, ERβF289L, with an amino acid change from phenylalanine to leucine at position 289 has also been described in African Americans. Compared to wtERβ this variant had reduced estrogen-binding affinity and impaired response to 17β-estradiol-induced transactivation, leading the authors to conclude that it might confer genetic susceptibility to particular endocrine-related diseases in African Americans [71].

Single nucleotide polymorphism (SNP) genotyping has identified eight ERβ sequence variants in a cohort of 30 Chinese women where increased breast cancer risk was associated with a CG or GG genotype in SNP [C(33390)G] combined with high levels of systemic steroid sex hormones or low levels of sex hormone-binding globulins [72]. Potential synergistic effects between SNP [C(33390)G] and levels of sex steroid hormones were also seen. In Scandinavian populations there does not appear to be any clear association of ERβ polymorphisms in familial or sporadic breast cancer [73, 74], also reported in a Greek population [75]. Overall, genetic modifications to ERβ might alter receptor–ligand affinities and endogenous estrogen exposure could impact on breast cancer development in these different ethnic groups. However, data so far do not indicate any definite association between ERβ gene polymorphisms and the risk of breast cancer.

Detailed mutational analysis of the entire coding region of ERβ was done on 93 breast carcinomas using single-strand conformational polymorphisms. One missense mutation and three silent mutations were identified in breast tumors and in constitutional DNA with a similar frequency to healthy individuals. The authors concluded that all those mutations were single nucleotide polymorphisms (SNP) that were not related to breast cancer risk and that ERβ does not act as a classic tumor suppressor gene [76 and supported by LOH data from our group, 77].

Prospects for Therapy

Epigenetic Targeting

Epigenetic gene silencing through aberrant methylation of promoter CpG islands is a common event in cancer. There is good evidence that ERβ is a methylation target as there are CpG islands within its promoter [78]. A mechanism can be envisaged whereby methylated ERβ CpG islands could progressively accumulate during tumor development, resulting in CpG island hypermethylation, eventually leading to gene silencing. The anti-proliferative effects of ERβ described above would then be lost in these cells, leading to a growth advantage.

In breast cancer cell lines and in clinical breast cancer, a significant correlation between promoter hypermethylation and loss of ERβ mRNA expression has been shown [79]. Methylation-linked silencing of ERβ means this gene represents a potential target for therapeutic strategies based on reversal of epigenetic silencing since the DNA of epigenetically inactivated genes is not mutated. In vitro data showed ERβ expression can be reversibly modified via DNA methyltransferase inhibitors such as 5′ -aza-deoxycytidine (DAC) [57, 79]. As ERβ expression is lost or reduced in many breast tumors, using these agents to induce its re-expression might be a good prospect for breast cancer patients. This may have clinical impact as it has been demonstrated that re-introduction of ERβ protein with adenoviral vectors in breast cancer cells in vitro inhibited cell proliferation, invasion and motility [20, 22]. Re-expression of

ERβ in ERβ-negative tumors by agents such as DAC may lead to suppression of tumor growth or even sensitization to anti-cancer therapies, which are being developed specifically to target ERβ.

This feature of ERβ may also impact on current hormone therapies as recent experimental evidence has shown that while ERβ expression is increased by DAC, ERα expression is actually decreased [80]. In breast cancer cell lines, when ERα and ERβ are co-expressed, ERβ is anti-proliferative [22]. Therapeutic strategies could be designed to take advantage of this. In theory, in ERα + ERβ+ or ERα + ERβ− tumors an epigenetically targeted drug such as DAC would stimulate expression of ERβ and all the positive anti-proliferative effects this would give while at the same time downregulating ERα. This would be followed by conventional ER-targeted endocrine therapies, which theoretically should still be effective as most current ER antagonists have similar affinity for ERα and ERβ [81]. This selective approach remains to be tested in patients but preliminary in vitro work suggests it is feasible [80] and is illustrated schematically in Fig. 4. Clinical trials of epigenetic therapies are now underway and the histone deacetylase inhibitor suberoylanilide hydroxamic acid (SAHA) is in phase I/II clinical trials and has already shown anti-tumor activity in solid tumors including breast at well-tolerated doses [82]. It remains possible that these new epigenetically

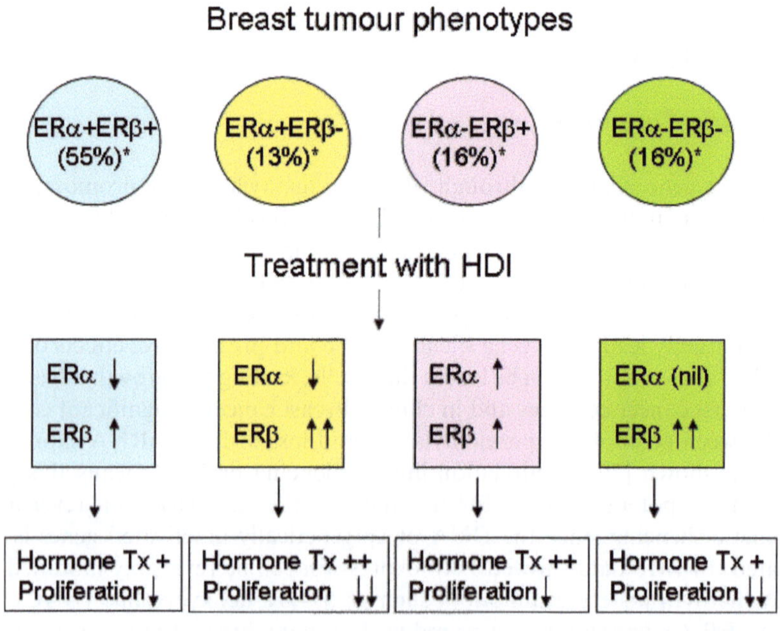

Fig. 4 Hypothetical outcome of the use of histone deacetylase inhibitors (HDI) in breast cancers of defined ER phenotype. In theory, HDIs would modulate activity of ERα and ERβ in breast tumors as illustrated. The predicted response of these tumors to conventional ER-targeted endocrine therapies following HDI treatment is also shown. *Figures adapted from Saji et al. [39]

targeted agents could be used in conjunction with conventional endocrine therapies to achieve maximum benefit from selective ER expression, thus giving breast cancer patients the best possible chance of hormone response and is interesting to note that an AACR Task Force Report has listed ERβ as a possible target for molecular chemoprevention via epigenetic modulation [83].

ERβ-Selective Agents

Development of novel ERβ-specific drugs, akin to "designer estrogens" [84] is an attractive prospect and the possibility now exists for their synthesis which could maintain the positive benefits of endocrine therapy but without some of the associated risks, i.e., uterine and breast stimulation. The oral steroidal anti-estrogen TAS-108, currently in phase II trials for breast cancer, is one such compound which is a pure antagonist on ERα and a partial agonist on ERβ and has little uterotrophic effect [85]. Many new non-steroidal compounds such as aryl benzthiophenes [86], aryl diphenolic azoles [87] and indazole compounds [88] have been developed as potential ERβ-selective ligands and their ERβ selectivity could lead to the design of pharmacologically useful ERβ-selective agonists or antagonists. The dihydrotestosterone metabolite 5a-androstane-3b,17b-diol was shown to potently inhibit migration of prostate cancer cells in vitro via ERβ [89] and this could have potential in other ERβ-expressing tumors.

Trials of a 3β-hydroxysteroid dehydrogenase inhibitor, trilostane (Modrenal), which is believed to function through ERβ-mediated pathways [90], have just been completed in the UK for advanced breast cancer patients who relapsed after initial hormone therapy. Dietary phytoestrogens share structural similarity with 17β-estradiol (E2) and have high affinity for ERβ [81]. Isocoumarin analogues structurally related to the phytoestrogens daidzein, genistein and coumestrol have been developed and show promise in vitro [91].

Of note, a recent AACR Task Force Report has identified resveratrol (a red wine polyphenol) and TAS-108 (discussed above) as two potential agents that are currently being tested for breast cancer chemoprevention [83]. This offers the exciting possibility of a potential new role for ERβ as a chemopreventative target.

Conclusions

From the data accumulated thus far it is clear that expression of ERβ and its isoforms is widespread in male and female breast cancer. In addition to their ability to modulate hormone action through heterodimerization, these isoforms are likely to have distinct distribution and functions, however, we still are some way off fully understanding their individual and collective role. This could be addressed through microarray analysis. Indeed, a custom-made gene microarray designed to detect estrogen-regulated genes revealed that MCF-7 cells stably transfected with ERβ2 had a unique gene expression profile compared to wtMCF-7 cells or those transfected with ERβ1, whose gene profiles were similar [92]. This suggests that ERβ2 regulates a distinct set of genes. This type of approach could be used to more fully define the role of ERβ isoforms and identify pathways activated by them, which could eventually have therapeutic potential.

Although clinical data regarding the prognostic significance of ERβ have been conflicting, the emerging view indicates that ERβ, particularly the ERβ2 isoform, is likely to be associated with favorable prognosis in breast cancer. With this in mind, it is perhaps time to think about incorporating ERβ1 and ERβ2 immunohistochemistry into histopathological review of breast cancer, especially now that robust antibodies are available. This may be even more important with the development of new endocrine agents and implementation of patient-specific therapies, which will only increase the need for detailed hormone receptor profiles. ERβ-selective agents have tremendous potential, and ongoing trials are likely to shed light on the functional role of ERβ.

In conclusion, ERβ and its isoforms may have functional implications in breast cancer and could have important and perhaps complementary roles to ERα in terms of predicting endocrine response and clinical outcome. Once these roles are established, routine testing for ERβ, in conjunction with ERα, could be justified.

Acknowledgments We gratefully acknowledge Yorkshire Cancer Research, Breast Cancer Campaign, Breast Cancer Research Trust, Breast Cancer Research Action Group, Liz Dawn Breast Cancer Appeal and the Leeds Teaching Hospitals NHS Trust for supporting our ERβ research program.

References

1. Kuiper GG, Enmark E, Pelto-Huikko M, et al. Cloning of a novel receptor expressed in rat prostate and ovary. Proc Natl Acad Sci USA. 1996;93:5925–30.
2. Mosselman S, Polman J, Dijkema R. ER beta: identification and characterization of a novel human estrogen receptor. FEBS Lett. 1996;392:49–53.
3. Tremblay GB, Tremblay A, Copeland NG, et al. Cloning, chromosomal localization, and functional analysis of the murine estrogen receptor beta. Mol Endocrinol. 1997;11:353–65.
4. Enmark E, Pelto-Huikko M, Grandien K, et al. Human estrogen receptor beta-gene structure, chromosomal localization, and expression pattern. J Clin Endocrinol Metab. 1997;82:4258–65.
5. Menasce LP, White GR, Harrison CJ, et al. Localization of the estrogen receptor locus (ESR) to chromosome 6q25.1 by FISH and a simple post-FISH banding technique. Genomics 1993;17:263–5.
6. Leygue E, Dotzlaw H, Watson PH, et al. Expression of estrogen receptor beta1, beta2, and beta5 messenger RNAs in human breast tissue. Cancer Res. 1999;59:1175–9.
7. Tong D, Schuster E, Seifert M, et al. Expression of estrogen receptor beta isoforms in human breast cancer tissues and cell lines. Breast Cancer Res Treat. 2002;71:249–55.
8. Iwao K, Miyoshi Y, Egawa C, et al. Quantitative analysis of estrogen receptor-beta mRNA and its variants in human breast cancers. Int J Cancer. 2000;88:733–6.

9. Poola I, Abraham J, Baldwin K, et al. Estrogen receptors beta4 and beta5 are full length functionally distinct ERbeta isoforms: cloning from human ovary and functional characterization. Endocrine 2005;27:227–38.
10. Chu KC, Lamar CA, Freeman HP. Racial disparities in breast carcinoma survival rates: separating factors that affect diagnosis from factors that affect treatment. Cancer 2003;97:2853–60.
11. Ogawa S, Inoue S, Watanabe T, et al. The complete primary structure of human estrogen receptor beta (hER beta) and its heterodimerization with ER alpha in vivo and in vitro. Biochem Biophys Res Commun. 1998;243:122–6.
12. Wilkinson HA, Dahllund J, Liu H, et al. Identification and characterization of a functionally distinct form of human estrogen receptor beta. Endocrinology 2002;143:1558–61.
13. Xu L, Pan-Hammarstrom Q, Forsti A, et al. Human estrogen receptor β 548 is not a common variant in three distinct populations. Endocrinology 2003;144:3541–6.
14. Peng B, Lu B, Leygue E, Murphy LC. Putative functional characteristics of human estrogen receptor-beta isoforms. J Mol Endocrinol. 2003;30:13–29.
15. Pike AC, Brzozowski AM, Hubbard RE, et al. Structure of the ligand-binding domain of oestrogen receptor beta in the presence of a partial agonist and a full antagonist. EMBO J. 1999;18:4608–18.
16. Klinge CM. Estrogen receptor interactions with co-activators and co-repressors. Steroids 2000;65: 227–51.
17. Moore JT, McKee DD, Slentz-Kesler K, et al. Cloning and characterization of human estrogen receptor beta isoforms. Biochem Biophys Res Commun. 1998;247:75–8.
18. Paech K, Webb P, Kuiper GGJM, et al. Differential Ligand Activation of Estrogen Receptors ERα and ERβ at AP1 Sites. Science 1997;277:1508–10.
19. Barkhem T, Nilsson S, Gustafsson JA. Molecular mechanisms, physiological consequences and pharmacological implications of estrogen receptor action. Am J Pharmacogenomics. 2004;4:19–28.
20. Lazennec G, Bresson D, Lucas A, et al. ER beta inhibits proliferation and invasion of breast cancer cells. Endocrinology 2001;142:4120–30.
21. Murphy LC, Peng B, Lewis A, et al. Inducible upregulation of oestrogen receptor-β1 affects oestrogen and tamoxifen responsiveness in MCF7 human breast cancer cells. J Mol Endocrinol. 2005;34:553–66.
22. Paruthiyil S, Parmar H, Kerekatte V, et al. Estrogen receptor beta inhibits human breast cancer cell proliferation and tumor formation by causing a G2 cell cycle arrest. Cancer Res. 2004;64:423–8.
23. Speirs V, Carder PJ, Lane S, et al. Oestrogen receptor β: what it means for patients with breast cancer. Lancet Oncol. 2004;5:174–81.
24. Bardin A, Boulle N, Lazennec G, et al. Loss of ERbeta expression as a common step in estrogen-dependent tumor progression. Endocr Relat Cancer. 2004;11:537–51.
25. Ogawa S, Inoue S, Watanabe T, et al. Molecular cloning and characterization of human estrogen receptor βcx: a potential inhibitor of estrogen action in human. . Nucleic Acids Res. 1998;26:3505–12.
26. Pettersson K, Delaunay F, Gustafsson JA. Estrogen receptor beta acts as a dominant regulator of estrogen signaling. Oncogene 2000;19:4970–8.
27. Chi A, Chen X, Chirala M, et al. Differential expression of estrogen receptor beta isoforms in human breast cancer tissue. Anticancer Res. 2003;23:211–6.
28. Girault I, Andrieu C, Tozlu S, et al. Altered expression pattern of alternatively spliced estrogen receptor beta transcripts in breast carcinoma. Cancer Lett. 2004;215:101–12.
29. Poola I, Abraham J, Baldwin K, et al . Estrogen receptors beta4 and beta5 are full length functionally distinct ERbeta isoforms: cloning from human ovary and functional characterization. Endocrine 2005;27:227–38.
30. Herynk MH, Fuqua SAW. Estrogen Receptor Mutations in Human Disease. Endocr Rev. 2004;25:869–98.

31. Poola I, Abraham J, Baldwin K. Identification of ten exon deleted ER[beta] mRNAs in human ovary, breast, uterus and bone tissues: alternate splicing pattern of estrogen receptor β mRNA is distinct from that of estrogen receptor α. FEBS Lett. 2002;516:133–38.
32. Poola I, Abraham J, Liu A. Estrogen receptor beta splice variant mRNAs are differentially altered during breast carcinogenesis. J Steroid Biochem Mol Biol. 2002;82:169–79.
33. Inoue S, Ogawa S, Horie K, et al. An Estrogen Receptor [beta] Isoform That Lacks Exon 5 Has Dominant Negative Activity on both ERα and ERβ. Biochem Biophys Res Commun. 2000;279:814–19.
34. Speirs V, Adams IP, Walton DS, et al. Identification of Wild-Type and Exon 5 Deletion Variants of Estrogen Receptor β in Normal Human Mammary Gland. J Clin Endocrinol Metab. 2000;85:1601–05.
35. Speirs V, Skliris GP, Burdall SE, et al. Distinct expression patterns of ER α and ER β in normal human mammary gland. J Clin Pathol. 2002;55:371–4.
36. Shaaban AM, O'Neill PA, Davies MP, et al. Declining estrogen receptor-beta expression defines malignant progression of human breast neoplasia. Am J Surg Pathol. 2003; 27:1502–12.
37. Shaaban AM, Speirs V. The estrogen receptors α, β, and βcx. Clin Cancer Res. 2005;11:8222;author reply 8222–3.
38. Taylor AH, Al-Azzawi F. Immunolocalisation of oestrogen receptor beta in human tissues. J Mol Endocrinol. 2000;24:145–55.
39. Saji S, Hirose M, Toi M. Clinical significance of estrogen receptor beta in breast cancer. Cancer Chemother Pharmacol. 2005;56 Suppl 1:21–6.
40. Skliris GP, Parkes AT, Limer JL, et al . Evaluation of seven oestrogen receptor β antibodies for immunohistochemistry, western blotting, and flow cytometry in human breast tissue. J Pathol. 2002;197:155–62.
41. Weitsman GE, Skliris G, Ung K, et al. Assessment of multiple different estrogen receptor-beta antibodies for their ability to immunoprecipitate under chromatin immunoprecipitation conditions. Breast Cancer Res Treat. 2006.
42. Carder PJ, Murphy C, Dervan P, et al. A Multi-Centre Investigation Towards Reaching a Consensus on the Immunohistochemical Detection of ERβ in Archival Formalin-fixed Paraffin Embedded Human Breast Tissue. Breast Cancer Res Treat. 2005; 92:287–293.
43. Iwase H, Zhang Z, Omoto Y, et al. Clinical significance of the expression of estrogen receptors alpha and beta for endocrine therapy of breast cancer. Cancer Chemother Pharmacol. 2003;52 Suppl 1:S34–8.
44. Jarvinen TA, Pelto-Huikko M, Holli K, et al. Estrogen receptor beta is coexpressed with ERalpha and PR and associated with nodal status, grade, and proliferation rate in breast cancer. Am J Pathol. 2000;156:29–35.
45. Mann S, Laucirica R, Carlson N, et al. Estrogen receptor beta expression in invasive breast cancer. Hum Pathol. 2001;32:113–8.
46. Skliris GP, Carder PJ, Lansdown MR, et al. Immunohistochemical detection of ERbeta in breast cancer: towards more detailed receptor profiling? Br J Cancer. 2001;84:1095–8.
47. Hopp TA, Weiss HL, Parra IS, et al. Low levels of estrogen receptor beta protein predict resistance to tamoxifen therapy in breast cancer. Clin Cancer Res. 2004;10:7490–9.
48. Nakopoulou L, Lazaris AC, Panayotopoulou EG, et al. The favourable prognostic value of oestrogen receptor beta immunohistochemical expression in breast cancer. J Clin Pathol. 2004;57:523–8.
49. Myers E, Fleming FJ, Crotty TB, et al. Inverse relationship between ER-beta and SRC-1 predicts outcome in endocrine-resistant breast cancer. Br J Cancer. 2004;91:1687–93.
50. Omoto Y, Inoue S, Ogawa S, et al. Clinical value of the wild-type estrogen receptor beta expression in breast cancer. Cancer Lett. 2001;163:207–12.

51. Esslimani-Sahla M, Kramar A, Simony-Lafontaine J, et al. Increased estrogen receptor betacx expression during mammary carcinogenesis. Clin Cancer Res. 2005;11:3170–4.
52. Iwao K, Miyoshi Y, Egawa C, et al, Quantitative analysis of estrogen receptor $-\alpha$ and $-\beta$ messenger RNA expression in breast carcinoma by real-time polymerase chain reaction. Cancer 2000;89:1732–38.
53. Omoto Y, Kobayashi S, Inoue S, et al. Evaluation of oestrogen receptor beta wild-type and variant protein expression, and relationship with clinicopathological factors in breast cancers. Eur J Cancer. 2002;38:380–6.
54. Park BW, Kim KS, Heo MK, et al. The changes of estrogen receptor-? variants expression in breast carcinogenesis: decrease of estrogen receptor-?2 expression is the key event in breast cancer development. J Surg. Oncol. 2006;93:504–10.
55. Murphy CE, Carder PJ, Lansdown MRJ, et al. Steroid hormone receptor expression in male breast cancer. Eur J Surg. Oncol 2006;32:44–7.
56. Roger P, Sahla ME, Makela S, et al Decreased expression of estrogen receptor beta protein in proliferative preinvasive mammary tumors. Cancer Res. 2001;61:2537–41.
57. Skliris GP, Munot K, Bell SM, et al. Reduced expression of oestrogen receptor beta in invasive breast cancer and its re-expression using DNA methyl transferase inhibitors in a cell line model. J Pathol. 2003;201:213–20.
58. Rody A, Diallo R, Poremba C, et al. Estrogen receptor alpha and beta, progesterone receptor, pS2 and HER-2/neu expression delineate different subgroups in ductal carcinoma in situ of the breast. Oncol Rep. 2004;12:695–9.
59. Zhao C, Lam EW, Sunters A, et al. Expression of estrogen receptor beta isoforms in normal breast epithelial cells and breast cancer: regulation by methylation. Oncogene 2003;22:7600–6.
60. Shaaban AM, Jarvis C, Moore F, et al. Prognostic significance of estrogen receptor Beta in epithelial hyperplasia of usual type with known outcome. Am J Surg Pathol. 2005;29:1593–9.
61. Cappelletti V, Celio L, Bajetta E, et al. Prospective evaluation of estrogen receptor-beta in predicting response to neoadjuvant antiestrogen therapy in elderly breast cancer patients. Endocr Relat Cancer. 2004;11:761–70.
62. Knowlden JM, Gee JM, Robertson JF, et al A possible divergent role for the oestrogen receptor alpha and beta subtypes in clinical breast cancer. Int J Cancer. 2000;89:209–12.
63. Davies MP, O'Neill PA, Innes H, et al. Correlation of mRNA for oestrogen receptor beta splice variants ERbeta1, ERbeta2/ERbetacx and ERbeta5 with outcome in endocrine-treated breast cancer. J Mol Endocrinol. 2004;33:773–82.
64. Murphy LC, Leygue E, Niu Y, et al Relationship of coregulator and oestrogen receptor isoform expression to de novo tamoxifen resistance in human breast cancer. Br J Cancer. 2002;87 1411–16.
65. Miller WR, Anderson TJ, Dixon JM, et al. Oestrogen receptor beta and neoadjuvant therapy with tamoxifen: prediction of response and effects of treatment. Br J Cancer. 2006;94:1333–8.
66. Saji S, Omoto Y, Shimizu C, et al. Expression of estrogen receptor (ER) (beta)cx protein in ER(alpha)-positive breast cancer: specific correlation with progesterone receptor. Cancer Res. 2002;62:4849–53.
67. Palmieri C, Lam EW, Mansi J, et al. The expression of ER beta cx in human breast cancer and the relationship to endocrine therapy and survival. Clin Cancer Res. 2004;10:2421–8.
68. Esslimani-Sahla M, Simony-Lafontaine J, Kramar A, et al. Estrogen receptor beta (ER beta) level but not its ER beta cx variant helps to predict tamoxifen resistance in breast cancer. Clin Cancer Res. 2004;10:5769–76.
69. Chang HG, Kim SJ, Chung KW, et al. Tamoxifen-resistant breast cancers show less frequent methylation of the estrogen receptor beta but not the estrogen receptor alpha gene. J Mol Med. 2005;83:132–9.
70. Murphy LC, Watson PH. Is oestrogen receptor- {beta} a predictor of endocrine therapy responsiveness in human breast cancer? Endocr Relat Cancer. 2006;13:327–334.

71. Zhao C, Gustafsson JA, Dahlman-Wright K. Functional characterization of a novel variant of estrogen receptor beta identified in screening of DNA derived from African Americans. Pharmacogenet Genomics 2006;16:379–83.
72. Zheng SL, Zheng W, Chang BL, et al. Joint effect of estrogen receptor beta sequence variants and endogenous estrogen exposure on breast cancer risk in Chinese women. Cancer Res. 2003;63:7624–9.
73. Forsti A, Zhao C, Israelsson E, et al. Polymorphisms in the estrogen receptor beta gene and risk of breast cancer: no association. Breast Cancer Res Treat. 2003;79:409–13.
74. Maguire P, Margolin S, Skoglund J, et al. Estrogen Receptor Beta (ESR2) Polymorphisms in Familial and Sporadic Breast Cancer. Breast Cancer Res Treat. 2005;94:145–52.
75. Georgopoulos NA, Adonakis GL, Fotopoulos A, et al. Estrogen receptor polymorphisms in tamoxifen-treated women with breast cancer. Gynecol Endocrinol. 2006;22:185–9.
76. Hasegawa S, Miyoshi Y, Ikeda N, et al. Mutational analysis of estrogen receptor-beta gene in human breast cancers. Breast Cancer Res Treat. 2003;78:133–4.
77. Parker HD, Hanby AM, Bell SM, et al. Loss of heterozygosity at 14q does not correlate with estrogen receptor beta negative breast cancer. Breast Cancer Res Treat. 2005;94 (suppl 1):S245.
78. Nojima D, Li LC, Dharia A, et al. CpG hypermethylation of the promoter region inactivates the estrogen receptor-β gene in patients with prostate carcinoma. Cancer 2001;92:2076–2083.
79. Zhao C, Lam E, W-F., et al. Expression of estrogen receptor β isoforms in normal breast epithelial cells and breast cancer: regulation by methylation. Oncogene 2003;22: 7600–06.
80. Duong V, Licznar A, Margueron R, et al. ERα and ERβ expression and transcriptional activity are differentially regulated by HDAC inhibitors. Oncogene 2005;25:1799–06.
81. Kuiper GGJM, Carlsson B, Grandien K, et al. Comparison of the Ligand Binding Specificity and Transcript Tissue Distribution of Estrogen Receptors α and β. Endocrinology 1997;138:863–870.
82. Kelly WK, O'Connor OA, Krug LM, et al. Phase I Study of an Oral Histone Deacetylase Inhibitor, Suberoylanilide Hydroxamic Acid, in Patients With Advanced Cancer. J Clin Oncol. 2005;23:3923–31.
83. Kelloff GJ, Lippman SM, Dannenberg AJ, et al. Progress in chemoprevention drug development: the promise of molecular biomarkers for prevention of intraepithelial neoplasia and cancer – a plan to move forward. Clin Cancer Res. 2006.
84. Jordan V. Designer estrogens. Sci Am. 1998;279:60–7.
85. Yamamoto Y, Shibata J, Yonekura K, et al. TAS-108, a novel oral steroidal antiestrogenic agent, is a pure antagonist on estrogen receptor alpha and a partial agonist on estrogen receptor beta with low uterotrophic effect. Clin Cancer Res. 2005;11:315–22.
86. Schopfer U, Schoeffter P, Bischoff SF, et al. Toward selective ERbeta agonists for central nervous system disorders: synthesis and characterization of aryl benzthiophenes. J Med Chem. 2002;45:1399–401.
87. Malamas MS, Manas ES, McDevitt RE, et al. Design and synthesis of aryl diphenolic azoles as potent and selective estrogen receptor-beta ligands. J Med Chem. 2004;47:5021–40.
88. De Angelis M, Stossi F, Carlson KA, et al. Indazole estrogens: highly selective ligands for the estrogen receptor beta. J Med Chem. 2005;48:1132–44.
89. Guerini V, Sau D, Scaccianoce E, et al. The androgen derivative 5alpha-androstane-3beta,17beta-diol inhibits prostate cancer cell migration through activation of the estrogen receptor beta subtype. Cancer Res. 2005;65:5445–53.
90. Puddefoot JR, Barker S, Glover HR, et al. Non-competitive steroid inhibition of oestrogen receptor functions. Int J Cancer. 2002;101:17–22.
91. De Angelis M, Stossi F, Waibel M, et al. Isocoumarins as estrogen receptor beta selective ligands: isomers of isoflavone phytoestrogens and their metabolites. Bioorg Med Chem. 2005;13:6529–42.

92. Omoto Y, Eguchi H, Yamamoto-Yamaguchi Y et al. Estrogen receptor (ER) beta1 and ERbetacx/beta2 inhibit ERalpha function differently in breast cancer cell line MCF7. Oncogene. 2003;22:5011–20.
93. Fuqua SAW, Schiff R, Parra I, et al. Estrogen receptor β protein in human breast cancer: correlation with clinical tumour parameters. Cancer Res. 2003;63: 2343–439.
94. Koda M, Sulkowski S, Kanczuga-Koda L, et al. Expression of ERalpha, ERbeta and Ki-67 in primary tumors and lymph node metastases in breast cancer. Oncol Rep. 2004;11: 753–59.
95. Stefanou D, Batistatou A, Briasoulis E et al. Estrogen receptor beta (ERbeta) expression in breast carcinomas is not correlated with estrogen receptor alpha (ERalpha) and prognosis: the Greek experience. Eur J Gynaecol Oncol. 2004;25:457–61.
96. Jensen EV, Cheng G, Palmieri C et al. Estrogen receptors and proliferation markers in primary and recurrent breast cancer. Proc Natl Acad Sci USA. 2001;98: 15197–02.
97. Jarzabek K, Koda M, Kozloski L et al. Distinct mRNA, protein expression patterns and distribution of oestrogen receptors alpha and beta in human primary breast cancer: correlation with proliferation marker Ki-67 and clinicopathological factors. Eur J Cancer. 2005;41:2924–94.
98. Miyoshi Y, Taguchi T, Gustafsson JA, et al. Clinicopathological characteristics of estrogen receptor-beta-positive human breast cancers. Jpn J Cancer Res. 2001;92: 1057–61.
99. Papadaki I, Mylona E, Giannopouloui I, et al. PPARgamma expression in breast cancer: clinical value and correlation with ERbeta. Histopathology. 2005;46: 37–42.
100. O'Neill PA, Davies MP, Shaaban AM et al. Wild-type oestrogen receptor beta (ERbeta1) mRNA and protein expression in Tamoxifen-treated post-menopausal breast cancers. Br J Cancer. 2004;91:1694–102.
101. Fleming FJ, Hill AD, McDermott EW et al. Differential recruitment of coregulator proteins steroid receptor coactivator-1 and silencing mediator for retinoid and thyroid receptors to the estrogen receptor-estrogen response element by beta-estradiol and 4-hydroxytamoxifen in human breast cancer. J Clin Endocrinol Metab. 2004;89: 375–83.
102. Saunders PT, Millar MR, Williams K et al. Expression of oestrogen receptor beta (ERbeta1) protein in human breast cancer biopsies. Br J Cancer. 2002;86: 250–56.
103. Choi Y, Pinto M. Estrogen receptor beta in breast cancer: associations between ERbeta, hormonal receptors, and other prognostic biomarkers. Appl Immunohistochem Mol Morphol. 2005;13:19–24.
104. Gruvberger-Saal SK, Bendahl PO, Saal LH et al. Estrogen receptor beta expression is associated with tamoxifen response in ERalpha-negative breast carcinoma. Clin Cancer Res. 2007; 13: 1987–1994.
105. Novelli F, Milella M, Melucci E et al. A divergent role for estrogen receptor beta in node-positive and node-negative breast cancer classified according to molecular subtypes: an observational prospective study. Breast Cancer Res. 2008; 10: R74.
106. Vinayagam R, Sibson DR, Holcombe C, et al. Association of oestrogen receptor beta 2 (ER beta 2/ER beta cx) with outcome of adjuvant endocrine treatment for primary breast cancer - a retrospective study. BMC Cancer. 2007; 7: 131–140.
107. Sugiura H, Toyama T, Hara Y et al. Expression of estrogen receptor beta wild-type and its variant ERbetacx/beta2 is correlated with better prognosis in breast cancer. Jpn J Clin Oncol. 2007; 37: 820–828.
108. Skliris GP, Leygue E, Curtis-Snell L et al. Expression of oestrogen receptor-beta in oestrogen receptor-alpha negative human breast tumours. Br J Cancer. 2006; 95: 616–626.
109. Honma N, Horii R, Iwase T, et al. Clinical importance of estrogen receptor-beta evaluation in breast cancer patients treated with adjuvant tamoxifen therapy. J Clin Oncol. 2008; 26:3727–3734.

110. Shaaban AM, Green AR, Karthik S et al. Nuclear and cytoplasmic expression of ERbeta1, ERbeta2, and ERbeta5 identifies distinct prognostic outcome for breast cancer patients. Clin Cancer Res. 2008; 14: 5228–5235.
111. Skliris GP, Leygue E, Watson PH et al. Estrogen receptor alpha negative breast cancer patients: estrogen receptor beta as a therapeutic target. J Steroid Biochem Mol Biol. 2008; 109: 1–10.

Hormone Action and Breast Cancer

Ellis R. Levin

Estrogen Receptors

The two major sex steroids in women, estrogen and progesterone, have each been implicated to act in various ways to promote the development of breast cancer. The major form of estrogen produced in the ovary and adrenal is 17-β-estradiol (E2), and this hormone appears to act exclusively via estrogen-binding proteins (receptors) in breast cancer.

The overwhelming consensus from many studies is that estrogen acts through the conventional estrogen receptor, ERα, to promote tumor cell biology [1, 2]. This receptor is highly expressed in human breast epithelial cells and the approximate two-thirds of human breast cancers that arise from transformed epithelial cells [3]. Furthermore, there is evidence that early tumor progenitor cells (perhaps tumor stem cells) express ER [4]. E2 binding to ERα also occurs to an extent in stroma surrounding the breast/breast cancer epithelial cells [5], suggesting a paracrine mode of action in addition to the direct action of the sex steroid on the cancer cell [6]. This mechanism may be particularly applicable to rodent breast, but the precise contributions of stromal ER to the pathogenesis of human breast cancer remain to be defined.

Recent studies have implied that E2 binding to an orphan G-protein-coupled receptor, GPR30 [7, 8], is functionally important. However, these studies have primarily been carried out in ER-negative breast cancer cell lines. Estrogen effects on the biology of ER null breast tumors in vitro, or in women with ER-negative tumors in vivo [9], have not been demonstrated. Thus, the importance of GPR30 for estrogen action in this malignancy remains unsupported.

Understanding the mechanisms of ER action is therefore important to understand the biology of this malignancy. ER participation occurs either in response to binding by E2 or through activation from growth factor signaling to

E.R. Levin (✉)
Division of Endocrinology and Metabolism, University of California, Irvine and the Long Beach VA Medical Center, Long Beach, CA, USA
e-mail: ellis.levin@va.gov

S.A.W. Fuqua (ed.), *Hormone Receptors in Breast Cancer*,
Cancer Treatment and Research 312, DOI 10.1007/978-0-387-09463-2_3,

phosphorylation of the receptor. The latter does not require E2 presence [10, 11]. Estrogen metabolites may also contribute to the development of breast cancer [12], and this most often occurs through activating ER. In most forms of human breast cancer or cell lines derived from human tumors, ERα is the predominant receptor. However, it is clear that a small amount of ERβ is also present in breast tumors and cell lines, and some studies suggest that ERβ RNA expression correlates to tamoxifen resistance [13, 14]. Little is currently known, however, about the functions of this ER isoform that might affect the development of mammary gland malignancy.

ERα

Downregulation of the estrogen receptor number or function has historically been the single most effective adjuvant therapy for the treatment of sex steroid receptor positive breast cancers in women. Current approaches include aromatase inhibitors to prevent estrogen formation from androgen precursors [15, 16], receptor inhibition with faslodex, a drug that causes the loss of ER in tumor cells [17], or SERMS such as tamoxifen or raloxifene that have various functions to prevent the tumor-promoting actions of ER [2]. Growth factor receptor tyrosine kinase inhibitors and inhibitory antibodies, such as Iressa and Herceptin, may prevent the cross talk of EGFR/ErbB2 to enhance nuclear ER transactivation of genes implicated in breast cancer [18, 19]. Additionally, signaling from ErbB2 probably contributes to tamoxifen resistance [20].

Nuclear ER

ERα resides in the cytoplasm after synthesis on the ribosome, but translocates to the nucleus through unclear transport mechanisms. A nuclear localization sequence largely in the D domain (mid-molecule) facilitates transport. Upon ligation by the lipophilic sex steroid, ERα is imported into the nucleus, Hsp 70 dissociates from ER, and the receptor localizes to histones/DNA found in various nuclear compartments. Nucleotides that are present mainly in the E domain of the receptor mediate homodimerization, a post-translational requirement for optimal transcription promotion [21]. E2 promotes homodimerization, thus facilitating ER function.

In contrast, the N-terminus region (A/B) of ERα including the activator function 1 (AF-1) sequence promotes target gene transactivation in a steroid-independent manner [22]. This may arise from the phosphorylation of ERα at ser 118 and other critical residues upon growth factor receptor signaling through ERK and PI3 kinase [9]. ERα phosphorylation upregulates the activity of ERα in transcribing some genes in breast cancer cell lines [11, 23], but the relevance of this for the in vivo tumor biology is not well supported at present. The ability of the AF-1 region to augment target gene transcription has been reported to be independent of co-activator recruitment but may be relevant to E2 action in highly differentiated cells [22]. The precise functions of this region of the steroid receptor for tumor biology are undergoing continued investigation. There is some evidence that this region contributes to tamoxifen resistance [23].

The ability of ERα to increase gene transcription is the fundamental and perhaps only known function of the nuclear receptor pool that promotes the biology of the tumor. Thus, the mechanisms by which E2-bound steroid receptors induce transcription are important to understanding tumor pathogenesis. ER binds directly to DNA at estrogen response elements through the receptor's DNA-binding domain (C domain), or facilitates the ability of transcription factors such as AP-1 or SP-1 to bind their cognate DNA sequences [24]. This promotes co-activator recruitment and subsequent transcription, thereby expanding the repertoire of genes that are targets for steroid hormone action.

Important to transcription is the E domain of the receptor, a region comprised of both the ligand-binding domain and the activator function 2 (AF-2) region. AF-2 appears to be important for the upregulation of genes that promote breast tumor cell cycle progression (c-myc, cyclin D1) [25]. It is at AF-2, largely, that P160 family co-activator proteins such as SRC-1 and SRC-3/AIB1 are recruited to the transcriptosome [24, 26]. This occurs at least in part through the phosphorylation of discrete residues of co-activators by kinases such as protein kinase C [27]. Signaling by growth factor receptors including IGF-1R and the ErbB family at the surface of the transformed epithelial cell is likely to be important in this regard. However, E2 action at a second pool of receptors localized to the plasma membrane may also contribute in this regard [27, 28] (see below). Recent work has defined the kinetics of transcription in breast cancer cells. This involves sequential on–off cycling of ER, co-activators, and co-repressors, directing both activating and suppressive phases of chromatin remodeling [29]. It appears that both aspects are required for gene transcription.

Membrane ER

A small pool of ERα localizes to the plasma membrane of breast cancer cells, probably contained within membrane raft domains (caveolar and non-caveolar rafts) or tethered to the cytoplasmic face of the membrane bi-layer (reviewed in [30]). In conjunction with scaffold proteins (MNAR, caveolin), adaptor proteins (Shc), G proteins, receptor tyrosine kinases (EGFR, ErbB2, IGF1R), and non-receptor kinases (Src, PKC, PI3 kinase), ER forms a highly plastic signalsome. Although the kinetics of recruitment and activation are unknown, E2-induced second messenger generation (cAMP, cGMP), kinase activation

(PI3K, ERK, p38), and calcium signaling result. This generates further cascades of signaling through kinase networks, stimulating breast cancer cell proliferation [31], and survival [32].

Membrane-initiated steroid signaling (MISS) impacts both genomic and non-genomic functions of E2 [33]. Modulation of cytoskeletal protein function results from post-translational modifications through phosphorylation [34, 35]. The restraint of ER signaling by intact but not mutant BRCA1 is the result of phosphatase/kinase activity, regulated jointly by the tumor suppressor and the liganded steroid receptor [36]. This provides a plausible understanding of the interactions of BRCA1 mutations and sex steroids to promote breast cancer development [37]. Signaling through PI3 kinase restrains transcription factors (e.g., Forkhead family members) from entering the nucleus, thereby preserving cell viability [38]. Finally, the ability of membrane-localized ER/E2 to transactivate typical growth factor receptors in breast cancer (EGFR,ErbB2, IGFR1) leads to downstream kinase signaling. This probably contributes to the overall actions of the sex steroid (reviewed in [30]).

In addition, membrane ER signaling through PI3 kinase and ERK stimulates the transcription of relevant genes, such as cyclin D1, and promotes cell proliferation [32, 37, 39]. This occurs through several mechanisms. Membrane ER/E2 transactivates growth factor receptor signaling, required for kinase activation in breast cancer cells. ERK, PI3K, and other kinases phosphorylate the nuclear ER, leading to enhanced transcription. The importance of this is seen in that phosphorylation of ERα at serine 305 changes tamoxifen from an antagonist to an agonist in vivo [40], contributing to tamoxifen resistance. Recruitment of co-activator proteins to the promoter of genes enhances target gene transcription in this malignancy, and recruitment is stimulated in part by phosphorylation [27]. In addition, kinase signaling activates transcription factors such as AP-1 and sp-1, leading to the upregulation of cell survival and proliferation-inducing genes in breast cancer [41, 42]. This may be either nuclear ER dependent or independent.

Progesterone Receptors

A second female sex steroid, progesterone (P), is primarily formed in the ovary and adrenal and binds to two known receptor isoforms [43]. Progesterone receptors A and B (PR-A and PR-B) are products of a single gene and are differentially expressed in target tissues. The ratio and singular expression of the two isoforms in discrete cell types dictate the hormonal response. Ablation of PR-A in mice leads to the loss of normal uterine and ovarian function, producing infertility [44]. In contrast, PR-B has little discernible function in these target organs, but significantly contributes to normal mammary duct and alveolar formation, the latter prominent during pregnancy [45]. PR translocates to the nucleus and dissociates from chaperone/folding proteins such as heat shock proteins in response to ligand. In both ligand-dependent and ligand-independent fashion, PR modulates gene transcription, through multiple mechanisms, comparably to ER.

Structure/Function of PR

It is proposed that the PR isoforms are generated by alternative initiation translation sites from a single mRNA or by transcription arising from two separate promoters [46, 47]. PR structural organization is very similar to other steroid receptors (including ER), with specified domains for DNA binding, nuclear localization, ligand binding and dimerization, and transactivation of target genes. Dynamic recruitment/displacement of co-activators or co-repressors helps assemble the mature transcriptosome at target promoters and is important for function.

Distinct co-activators interact with the transactivation domains (AF-1 and AF-3) contained in the N-terminus, A/B region of the receptor (reviewed in [48]). This is in contrast to other co-activators that interact with the AF-2 (helix 12) region of PR, or to the DNA-binding domain of the receptor. Recruitment of co-repressors leading to gene inhibition is importantly mediated through the A/B domain. Differential recruitment of co-modulators provides plasticity to transcription and expands the potential responses to P or other activators of PR (dopamine, growth factor signaling) (reviewed in [49]). Active areas of PR research involve defining the mechanisms of differential co-activator recruitment and identifying the resulting gene targets that mediate the cell biology.

AF-3 is contained within the 164-amino acid, N-terminal-extended, PR-B isoform. This partly explains the differential gene transcription between PR-A and PR-B. Different genes are potentially activated depending on the formation of PRA or PRB homodimers, and/or the PRA/PRB heterodimer, but the importance of multiple dimer(s) expression for cell biology is largely undetermined. PR-B expressing breast tumors growing in ovariectomized mice are much larger than PR-A expressing tumors [50]. When PR-A is transfected/expressed, it represses PR-B (and ERα)-mediated transcription [51]. However, in a breast cell line, PR-A upregulates the survival gene, BCL-xl, perhaps providing protection against apoptotic cell death [52]. The precise roles of each isoform as contributing to the pathogenesis of breast cancer are unknown.

Variants of PR have been identified in normal cells and transformed breast epithelial cells (reviewed in [48]). This includes an N-terminal truncated form of PR, PR-C. Mutant PR that confer a growth or survival advantage to breast cancer cells are not established in this human malignancy. PR upregulation also results from ERα or ERβ signaling, perhaps providing synergy for the observation that estrogen plus progesterone treatment after the menopause stimulates breast cancer development more effectively than E2 alone [53].

PR Phosphorylation

Just as with ER, PR can be activated by serine phosphorylation induced by growth factor signaling (reviewed in [49]). This occurs independently of steroid ligand and leads to transcriptional regulation of cell proliferation genes in breast cancer, such as cyclin D1, and c-fos [54]. Growth factor signaling from the MAPK, ERK, to the transcription factors ETS or the AP-1 heterodimer also contributes to the upregulation of proliferation-related genes; it is unclear whether this requires the nuclear PR. Serine 294 of PR is phosphorylated by ERK, and augments the P-induced transcriptional response, in concert with growth factor signaling. In part, this may be mediated by promoting rapid degradation of PR through the ubiquitin-proteosome pathway, now known to be necessary for the kinetics of nuclear receptor function [55]. Other sites of phosphorylation (e.g., Ser400) are targets for kinases such as the G1/S cell cycle regulator, CDK2, potentially augmenting transcription [56]. P-independent downregulation of PR results from growth factor signaling through the PI3-kinase modulated, serine/threonine kinase, AKT [57]. PR downregulation is associated with tamoxifen resistance [58], but the importance of PR loss for this clinically important issue is unclear. The roles of discrete residue phosphorylation require further understanding in relation to participation of PR in breast cancer.

Membrane PR

Rapid signaling by P to the modulation of various kinases has been best documented in xenopus oocytes [59, 60]. These cells lack nuclear PR, but respond to P with inhibition of cAMP, JNK, and ERK activation, leading to meiosis. Steroid engagement of the receptor results in the physical association of PR with ERK and PI3 kinase, leading to M-phase transition of meiosis I. These results suggest that a membrane-localized PR mediates this rapid signaling, independently of the receptor's transcriptional functions (reviewed in [49]).

The nature of this receptor is unclear, as some data suggests that the receptor is the nuclear PR localized to the membrane [60, 61]. Recently, a novel family of PRs that are typical heptahelical, G-protein-coupled receptors have been isolated from fish and mammalian cells [62]. These mPR are products of genes distinct from the classical PR gene, are differentially distributed in different cell types, and signal to various downstream second messengers and kinases. The importance of these mPR genes for rapid signaling in breast cancer awaits demonstration of their existence. As defined initially by Aurrichio and colleagues, PR-B signaling from the membrane may require physical association with membrane ER, transmitting G-protein activation and signaling through Src to kinases such as ERK [63]. However, the interaction of ER and PR for P-rapid signaling has not been found necessary by another laboratory [64].

References

1. Ali S, Coombes RC. Estrogen receptor alpha in human breast cancer: occurrence and significance. J Mammary Gland Biol Neoplasia. 2000;5:271–281.
2. Jordan VC. Selective estrogen receptor modulation: concept and consequences in cancer. Cancer Cell 2004;5(3):207–213.
3. Nandi S, Guzman RC, Yang J. Hormones and mammary carcinogenesis in mice, rats, and humans: a unifying hypothesis. Proc Natl Acad Sci USA. 1995;92(9):3650–3657
4. Bontu G, El-Ashry D, Wicha MS. Breast cancer, stem/progenitor cells and the estrogen receptor. Trends Endocrinol Metab. 2004;15(5):193–207.
5. Haslam SZ, Woodward TL. Host microenvironment in breast cancer development: epithelial-cell-stromal-cell interactions and steroid hormone action in normal and cancerous mammary gland. Breast Cancer Res. 2003;5(4):208–215.
6. Wiseman BS, Werb Z. Stromal effects on mammary gland development and breast cancer. Science 2002;296(5570):1046–1049.
7. Filardo EJ, Quinn JA, Bland KI, Frackelton AR. Estrogen-induced activation of Erk-1 and Erk-2 requires the G-protein-coupled receptor homolog, gpr30, and occurs via transactivation of the epidermal growth factor receptor through release of HB-EGF. Mol Endocrinol. 2000;14:1649–1660.
8. Revankar CM, Cimino DF, Sklar LA, Arterburn JB, Prossnitz ER A transmembrane intracellular estrogen receptor mediates rapid cell signaling. Science 2005;307:1625–1630.
9. Howell A, Cuzick J, Baum M, Buzdar A, Dowsett M, Forbes JF, Hoctin-Boes G, Houghton J, Locker GY, Tobias JS, ATAC Trialists' Group Results of the ATAC (Arimidex, Tamoxifen, Alone or in Combination) trial after completion of 5 years' adjuvant treatment for breast cancer. Lancet 2005;365:60–62.
10. Kato S, Endoh H, Masuhiro Y, Kitamoto T, Uchiyama S, Sasaki H, Masushige S, Gotoh Y, Nishida E, Kawashima H, et al. Activation of the estrogen receptor through phosphorylation by mitogen-activated protein kinase. Science 1995;270:1491–1494.
11. Balasenthil S, Barnes CJ, Rayala SK, Kumar R Estrogen receptor activation at serine 305 is sufficient to upregulate cyclin D1 in breast cancer cells. FEBS Lett. 2004;567: 243–247.
12. Russo J, Hasan Lareef M, Balogh G, Guo S, Russo IH. Estrogen and its metabolites are carcinogenic agents in human breast epithelial cells. J Steroid Biochem Mol Biol. 2003;87(1):1–25.
13. Speirs V, Malone C, Walton DS, Kerin MJ, Atkin SL. Increased expression of estrogen receptor beta mRNA in tamoxifen-resistant breast cancer patients. Cancer Res. 1999;59(21):5421–5424.
14. Hopp TA, Weiss HL, Parra IS, Cui Y, Osborne CK, Fuqua SAW. Low levels of estrogen receptor beta protein predict resistance to tamoxifen therapy in breast cancer. Clin Can Res. 2004;10:7490–7499.
15. Thurlimann B, Keshaviah A, Coates AS, Mouridsen H, Mauriac L, Forbes JF, Paridaens R, Castiglione-Gertsch M, Gelber RD, Rabaglio M, Smith I, Wardly A, Price KN, Goldhirsch A; Breast International Group (BIG) 1–98 Collaborative Group.A comparison of letrozole and tamoxifen in postmenopausal women with early breast cancer. N Engl J Med. 2005;353(26):2747–2757.
16. Howell A, Cuzick J, Baum M, Buzdar A, Dowsett M, Forbes JF, Hoctin-Boes G, Houghton J, Locker GY, Tobias JS; ATAC Trialists' Group. Results of the ATAC (Arimidex, Tamoxifen, Alone or in Combination) trial after completion of 5 years' adjuvant treatment for breast cancer. Lancet 2005;365(9453):60–62.
17. Bundred N, Howell A. Fulvestrant (Faslodex): current status in the therapy of breast cancer. Expert Rev Anticancer Ther. 2002;2(2):151–160.
18. Martin MB, Franke TF, Stoica GE, Chambon P, Katzenellenbogen BS, Stoica BA, McLemore MS, Olivo SE, Stoica A. A role for Akt in mediating the estrogenic functions

of epidermal growth factor and insulin-like growth factor I. Endocrinology 2000;141(12):4503–4511.
19. Slamon DJ, Leyland-Jones B, Shak S, Fuchs H, Paton V, Bajamonde A, Fleming T, Eiermann W, Wolter J, Pegram M, Baselga J, Norton L. Use of chemotherapy plus a monoclonal antibody against HER2 for metastatic breast cancer that overexpresses HER2. N Engl J Med. 2001;344(11):783–792.
20. Osborne CK, Shou J, Massarweh S, Schiff R. Crosstalk between estrogen receptor and growth factor receptor pathways as a cause for endocrine therapy resistance in breast cancer. Clin Cancer Res. 2005;11(2 Pt 2):865s–870s.
21. Tamrazi A, Carlson KE, Daniels JR, Hurth KM, Katzenellenbogen JA Estrogen receptor dimerization: ligand binding regulates dimer affinity and dimer dissociation rate. Mol Endocrinol. 2002;16:2706–2719.
22. Merot Y, Metivier R, Penot G, Manu D, Saligaut C, Gannon F, Pakdel F, Kah O, Flouriot G. The relative contribution exerted by AF-1 and AF-2 transactivation functions in estrogen receptor alpha transcriptional activity depends upon the differentiation stage of the cell. J Biol Chem. 2004;279(25):26184–26191.
23. Bunone G, Briand PA, Miksicek RJ, Picard D. Activation of the unliganded estrogen receptor by EGF involves the MAP kinase pathway and direct phosphorylation. EMBO J. 1996;15(9):2174–2183.
24. Halachmi S, Marden E, Martin G, MacKay H, Abbondanza C, Brown M. Estrogen receptor-associated proteins: possible mediators of hormone-induced transcription. Science 1994;264:1455–1458.
25. Doisneau-Sixou SF, Sergio CM, Carroll JS, Hui R, Musgrove EA, Sutherland RL. Estrogen and antiestrogen regulation of cell cycle progression in breast cancer cells. Endocr Relat Cancer. 2003;10(2):179–186.
26. Font de Mora J, Brown M. AIB1 is a conduit for kinase-mediated growth factor signaling to the estrogen receptor. Mol Cell Biol. 2000;20(14):5041–5047.
27. Wu RC, Qin J, Yi P, Wong J, Tsai SY, Tsai MJ, O'Malley BW. Selective phosphorylations of the SRC-3/AIB1 coactivator integrate genomic reponses to multiple cellular signaling pathways. Mol Cell. 2004;15(6):937–949.
28. Marquez DC, Chen HW, Curran EM, Welshons WV, Pietras RJ. Estrogen receptors in membrane lipid rafts and signal transduction in breast cancer. Mol Cell Endocrinol. 2005 Dec 30; [Epub ahead of print].
29. Metivier R, Penot G, Hubner MR, Reid G, Brand H, Kos M, Gannon F. Estrogen receptor-alpha directs ordered, cyclical, and combinatorial recruitment of cofactors on a natural target promoter. Cell 2003;115(6):751–763.
30. Levin, ER. Integration of the extra-nuclear and nuclear actions of estrogen. Mol Endocrinol. 2005;19(8):1951–1959.
31. Razandi, M, Pedram, A, Levin, ER. Plasma membrane estrogen receptors signal to anti-apoptosis in breast cancer. Mol Endocrinol. 2000;14(9):1434–1447.
32. Marquez DC, Pietras RJ. Membrane-associated binding sites for estrogen contribute to growth regulation of human breast cancer cells. Oncogene 2001;20:5420–5430.
33. Song RX, McPherson RA, Adam L, Bao Y, Shupnik M, Kumar R, Santen RJ. Linkage of rapid estrogen action to MAPK activation by ERalpha-Shc association and Shc pathway activation. Mol Endocrinol. 2002;16(1):116–127.
34. Nemere I, Pietras RJ, Blackmore PF. Membrane receptors for steroid hormones: signal transduction and physiological significance. J Cell Biochem. 2003;88(3):438–445.
35. Meyer G, Feldman EL. Signaling mechanisms that regulate actin-based motility processes in the nervous system. J Neurochem. 2002;83:490–503.
36. Razandi M, Pedram A, Rosen E, Levin ER. BRCA1 inhibits membrane estrogen and growth factor receptor signaling to cell proliferation in breast cancer. Mol Cell Biol. 2004;24:5900–5913

37. Kauff ND, Satagopan JM, Robson ME, Scheuer L, Hensley M, Hudis CA, Ellis NA, Boyd J, Borgen PI, Barakat RR, Norton L, Castiel M, Nafa K, Offit K. Risk-reducing salpingo-oophorectomy in women with a BRCA1 or BRCA2 mutation. N Engl J Med. 2002;346(21):1609–1615.
38. Brunet A, Bonni A, Zigmond MJ, Lin MZ, Juo P, Hu LS, Anderson MJ, Arden KC, Blenis J, Greenberg ME. Akt promotes cell survival by phosphorylating and inhibiting a Forkhead transcription factor. Cell 1999;96:857–868
39. Butt AJ, McNeil CM, Musgrove EA, Sutherland RL. Downstream targets of growth factor and oestrogen signalling and endocrine resistance: the potential roles of c-Myc, cyclin D1 and cyclin E. Endocr Relat Cancer. 2005;12 Suppl 1:S47-S59.
40. Michalides R, Griekspoor A, Balkenende A, Verwoerd D, Janssen L, Jalink K, Floore A, Velds A, van't Veer L, Neefjes J. Tamoxifen resistance by a conformational arrest of the estrogen receptor alpha after PKA activation in breast cancer. Cancer Cell 2004;5(6):597–605.
41. Duan R, Xie W, Li X, McDougal A, Safe S. Estrogen regulation of c-fos gene expression through phosphatidylinositol-3-kinase-dependent activation of serum response factor in MCF-7 breast cancer cells. Biochem Biophys Res Commun. 2002;294:384–394.
42. Dong L, Wang W, Wang F, Stoner M, Reed JC, Harigai M, Samudio I, Kladde MP, Vyhlidal C, Safe S. Mechanisms of transcriptional activation of bcl-2 gene expression by 17beta-estradiol in breast cancer cells. J Biol Chem. 1999;274(45):32099–32107.
43. Conneely OM, Lydon JP. Progesterone receptors in reproduction: functional impact of the A and B isoforms. Steroids 2000;65(10–11):571–577.
44. Conneely OM, Mulac-Jericevic B, Lydon JP, De Mayo FJ. Reproductive functions of the progesterone receptor isoforms: lessons from knock-out mice. Mol Cell Endocrinol. 2001;179(1–2):97–103.
45. Mulac-Jericevic B, Lydon JP, DeMayo FJ, Conneely OM. Defective mammary gland morphogenesis in mice lacking the progesterone receptor B isoform. Proc Natl Acad Sci USA. 2003;100(17):9744–9749.
46. Conneely OM, Maxwell BL, Toft DO, Schrader WT, and O'Malley BW. The A and B forms of the chicken progesterone receptor arise by alternative initiation of translation of a unique mRNA Biochem Biophys Res Commun. 1987;149:493–501.
47. Kastner P, Krust A, Turcotte B, Stropp U, Tora L, Gronemeyer H, Chambon P. Two distinct estrogen-regulated promoters generate transcripts encoding the two functionally different human progesterone receptor forms A and B. EMBO J. 1990;9(5):1603–1614.
48. Li X, O'Malley BW. Unfolding the action of progesterone receptors. J Biol Chem. 2003;278(41):39261–39264.
49. Lange CA. Making sense of cross-talk between steroid hormone receptors and intracellular signaling pathways: who will have the last word? Mol Endocrinol. 2004;18(2): 269–278.
50. Jacobsen BM, Richer JK, Sartorius CA, Horwitz KB. Expression profiling of human breast cancers and gene regulation by progesterone receptors. J Mammary Gland Biol Neoplasia. 2003;8(3):257–268.
51. Vegeto E, Shahbaz MM, Wen DX, Goldman ME, O'Malley BW, McDonnell DP. Human progesterone receptor A form is a cell- and promoter-specific repressor of human progesterone receptor B function. Mol Endocrinol. 1993;7(10):1244–1255.
52. Shyamala G, Yang X, Silberstein G, Barcellos-Hoff MH, Dale E. Transgenic mice carrying an imbalance in the native ratio of A to B forms of progesterone receptor exhibit developmental abnormalities in mammary glands. Proc Natl Acad Sci USA. 1998;95(2): 696–701.
53. Rossouw JE, Anderson GL, Prentice RL, LaCroix AZ, Kooperberg C, Stefanick ML, Jackson RD, Beresford SA, Howard BV, Johnson KC, Kotchen JM, Ockene J. Writing Group for the Women's Health Initiative Investigators. Risks and benefits of estrogen

plus progestin in healthy postmenopausal women: principal results from the Women's Health Initiative randomized controlled trial. JAMA 2002;288(3):321–333.
54. Albanese C, Johnson J, Watanabe G, Eklund N, Vu D, Arnold A, Pestell RG. Transforming p21ras mutants and c-Ets-2 activate the cyclin D1 promoter through distinguishable regions. J Biol Chem. 1995;270(40):23589–23597.
55. Dennis AP, Haq RU, Nawaz Z. The regulation of nuclear receptor degradation. Front Biosci. 2001;6:D954–D959.
56. Pierson-Mullany LK, Lange CA. Phosphorylation of progesterone receptor serine 400 mediates ligand-independent transcriptional activity in response to activation of cyclin-dependent protein kinase 2. Mol Cell Biol. 2004;24(24):10542–10557.
57. Cui X, Zhang P, Deng W, Oesterreich S, Lu Y, Mills GB, Lee AV. Insulin-like growth factor-I inhibits progesterone receptor expression in breast cancer cells via the phosphatidylinositol 3-kinase/Akt/mammalian target of rapamycin pathway: progesterone receptor as a potential indicator of growth factor activity in breast cancer. Mol Endocrinol. 2003;17(4):575–588.
58. Cui X, Schiff R, Arpino G, Osborne CK, Lee AV. Biology of progesterone receptor loss in breast cancer and its implications for endocrine therapy. J Clin Oncol. 2005;23(30):7721–7735.
59. Andresson T, Ruderman JV. The kinase Eg2 is a component of the Xenopus oocyte progesterone-activated signaling pathway. EMBO J. 1998;17(19):5627–37.
60. Lutz LB, Kim B, Jahani D, Hammes SR. G protein beta gamma subunits inhibit nongenomic progesterone-induced signaling and maturation in Xenopus laevis oocytes. Evidence for a release of inhibition mechanism for cell cycle progression. J Biol Chem. 2000;275(52):41512–41520.
61. Bayaa, M, Ronald A. Booth, RA., Yinglun, S., and Liu, XJ. The classical progesterone receptor mediates Xenopus oocyte maturation through a nongenomic mechanism. Proc Natl Acad Sci USA. 2000;97(23):12607–12612
62. Zhu Y, Bond J, Thomas P. Identification, classification, and partial characterization of genes in humans and other vertebrates homologous to a fish membrane progestin receptor. Proc Natl Acad Sci USA. 2003;100(5):2237–2242.
63. Migliaccio A, Piccolo D, Castoria G, Di Domenico M, Bilancio A, Lombardi M, Gong W, Beato M, Auricchio F. Activation of the Src/p21ras/Erk pathway by progesterone receptor via cross-talk with estrogen receptor. EMBO J. 1998;17(7):2008–2018.
64. Boonyaratanakornkit V, Scott MP, Ribon V, Sherman L, Anderson SM, Maller JL, Miller WT, Edwards DP. Progesterone receptor contains a proline-rich motif that directly interacts with SH3 domains and activates c-Src family tyrosine kinases. Mol Cell. 2001;(2):269–280.

Estrogen Receptors in Breast Tumors of African American Patients

Indira Poola

It is now fairly well recognized that African American women (AAW) develop aggressive breast tumors and experience higher mortality rate than women in other population [1–10]. The higher mortality rate in AA population has been assumed to be due to, in part, late stage of disease at diagnosis, low socioeconomic status, and limited access to medical facilities and services [11–20]. When the above factors were controlled the high mortality rate appears to be due to differences in tumor biology observed in AAW [21]. Several studies have established that breast tumors in AAW are poorly differentiated with increased frequency of nuclear atypia, higher mitotic activity, higher S-phase fraction, and tumor necrosis [22–27]. Another characteristic of breast tumors in AAW is the frequency of expression of estrogen receptor (ER) and progesterone receptor (PR); the presence of these indicate a good prognosis and response to anti-estrogen and other therapies. Several reports have shown that the presence of ER and PR in AA patient tumors is lower compared to breast cancer patients in other populations. Reports show that less than 50% of patients are positive for ER whereas in other population, more than 65% are positive for ER after adjusting for menopausal state and age [28–32].

The ER positivity in tumors was traditionally determined based on immunohistochemical assessment of the presence of the major ER protein, ERalpha (ERα), using monoclonal antibodies. However, it is now well established that breast tumor samples express a number of splice variants of ERα in addition to wild-type ERα and the second structurally and functionally related but genetically distinct receptor, ERβ, and a number of its splice variants. Because estrogen signaling through ERs is known to drive the progression of majority of breast tumors, we thought that the qualitative and quantitative differences in the molecular composition of ER isoforms in AAW could, in part, account for the aggressive tumor biology and lower overall survival observed in this

I. Poola (✉)
Department of Surgery and Breast Center, Howard University College of Medicine, Washington, DC 20059, USA
e-mail: ipoola@howard.edu

S.A.W. Fuqua (ed.), *Hormone Receptors in Breast Cancer*,
Cancer Treatment and Research 312, DOI 10.1007/978-0-387-09463-2_4,

population. To determine the above, we studied the two ERs, wild-type ERα and ERβ, and an abundantly expressed variant of ERβ, ERβ5, in breast tumors of AAW in comparison with Caucasian patient tumors.

African American Patient Breast Tumors Are Not Significantly Different from Caucasian Patient Tumors in the Levels of Wild-Type ERα

To test if AAW breast tumors are different with respect to ERα expression, the ERα wild-type levels were determined in 40 immunohistochemically ERα-positive tumors from AAW and 34 tumor samples from Caucasian patients at mRNA levels by established Q real-time PCR methods that can precisely determine its exact mRNA copy numbers [33]. The ERα mRNA copy numbers in tumors of both racial groups were profiled with reference to the mRNA copy numbers of the housekeeping gene, glyceraldehyde 3-phosphate dehydrogenase (GAPDH). The expression data between the tumors of two racial groups was analyzed using two-sided Wilcoxon rank sum test for any differences. By the above approach, no statistically significant difference in the expression of ERα in the tumors between the two racial groups was observed [34]. The expression levels of ERα mRNA copy numbers in each racial group with reference to GAPDH mRNA copy numbers are shown schematically in Fig. 1. The mean values of ERα mRNA levels and standard deviation in each racial group are also shown in Table 1.

The Wild-Type ERβ, the ERβ1, Levels Are Significantly Higher in Both Immunohistochemically ERα -Positive and Negative Breast Tumors of African American Patients Compared to Caucasian Patient Tumors

To determine if the AA patient tumors may be different with respect to ERβs levels, the expression levels of this receptor at mRNA were compared in 40 immunohistochemcially ERα-positive and 40 negative samples with 34 positive and 20 negative tumor samples from Caucasian patients by Q real-time PCR and with reference to GAPDH mRNA copy numbers [35]. The ERβ mRNA levels between two racial groups and in between ERα-positive and ERα-negative tumors were compared by two-sided Wilcoxon rank sum test. By this approach, statistically significant differences between the two racial groups in the levels of this receptor were found in the mRNA levels of ERβ1. The expression of ERβ1 was significantly higher in both ERα-positive and ERα-negative tumors from African American patients in comparison with Caucasian patients (ERα-positive

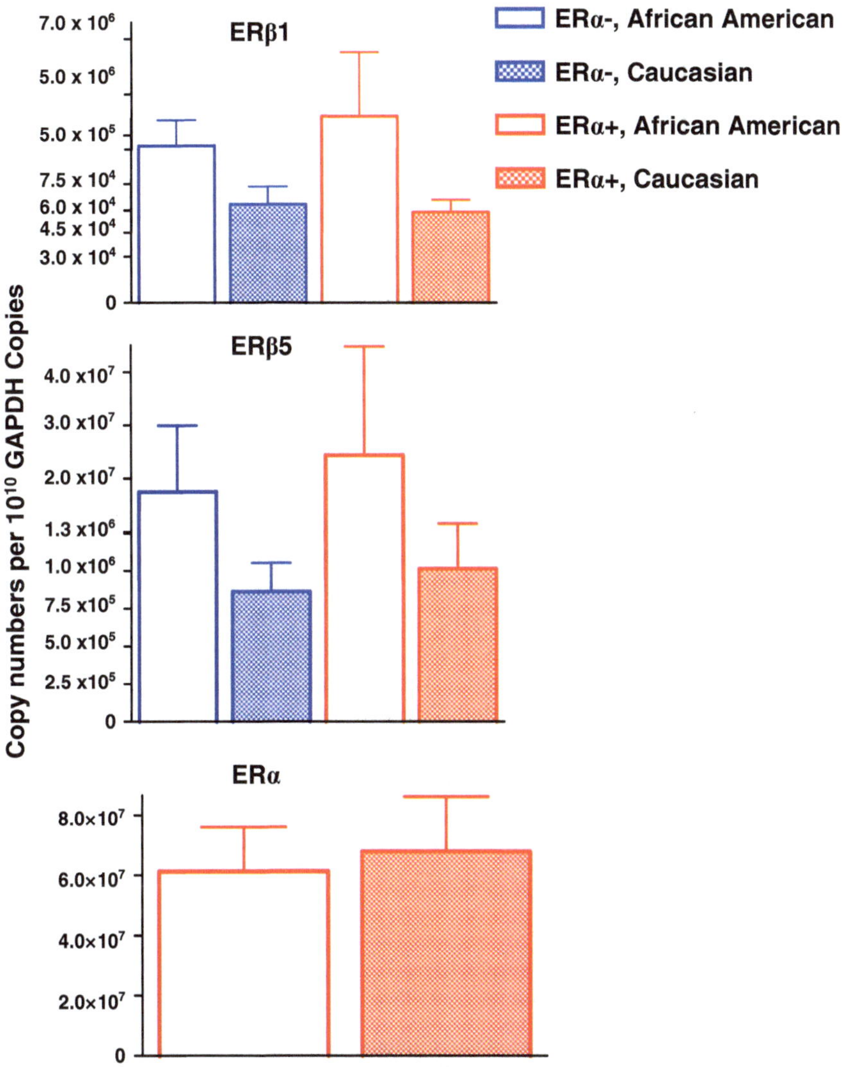

Fig. 1 Expression levels of ERβ1 and ERβ5 transcripts in ERα-negative and ERα-positive tissues from African American and Caucasian patient tumors

Table 1 Expression levels of ERβ1 and ERβ5 (mean and standard deviation) in ERα-negative and ERα-positive breast cancer tissues (mRNA copies per 10^{10} mRNA copies of GAPDH)

	ERα negative		ERα positive	
Isoform	African American	Caucasian	African American	Caucasian
ERβ1	5×10^5 and 1×10^5	6×10^4 and 1×10^4	1×10^6 and 3×10^5	6×10^4 and 8×10^3
ERβ5	2×10^7 and 1×10^7	9×10^5 and 2×10^5	3×10^7 and 2×10^7	1×10^6 and 3×10^5
ERα	NA	NA	6×10^7 and 1×10^7	7×10^7 and 2×10^7

NA, not applicable.

tumors, $p = 0.0004$, and ERα-negative tumors, $p = 0.0048$). However, the expression levels of ERβ1 mRNA are not associated with tumor grade, stage of the cancer, histological type, menopausal status, progesterone receptor, or nodal status by ANOVA [34]. The mean expression levels in both racial groups and standard deviation are shown in Table 1 and Fig. 1.

An Isoform of ERβ, an Estrogen-Independent Transcription Factor, ERβ5, Is Abundantly Expressed in Both ERα-Positive and Negative Breast Tumors of African American Patients Compared to Caucasian Patient Tumors

Although breast tumors are shown to express a number of splice variants of both ERα and ERβ, ERβ5 is by far the most abundant isoform of all the splice variants. It is a full-length receptor identical to wild-type ERβ except it has unique short nucleotide sequence arising from retention of an intron in the place of exon 8. Although it lacks estrogen-binding property, it gets internalized to nucleus, binds ERE sequences on DNA, and activates transcription [36]. This receptor is expressed at much higher levels in the breast tumors of African American patients compared to Caucasian patients in both ERα-positive and ERα-negative tumors (ERα-positive tumors, $p= 0.0002$, and ERα-negative tumors, $p = 0.0213$, by two-sided Wilcoxon rank sum test). However, the higher expression of this receptor is not related to stage, size, menopausal status, age, or metastasis to the nodes [34].

The significantly higher levels of ERβ1 and ERβ5 in ERα-negative tissues in African American patient tumors offer possibilities to design therapies targeted at these receptors to treat ERα-negative tumors.

References

1. Eley JW, Hill HA, Chen VW, et al. Racial differences in survival from breast cancer: results of the National Cancer Institute Black/White Cancer Survival study. JAMA 1994;272:947–954.
2. Moorimer J. Breast cancer in black women. Ann Internal Med. 1996;15:897–905.
3. Dignam H, Redmond CK, Fisher B, Costantino JP, Edwards BK. Prognosis among African women and white women with lymph node negative breast cancer. Cancer 1997;80:80–90.
4. Dignam JJ. Differences in breast cancer prognosis among African American and Caucasian women. CA Cancer J Clin. 2000;50:50–64.
5. Josylyn SA, West MM. Racial differences in breast carcinoma survival. Cancer 2000;88:114–123.
6. American Cancer Society. Cancer Facts and Figures- 2001. Atlanta, GA: American Cancer Society, 2001.
7. Chu KC, Lamar CA, Freeman HP. Racial disparities in breast carcinoma survival rates. Cancer 2003;97:2853–2860.

8. Field TS, Buist DSM, Doubeni C, Enger S, et al. Disparities and survival among breast cancer patients. J Natl Cancer Inst Monographs. 2005;(35).
9. Chlebowski RT, Chen Z, Anderson GL, et al. Ethnicity and breast cancer: factors influencing differences in incidence and outcome. J Natl Cancer Inst. 2005;97:439–448.
10. Jamal A, Siegel R, Ward E, Murry T, Xu J, Thun MJ. Cancer Statistics for 2007. CA Cancer J Clin. 2007;57:43–66.
11. Ayanian JZ, Kohler BA, Abe T, Epstein AM. The relation between health insurance coverage and clinical outcome among women with breast cancer. New England J Med. 1993;329:326–331.
12. Wojcik B, Spinks M, Otenberg S. Breast cancer survival analysis for African American and white women in an equal access health care system. Cancer 1998;82:1310–1318.
13. Lamin DR, Mathews HF, Mitchell J, Swanson MS, Swanson FH, Edwards MS. Influence of socio-economic and cultural factors on racial differences in late stage presentation of breast cancer. JAMA 1998;279:1801–1807.
14. Brawley OW. Disaggregating the effects of race and poverty on breast cancer outcome. J Natl Cancer Inst. 2002;94:471–473.
15. Bradley CI, Given CW, Roberts C. Race, socioeconomic status and breast cancer treatment and survival. J Natl Cancer Inst. 2002;94:90–96.
16. Newman LA, Mason I, Cote D, Vin Y, Caroline K, et al. African American ethnicity, socioeconomic status, and breast cancer survival. Cancer 2002;94:2844–2854.
17. Smedley BD, Stith A, Nelson AR (eds). Unequal treatment-confronting racial and ethnic disparities in health care. Washington, DC: Institute of Medicine, National Academy Press; 2002.
18. Shavers VL, Brown MI. Racial and ethnic disparities in the receipt of cancer treatment. J Natl Cancer Inst. 2002;94:334–357.
19. Li CI, Malone KE, Daling JR Differences in breast cancer stage, treatment, and survival by race and ethnicity. Arch Intern Med. 2003;163:49–56.
20. Newman LA, Griffith KA, Jatoi I, et al. Meta-analysis of survival in African American and white patients with breast cancer: ethnicity compared to socioeconomic status. J Clin Oncol. 2006;24:1342–1349.
21. Albain KS, Unger JM, Hutchins LF, Rivkin SE and others. Outcome of African American on Southwest Oncology group (SWOG) breast cancer adjuvanttherapy trials. Breast Cancer Res Treat. 2003;82(Suppl 1):A21.
22. Elledge RM, Clark GM, Chamness GC, Osborne CK. Tumor biologic factors and breast cancer prognosis among white, hispanic and black women in the United States. J Natl Cancer Inst. 1994;86:705–712.
23. Chen VW, Correa P, Kurman RJ, et al. Histological characteristics of breast carcinoma in blacks and whites. Cancer Epidemol Biomarkers Prev. 1994;3:127–35.
24. Furberg H, Millikan R, Dressler L, Newman B, Geradts J. Tumor characteristics in African American and white women. Breast Cancer Res Treat. 2001;68:33–43.
25. Middleton IP, Chen Y, Perkins GH, Pin V, Page D. Histopathology of breast cancer among African American women. Cancer 2003;97:253–257.
26. Ikpatt OF, Dignam J, et al. Breast tumor morphometry in relation to race reveals significant differences among Nigerian, African American Caucasian Americans. Proc Am Soc Clin Oncol. 2004;23:9567.
27. Amend K, Hicks D, Ambrosone CB. Breast cancer in African American women: differences in tumor biology from European – American women. Cancer Res. 2006;66:8327–8330.
28. Mohla S, Sampson CX, Khan T, Enterline JP, Leffall L, White JE. Estrogen and progesterone receptors in breast cancer in black Americans. Correlation of receptor data with tumor differentiation. Cancer 1982;50:552–559.
29. Pegorano PI, Karnam V, Nirmul D, Joubert SM. Estrogen and progesterone receptors in breast cancer among women of different racial groups. Cancer Res. 1986;46:2117–2120.

30. Beverly UN, Flanders D, et al. A comparison of estrogen and progesterone receptors in black and white breast cancer patients. Am J Public Health. 1987;77:351–353.
31. Gapstur, SM, Dupuis J, et al. Hormone receptor status of breast cancer in black, Hispanic and non-hispanic-white women. Cancer 1995;77:1465–1471.
32. Joslyn SA. Hormone receptors in breast cancer: racial differences in distribution and survival. Breast Cancer Res Treat. 2002;73:45–59.
33. Poola I. Molecular assay to generate expression profiles of eight estrogen receptor alpha isoform mRNA copy numbers in picogram amounts of total RNA from breast cancer tissues. Anal Biochem. 2003;314:217–226.
34. Poola I, Fuqua SAW, DeWitty RW, Abraham J, Marhsalleck J, Liu A. Estrogen receptor alpha negative breast cancer patients express significant levels of estrogen-independent transcription factors. ERbeta1 and ERbeta5: potential molecular targets for chemoprevention. Clinical Cancer Res. 2005;11:7579–7585.
35. Poola I. Molecular assays to distinguish and quantify ten estrogen receptor beta isoform mRNA copy numbers. Endocrine 2003;22:101–111.
36. Poola I, Abraham J, Baldwin K, Saunders A, Bhatnagar R. Estrogen receptor beta4 and beta5 are full length functionally active isoforms. Cloning from human ovary and functional characterization. Endocrine 2005;27:227–238.

BRCA1 Cross-Talk with Hormone Receptors

Eliot M. Rosen, Yongxian Ma, and Saijun Fan

Introduction

During the mid-1990s, two breast cancer susceptibility genes, BRCA1 [1] and BRCA2 [2, 3], were identified and cloned. Together, BRCA1 and BRCA2 mutations account for about 80% of all hereditary breast cancer cases, suggesting the existence of at least one more, as yet unidentified, BRCA genes. BRCA1 fits the definition of a classical Knudsen-type tumor suppressor gene, since nearly all BRCA1-mutant cancers show loss of the wild-type allele within the tumors [4]. In studies aimed at understanding why BRCA1 mutations lead to cancer development, a variety of functional roles for BRCA1 have been identified, including roles in several different DNA repair pathways (e.g., homology-directed DNA repair and Fanconi-type repair), DNA damage signaling, DNA damage-responsive cell cycle checkpoints, and apoptosis susceptibility (cell "fate" decisions) (reviewed in [5, 6]). Consistent with these findings, cultured cells and tumors deficient in BRCA1 show a characteristic pattern of genomic instability, including centrosomal amplification, aneuploidy, and chromosome aberrations [7–9]. Based on these considerations, it has been suggested that BRCA1 serves as a "caretaker" gene to protect cells against genotoxic damage and preserve genomic integrity.

While these functions generally fit with the idea that BRCA1 is a tumor suppressor gene, they do not explain the particular spectrum of tumor types observed in BRCA1 mutation carriers. Thus, a study of 699 BRCA1-mutant breast cancer families suggests that in addition to breast and ovarian cancers, BRCA1 mutation carriers also have a significantly increased risk for

E.M. Rosen (✉)
Department of Oncology, Lombardi Comprehensive Cancer Center, Georgetown University, 3970 Reservoir Road, NW, Box 571469, Washington, DC 20057-1469, USA
e-mail: emr36@georgetown.edu

S.A.W. Fuqua (ed.), *Hormone Receptors in Breast Cancer*,
Cancer Treatment and Research 312, DOI 10.1007/978-0-387-09463-2_5,

endometrial and cervical cancers in women and for prostate cancers in men younger than 65 years [10]. Interestingly, these are all tumor types that appear to be steroid hormone responsive, at least at some point during their development. Thus, breast and endometrial cancers are known to be estrogen responsive, while prostate cancer is an androgen-sensitive tumor type. Although a hormonal etiology is not as clearly established in cervical cancer as in the other tumor types, estrogen is thought to contribute to cell proliferation during the pathogenesis of cervical cancer [11–13]. BRCA2 mutations have been linked to ovarian, pancreatic, and prostatic cancers; but unlike BRCA1, BRCA2 mutations have not been linked to cervical and endometrial cancers [14, 15]. These considerations suggest that cross-talk with hormone receptor pathways may contribute to the development of BRCA1-dependent breast cancers.

Further evidence in support of a hormonal etiology for BRCA1-mutant breast cancer comes from clinical-epidemiological studies. Although studies of risk modifiers in BRCA1 mutation carriers have led to conflicting results [in part, due to the relatively small number of cases], reproductive history does appear to modify breast cancer risk in BRCA1 carriers. This evidence has been reviewed elsewhere [16, 17]. Importantly, bilateral oophorectomy, especially when performed at an early age, confers a significant reduction in the risk for breast cancer in BRCA1 mutation carriers [18, 19]. And as described below, animal models of BRCA1-mutant breast cancer suggest that hormonal manipulations can substantially alter the risk of mammary cancer. In this chapter, we will describe various aspects of BRCA1:hormonal interactions in cell culture and animal models that may shed some light on the question of how BRCA1 suppresses breast cancer development.

The BRCA1 Protein

The BRCA1 gene is located on human chromosome 17q21, contains 24 exons, and encodes an 1863 amino acid protein [1]. The BRCA1 protein does not exhibit significant structural homology to other known proteins (including BRCA2), with the exception of a conserved N-terminal ring finger domain (amino acids 20–64) and a carboxy-terminal acidic domain that can mediate transcriptional activation when linked to a suitable DNA-binding domain [20]. The N-terminal ring finger domain of BRCA1 interacts with another ring finger protein, BARD1 (BRCA1-associated ring domain protein 1); and the BRCA1:-BARD1 complex can function as an E3 ubiquitin ligase, an activity that may be important for tumor suppression [21–23]. The BRCA1 carboxy-terminal transcriptional activation domain contains a tandem repeat of 95 amino acids called a BRCA1-associated carboxy-terminal domain (BRCT) that is homologous to similar domains found in various DNA repair and cell cycle checkpoint proteins [24]. BRCA1 contains functional nuclear import and nuclear export signals, suggesting that it may shuttle back and forth between the nucleus and the cytoplasm [25, 26]. However, it appears that most, if not all, BRCA1 functions require its nuclear localization.

The BRCA1 protein is a 220 kDa nuclear phosphoprotein that is expressed and phosphorylated during the cell cycle, with maximum expression and phosphorylation in late G1 and early to mid-S-phase [27, 28]. BRCA1 appears to be expressed predominantly in proliferating cells; and quiescence induced by removal of serum causes down-regulation of its expression [27]. However, as described below, differentiating mammary epithelial cells express high levels of BRCA1. Many biological functions of BRCA1 appear to be due to its ability to regulate transcription (reviewed in [5, 29]). BRCA1 has not been identified as a sequence-specific DNA-binding transcription factor. It appears to regulate transcription primarily by binding to various sequence-specific transcription factors and either increasing (e.g., p53, STAT1, ATF1) or decreasing (e.g., c-Myc, ER-α) their activity. In addition, BRCA1 can bind to components of the RNA polymerase II holoenzyme [e.g., RNA helicase A], transcriptional co-regulators and chromatin-modifying proteins [e.g., p300/CBP, the retinoblastoma protein (RB1), several RB1-associated proteins (RbAp46 and RbAp48), histone deacetylases, the SWI/SNF-related transcriptional activator BRG1, the cofactor of BRCA1 (COBRA1)], and other transcriptional regulatory proteins [5, 29]. In addition to its carboxy-terminal transcriptional activation domain, a second transcriptional activation domain (called "AD1") has been identified, located just amino-terminal to the BCRT [30]. The precise function of AD1 is unclear, but its activity appears to be dependent upon an interaction between BRCA1 and JunB.

BRCA1 Regulation of Estrogen Receptor (ER-α)

The first demonstration of a functional interaction between BRCA1 and ER-α was the observation that BRCA1 over-expression inhibits ER-α transcriptional activity in cultured human breast and prostate carcinoma cell lines [31]. Curiously, in that study, BRCA1 failed to inhibit ER-α activity in several human cervical cancer cell lines. It was subsequently discovered that human papillomavirus oncoproteins E6 and E7, which are expressed in human cervical cancer cell lines, can bind directly to BRCA1 and block its ability to repress ER-α activity [32]. Transcriptional activity assays further revealed that BRCA1 blocked the activity of the conserved carboxy-terminal activation domain of ER-α [designated "activation function 2" (AF-2)], which is linked to the ligand-binding domain, but did not inhibit the constitutively active amino-terminal activation domain (AF-1) [31, 33]. And BRCA1 inhibited the ability of 17β-estradiol (E2) to stimulate expression of several estrogen-responsive genes (pS2 and cathepsin D) [34].

Two mechanisms have been identified for BRCA1-mediated repression of ER-α. The first involves a direct interaction of the BRCA1 and ER-α proteins, and the second involves down-regulation of p300, a co-activator of ER-α [33–37], as will be described below. In contrast to wild-type BRCA1 (wtBRCA1), expression of a set of cancer-associated BRCA1-mutant proteins either did not inhibit ER-α activity or showed a greatly reduced ability to do so, consistent with the idea that repression of ER-α contributes to the tumor suppressor function of BRCA1. Interestingly, unlike the binding of some cofactors to ER-α [e.g., steroid receptor co-activator 1 (SRC-1)], the BRCA1:ER-α interaction was not E2 dependent (i.e., occurred to a similar extent in the absence vs presence of E2).

The interacting domains of the BRCA1 and ER-α proteins have been mapped at a high level of resolution. Here, two contact sites for ER-α on BRCA1 were identified, one within amino acids 67–100 and the other within amino acids 101–134 [38]. The ability of BRCA1 to bind ER-α and repress its activity was found to be particularly dependent upon a conserved helical motif (amino acids 86–95) that resembles a previously identified nuclear co-repressor motif [Lxx(I/H)Ixxx(I/L), where x = any amino acid]. Mutation of this motif disrupted the ability of BRCA1 to both bind and repress ER-α [38]. Consistent with the observation that BRCA1 inhibits AF-2 activity, the binding sites for BRCA1 on ER-α were located within the AF-2 domain of ER-α. Two contact sites were identified, a major site within amino acids 338–379 and a minor site within amino acids 420–595. Based on these mapping studies, a partial three-dimensional structure of the BRCA1:ER-α complex was proposed [38]. In this model, BRCA1 heterodimerizes with ER-α via an anti-parallel α-helix domain, mainly using the third helix (amino acids 80–96) of BRCA1. The ER-α side of the interacting surface is an α-helix of ER-α (amino acids 338–379), which is at the opposite side of the ER-α homo-dimerization surface. Consistent with this model, two cancer-associated BRCA1 mutations at the interacting surface (L63F and I89T) significantly impaired the ability of BRCA1 to repress ER-α activity [38].

As described above, the BRCA1 amino-terminal ring domain (amino acids 20–64) interacts with another ring domain protein (BARD1 [39]); and the complex can function as an E3 ubiquitin ligase. It was proposed that this ubiquitin ligase activity is essential for BRCA1 tumor suppressor function; and it has been shown that the ubiquitin ligase activity is required for the function of BRCA1 in maintaining the normal state of cellular radiation resistance [40]. Interestingly, while the BRCA1 ring domain is not required for BRCA1 binding to ER-α, it is required for repression of ER-α activity by the full-length BRCA1 protein, since two cancer-associated BRCA1 point mutations that disrupt the ring domain structure (^{61}Cys $\rightarrow$ Gly and ^{64}Cys $\rightarrow$ Gly) did not inhibit ER-α activity [34]. Two issues that remain to be addressed are the mechanism by which the ring domain mutations inactivate the BRCA1 repression of ER-α and whether or not the BRCA1 ubiquitin ligase activity is required for repression of ER-α. While we have not adduced any evidence that BRCA1 directs the proteolytic degradation of ER-α, it has been reported recently that ER-α is a substrate for the ubiquitin ligase activity of the BRCA1/BARD1 complex, which functions, predominantly, to mono-ubiquitinate ER-α [41]. Interestingly, two residues within the AF-2 domain of ER-α that were found to be essential for BRCA1-mediated ubiquitination of ER-α, I358 and Q375 [41], fall within the previously identified region of ER-α (amino acids 338–379) that mediates binding to BRCA1 [38].

As noted above, over-expression of BRCA1 (but not cancer-associated mutant BRCA1 proteins) down-regulates the expression of p300, a nuclear receptor co-activator [33, 35]. This down-regulation occurs at the mRNA level and does not affect the CREB-binding protein (CBP), a functional homolog of BRCA1. Exogenous p300 or CBP rescued (i.e., reversed) the wtBRCA1-mediated inhibition of ER-α activity, suggesting that p300 plays a role in this process [33]. Interestingly, only a small portion of the p300 protein containing a conserved cysteine-histidine-rich region (CH_3) was both necessary and sufficient to rescue the BRCA1 repression of ER-α. Several other nuclear receptor co-activators, including the glucocorticoid receptor interacting protein 1 (GRIP1), p300/CBP-associated factor (PCAF), and amplified in breast cancer 1 (AIB1), failed to rescue the BRCA1 inhibition of ER-α activity. Since the rescue function of p300 did not require its histone acetyltransferase or SRC-1-binding domains, this function appears to be distinct from its function as an ER-α co-activator.

Recent studies suggest the existence of a distinct pool of ER-α localized at the plasma membrane and possibly other sites (reviewed in [42]). The membrane ER-α is G-protein coupled and signals, in part, via cross-talk with the epidermal growth factor receptor (EGFR) and insulin-like growth factor-1 receptor (IGF1R). With regard to BRCA1, it was found that in estrogen-responsive human breast carcinoma cell lines (MCF-7 and ZR-75-1), E2 caused a rapid and sustained activation of extracellular signal-related kinase (ERK) that was strongly inhibited by expression of exogenous wild-type but not cancer-associated mutant BRCA1 proteins [43]. Of additional note are the findings that the E2-stimulated proliferation of MCF-7 cells was blocked by either wtBRCA1 or ERK inhibitors in a manner that was dependent upon mitogen-activated kinase phosphatase 1, an ERK phosphatase. These findings suggest that BRCA1 may interact functionally with membrane-localized ER-α and that this interaction may contribute to its ability to suppress E2-stimulated cell proliferation.

Ligand-Independent Repression of ER-α Activity by BRCA1

Zheng and colleagues [44] observed constitutive activity of ER-α in Brca1 null mouse embryo fibroblasts (MEFs), suggesting that the endogenous BRCA1 protein may function to prevent activation of ER-α in the absence of estrogen. Consistent with this idea, they found that BRCA1 was present at the estrogen-response element (ERE) site on the promoter of cathepsin D (an estrogen-responsive gene) in MCF-7 human breast carcinoma cells before treatment with E2 but not after treatment. In agreement with these observations, it was found that knockdown of the endogenous BRCA1 protein using small interfering RNA (siRNA) caused about a 5- to 10-fold stimulation of ER-α activity in the absence of E2 and also significantly enhanced ER-α activity in the presence of E2 [45, 46]. In further studies, the ligand-independent activation of ER-α caused by BRCA1 knockdown was attributable, in part, to activation of the phosphatidylinositol-3 kinase (PI3K)/c-Akt signaling pathway, which results in phosphorylation of several key serine residues (S118 and S167) within the AF-1 domain of ER-α [46]. The mechanism by which loss of BRCA1 causes the activation of c-Akt is not totally clear, but it appears to involve, in part, the inhibition of protein phosphatase 2A, an enzyme that dephosphorylates and, thereby, inactivates c-Akt [46].

BRCA1 and ER-β

ER-β, a homolog of ER-α, is structurally similar to ER-α; but it exhibits a different tissue distribution and both similar and distinct functional properties relative to ligand selectivity, ligand-binding affinity, and transcriptional activation [47]. In some contexts (e.g., in the uterus), ER-β can inhibit ER-α activity due, in part, to the E2-stimulated formation of ER-α/ER-β [48, 49, 50]. The co-expression of ER-α and ER-β not only conferred a reduced sensitivity to E2 but also caused a decrease in the agonist activity and an increase in the antagonist activity of tamoxifen, a selective estrogen receptor modulator (SERM) [48, 51]. It is unclear, at present, if ER-β participates in the BRCA1-mediated repression of ER-α activity, but it is interesting to note that in cultured MCF-7 cells knockdown of BRCA1 stimulated the agonist activity of tamoxifen for ER-α [45].

BRCA1 and Aromatase

The enzyme aromatase (also called CYP19A1) is a cytochrome P450 enzyme that catalyzes the formation of estrogens from androgen precursors. The formation of estrogens from adrenal-derived androgens in peripheral adipose tissue is thought to be a major contributor to the development of post-menopausal breast cancer. Several recent studies suggest that BRCA1 negatively regulates aromatase expression in ovarian granulosa cells, adipocytes, mammary fibroblasts, and breast cancer cells [52–54]. These findings suggest that in addition to up-regulating ER-α activity, the inactivation of BRCA1 (see below) might also contribute to increased estrogen synthesis via aromatization.

BRCA1 Regulation of Progesterone Receptor (PR)

The PR plays an important role in normal mammary development; and while its role is not as well established as for ER-α, both experimental and clinical-epidemiological studies suggest that it also contributes to breast cancer development. In a recent study, it was found that BRCA1 binds to PR, inhibits its transcriptional activity, and blocks progesterone-stimulated gene expression and breast carcinoma cell proliferation [55]. Knockdown of BRCA1 caused about a 4-fold increase in progesterone-stimulated PR activity but did not confer ligand-independent activation of PR. Like ER-α, the BRCA1:PR interaction was ligand independent; but unlike ER-α, the interaction involved domains within the amino- and carboxyl termini of PR. And unlike ER-α, over-expression of p300 did not rescue the BRCA1-mediated repression of PR activity. It has also been reported that BRCA1 exerts control of PR protein levels through an indirect mechanism in which a wild-type (functional) BRCA1 is required to target PR for proteasomal degradation [56]. These findings such that the ability of BRCA1 to inhibit PR activity and/or cause its degradation might also contribute to its ability to suppress breast cancer formation. Animal model studies suggesting roles for both ER-α and PR in BRCA1-mutant mammary carcinogenesis are described below.

BRCA1 Stimulation of Androgen Receptor (AR) Activity

AR signaling plays a significant role in human prostate carcinogenesis [57]; and, in women, androgens counteract the ability of estrogen and progesterone to stimulate mammary epithelial cell growth [58]. In several studies, BRCA1 was found to bind to AR and stimulate its activity [59, 60]. In one study, BRCA1 up-regulated the AR-mediated expression of the cell cycle inhibitory protein p21^{WAF1} and enhanced dihydrotestosterone (DHT)-induced cell death in human prostate cancer cells [60]. In another study, BRCA1 was found to interact directly with both AR and the nuclear receptor co-activator GRIP1 and to stimulate AR activity through the AF-1 domain of AR [59]. The ability of BRCA1 to stimulate AR activity was augmented by several co-activators, including CBP, GRIP1, and the 55 and 70 kDa androgen receptor co-activators (ARA55 and ARA70). AR mutations have been associated with the development of male breast cancer, and as noted above, androgens can inhibit the proliferation of mammary epithelial cells, suggesting a possible role for AR in mammary carcinogenesis [58, 61]. AR exhibits polymorphisms in the number of poly-glutamine (CAG) repeats in its AF-1 domain, with the repeat length inversely correlated with p160 co-activator binding and AR activity. Some studies suggest an association between a long CAG repeat length and an early onset of breast cancer in BRCA1 mutation carriers; while other studies do not support a correlation [62].

Role of BRCA1 in Development

BRCA1 homozygous null mutations in mice confer early embryonic lethality (by day 7.5), while BRCA2 null mutations cause embryonic lethality by about 1 day later (day 8.5) (reviewed in [63]). These findings suggest that both breast cancer susceptibility genes are required for embryonic development and that, in this context, they have non-redundant functions (i.e., one cannot substitute for the other). BRCA1 null embryos exhibited widespread defects in cell proliferation attributable, in part, to the activation of p53, presumably due to genomic instability owing to the absence of functional BRCA1. Thus, the BRCA1 null phenotype was partially rescued by a deficiency of either p53 or G1 cell cycle inhibitor $p21^{WAF1}$, whose expression is induced by p53 [64].

Several studies examined the pattern of BRCA1 mRNA expression during normal development in mice. BRCA1 was highly expressed in many tissues, particularly in cell compartments containing rapidly proliferating cells and cells undergoing differentiation [65, 66]. In this regard, BRCA1 expression was significantly increased in mammary epithelial cells during puberty and pregnancy. BRCA1 expression was also found to be up-regulated in cultured mammary epithelial cells induced to differentiate by a hormonal cocktail [27]; and in several cell culture models, BRCA1 was shown to accelerate mammary epithelial differentiation [67, 68]. Interestingly, the developmental expression pattern of BRCA2 was similar to that of BRCA1, with a few exceptions, including endocrine tissues such as the testis during spermatogenesis and the breast during pregnancy [69]. These studies raise the possibility that BRCA1 expression during key windows of time [i.e., those in which mammary epithelial cells undergo differentiation (puberty and pregnancy)] is important for tumor suppression.

In general, the phenotype of mice heterozygous for BRCA1 in the germ-line was similar to that of wild-type mice. However, in studies of the endocrine responses to diethylstilbestrol (DES), a synthetic estrogen, the BRCA1 heterozygous mice showed reduced mammary ductal branching, as compared with the wild-type mice [70]. Most heterozygous mice showed ovarian atrophy, as compared with wild-type mice, which showed arrested follicular development. These findings suggest that BRCA1 is haplo-insufficient with respect to some endocrine tissue responses to the steroid DES.

Mouse Models of BRCA1-Dependent Tumorigenesis

Since mice homozygous for a germ-line BRCA1 null mutation died during embryogenesis and mice heterozygous for BRCA1 did not develop tumors, it was necessary to utilize mice with a homozygous mammary-targeted BRCA1 mutation to study BRCA1-mutant mammary tumorigenesis. The best-studied mouse model of BRCA1-deficient tumorigenesis features a conditional (cre-lox dependent) mammary epithelial cell-targeted homozygous deletion of BRCA1 exon 11, which codes for more than 60% of the BRCA1 protein [71]. These mice contained two floxed BRCA1 alleles and were transgenic for the mouse mammary tumor virus (MMTV) promoter up-stream of a cre recombinase gene. The mice developed mammary cancers with a low incidence and a long latency period (12 months). However, the incidence was increased and the latency period decreased in the setting of a heterozygous deletion of the p53 gene [71]. The requirement for p53 deficiency is analogous to human BRCA1-mutant tumor development, since about 80% of human BRCA1-mutant breast cancers exhibit p53 mutations [72, 73]. The mammary cancers that developed in these BRCA1/p53-deficient mice recapitulated some of the features of human BRCA1-mutant cancers, including a similar pattern of chromosomal rearrangements and p53 mutations [74, 75].

A study of the effect of tamoxifen on the BRCA1/p53-deficient mice revealed that tamoxifen caused a significant increase in the incidence of mammary carcinomas [45]. This finding was consistent with the above-cited observation that tamoxifen increased the ratio of ER-α agonist to antagonist activity in cultured MCF-7 cells [45]. In further studies, it was found that mice with the conditional mammary-targeted BRCA1 deletion exhibited longer mammary ductal extension during puberty than did wild-type mice [76]. Terminal end bud differentiation was impaired in these mice, prolactin-induced alveolar differentiation remained intact, providing evidence for an increased effect of endogenous estrogen. Normally, exposure of mice to exogenous estrogen causes a burst of mammary epithelial cell proliferation that subsides rapidly due to normal compensatory mechanisms. However, in BRCA1-deficient animals, exogenous 17β-estradiol caused an abnormal sustained mammary epithelial cell proliferative response and appearance of mammary preneoplasia. In a BRCA1/p53-deficient setting, exogenous E2 caused an increase in the proportion of mice with multiple hyperplastic alveolar nodules (HANs) [76]. Finally, mice harboring mammary-targeted conditional ER-α over-expression in combination with mammary-targeted BRCA1 deficiency and p53 heterozygosity exhibited an increased incidence of multiple HANs, invasive cancers, and tumor multiplicity [76].

As noted earlier, bilateral oophorectomy in women who carry germ-line BRCA1 mutations conferred a reduced incidence of breast cancer. In the above-described mice with mammary-targeted BRCA1 deficiency and a heterozygous p53 deletion, bilateral oophorectomy conferred a reduced incidence of mammary cancers after 4 months post-oophorectomy, as compared with sham-operated mice [77]. These mice also showed mammary gland regression associated with a decreased number of mammary epithelial cells after ophorectomy. These findings are consistent with the idea that in mice, as in humans, ovarian steroids are required during the early stages of mammary cancer development.

In a similar mouse model, this time featuring a mammary-targeted BRCA1 deletion coupled to a homozygous p53 deletion, the mammary glands of nulliparous animals exhibited increased lateral branching and alveolar morphogenesis, a phenotype that is normally characteristic of progesterone effect during pregnancy [56]. In this mouse model, PR was found to be over-expressed due to reduced degradation through the proteasomal pathway. Here, treatment with a selective progesterone receptor modulator (SPRM), RU-486 (mifepristone, the "morning after pill"), prevented the development of mammary cancers. These observations are consistent with the previous findings that BRCA1 inhibits PR function and that exposure of BRCA1-deficient mice to exogenous progesterone causes an abnormal sustained mammary epithelial cell proliferative response with increased tertiary branching of the mammary ducts [55]. Together, this research suggests that the ability of BRCA1 to regulate progesterone action through the PR contributes to the BRCA1-mutant mammary tumorigenesis.

BRCA1 as a Target for Dietary Factors, Environmental Exposures, and Breast Cancer Prevention

Epidemiologic evidence suggests that moderate ethanol consumption is a significant risk factor for breast cancer development and that ethanol synergistically stimulates breast cancer risk in conjunction with estrogen replacement therapy in post-menopausal women [78, 79]. While the molecular basis for the linkage of alcohol consumption and breast cancer risk is unclear, a study of cultured human breast cancer cells revealed that exposure to ethanol causes an increase in ER-α protein levels and ER-α activity associated with a large dose-dependent decrease in BRCA1 protein levels [80]. Persistent organochlorines (POCs) are environmental carcinogens that contaminate the food chain. Some of these agents are xeno-estrogens that inhibit ER-α activity and may contribute to breast cancer risk. Thus, polychlorinated biphenyls (PCBs) and 2,3,7,8-tetrachlorodibenzo-*p*-dioxin (TCDD, or toxiphene) were reported to down-regulate E2-stimulated BRCA1 mRNA expression in MCF-7 human breast cancer cells [81]. The polycyclic aromatic hydrocarbon benzo(a)pyrene (B[a]P), a suspected mammary carcinogen, inhibited BRCA1 expression in ER-α positive but not ER-α negative human breast cancer cell lines [82]. The inhibition of E2-inducible BRCA1 expression by B[a]P and TCDD was mediated through ligation of the arylhydrocarbon receptor (AhR), which targets xenobiotic response elements (XREs) within the BRCA1 promoter [83]. Conversely, BRCA1 appears to function as a co-activator for the AhR nuclear translocator (ARNT), suggesting that loss of BRCA1 expression could impair the ability of cells to mount a normal response to xenobiotic stress [84].

Indole-3-carbinol (I3C) is a micronutrient found in cruciferous vegetables (e.g., cabbage, cauliflower, broccoli) with cancer preventive activity, particularly for estrogen-dependent tumor types (i.e., breast, cervical, and endometrial cancers) [85]. Thus, dietary supplementation with cruciferous vegetables or with

I3C blocks the development of E2-dependent tumors in animals. Protection against mammary tumorigenesis due to I3C carcinogenesis appears to be due, in part, to enhanced metabolism of estrone via the 2-hydroxylation pathway, which yields inert products, and decreased 16-hydroxylation, which yields pro-carcinogenic metabolites [86]. Recent studies indicate that I3C, its major active metabolite DIM (3,3′-diindolylmethane), and genistein (a soy isoflavone with cancer prevention activity) up-regulate the expression of BRCA1 in breast, cervical, and prostate carcinoma cell lines [87–90]. The up-regulation of BRCA1 expression by I3C and genistein may be due, in part, to the ability of these agents to cause an endoplasmic reticulum stress-like response [90]. In addition, the ability of I3C and genistein to inhibit E2-stimulated ER-α activity was BRCA1 dependent, as demonstrated by the use of BRCA1-siRNA to knock down the BRCA1 protein levels [90].

A study of rat mammary tumorigenesis induced by 7,12-dimethylbenz[a]anthracene (DMBA) revealed that pre-pubertal exposure (age 1–3 weeks) of female rats to 17β-estradiol or genistein (which has mixed ER-α agonist/antagonist activity) reduced the risk of developing DMBA-induced mammary cancers [91]. Both E2 and genistein caused a persistent up-regulation of BRCA1 expression in the mammary gland that was still present at age 16 weeks. Genistein, which can both activate ER-α by itself and inhibit E2-stimulated ER-α activity, is a more selective ligand for ER-β than for ER-α, suggesting that its ability to inhibit E2-stimulated ER-α activity may be due, in part, to the formation of ER-α/ER-β heterodimers [92, 93]. At present, it is unclear if the ability of genistein stimulate BRCA1 expression is dependent upon ER-β. In addition to I3C and genistein, several other dietary agents that can influence mammary tumorigenesis in rats have also been found to modulate BRCA1 expression, including whole wheat flour and (n–3) polyunsaturated fatty acids (PUFAs) [94, 95]. It remains to be proven whether the ability of dietary factors to induce the expression of BRCA1 within the mammary glands of these animals contributes to development of resistance to tumorigenesis.

Loss of ER-α Expression in BRCA1-Deficient Breast Cancers

Approximately two-thirds of all sporadic (non-hereditary) human breast cancers are ER-α positive. In contrast, about 80% of breast cancers that develop in BRCA1 mutation carriers are ER-α negative [73, 96,97]. Most of these tumors are negative for PR and HER2/Neu amplification [73]. Thus, BRCA1-mutant human breast cancers exhibit the so-called triple-negative breast cancer phenotype, which is also characteristic of "basal-like" breast cancers that exhibit aggressive clinical behavior [98]. Like human BRCA1-mutant breast cancers, most mammary cancers that develop in the BRCA1-deficient mouse models are also ER-α negative [75]. Thus, any accounting of a role for hormonal factors in BRCA1-mutant breast carcinogenesis must explain the apparently conflicting observation that most of these tumors lack ER-α and PR expression.

In this regard, in mice harboring a mammary-targeted BRCA1 deletion, tamoxifen-induced mammary hyperplasias exhibited down-regulation of BRCA1 expression [45]. Furthermore, estrogen-induced preneoplastic lesions in BRCA1-deficient mice were found to be ER-α negative [76]. Even the preneoplasias and cancers that developed in mice with mammary-targeted ER-α over-expression and BRCA1 deficiency were mostly ER-α negative [76]. These findings suggest that the absence of ER-α observed in BRCA1-mutant breast cancers is an early and integral component of the tumorigenesis pathway rather than a random late event. The mechanism underlying the loss of BRCA1 expression is unclear. However, one study of human BRCA1-mutant breast cancers revealed increased CpG methylation of the ER-α gene in those tumors that were ER-α negative, suggesting that ER-α promoter methylation might contribute to the loss of ER-α expression in these tumors [99]. Finally, in a recent study, it was found that in human breast cancer cells, BRCA1 is recruited to the ER-α promoter by the transcription factor Oct-1 and that both BRCA1 and Oct-1 are required for ER-α expression [100].

Functional Inactivation of BRCA1 in Sporadic Breast Cancers

While inherited BRCA1 mutations can account for only a small minority (2.5–5%) of human breast cancers, various studies have revealed BRCA1 mRNA and protein are absent or significantly decreased in about 30–40% of sporadic breast cancer cases [101–104]. The decreased expression of BRCA1 in these tumors may be attributed to hypermethylation of the BRCA1 promoter on CpG islands and/or loss of one of the BRCA1 alleles [105–107]. Aberrant expression of the DNA methyl transferase DNMT3B and the CCCTC-binding factor (CTCF) may account for the loss of BRCA1 expression in some of these cases [108]. while negative transcriptional elements within the BRCA1 promoter may also contribute to decreased BRCA1 expression [109]. The regulation of BRCA1 expression is described elsewhere [5]. At present, it is not clear if these BRCA1-under-expressing sporadic breast cancers represent a phenotypically distinct subset of cancers or if they resemble BRCA1-mutant breast cancers in other characteristics, such as hormonal responsiveness.

It should be noted that even in the absence of BRCA1 mutation or down-regulation of its expression, BRCA1 may be functionally inactivated by other oncogenic pathways. For example, over-expression of cyclin D1, which is amplified in about 15–20% of breast cancer cases, can rescue the BRCA1-mediated repression of ER-α activity through a direct interaction of the BRCA1 and cyclin D1 proteins [110]. As noted earlier, the human papilloma virus oncoproteins E6 and E7 can also reverse the BRCA1 inhibition of ER-α activity [32]. In addition, c-Akt can rescue the BRCA1 repression of ER-α in a manner that is dependent upon its kinase activity [46]. These findings raise the possibility that functional inactivation of BRCA1 through oncogenic signaling pathways could contribute to de-repression of ER-α activity in breast cancers that express normal levels of wild-type BRCA1 protein.

Model for BRCA1 Cross-Talk with Hormone Receptor Pathways in Mammary Tumorigenesis

Figure 1 illustrates schematically some of the interactions between BRCA1 and steroid hormonal receptor signaling pathways that may contribute to mammary tumor suppression or tumorigenesis. Thus, in the model presented, under normal conditions, BRCA1 is postulated to function to limit mammary epithelial cell (MEC) proliferation by inhibiting the activity of ER-α, PR, and aromatase and, possibly, by stimulating AR activity. BRCA1 also serves to promote MEC differentiation and to maintain genomic stability in this cell type, both functions that may also contribute to tumor suppression. The loss of these activities of BRCA1, as may occur through an inherited BRCA1 mutation, environmental exposures, epigenetic silencing, functional inactivation by activation of oncogenic signaling pathways, or a combination of these factors tends to promote mammary tumorigenesis, while enhanced BRCA1 expression due to dietary factors such as I3C and genistein is expected to have the opposite effect.

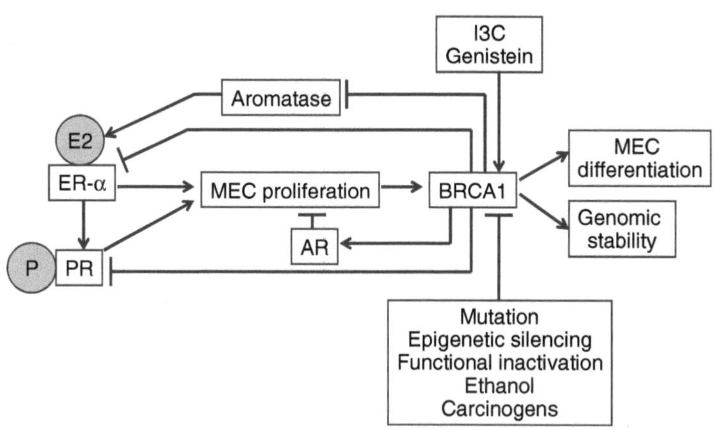

Fig. 1 Model for BRCA1 cross-talk with hormone receptors in mammary tumorigenesis. See text for description. MEC, mammary epithelial cell; P, progesterone. Other abbreviations, see text

As noted earlier, while BRCA1-mutant tumorigenesis in humans and mice is clearly hormone sensitive (at least in the early stages), the resultant tumors are usually ER-α negative. Theoretically, at least two models might account for this phenomenon. In one scheme, the same progenitor cell might undergo conversion from ER-α positivity to ER-α negativity during the process of tumorigenesis. In another scheme, BRCA1-deficient hormone receptor-positive MECs that are over-stimulated due to the loss of BRCA1-mediated repression of hormonal signaling might induce the proliferation of hormone receptor-negative MECs through a paracrine mechanism. Further research will be required to definitively identify the mechanism through which BRCA1-mutant tumors become ER-α negative.

Acknowledgments Dr. Rosen has been supported, in part, by USPHS grants R01-CA82599, RO1-CA80000, and RO1-CA104546.

References

1. Miki Y, Swensen J, Shattuck-Eidens D, Futreal PA, Harshman K, Tavtigian S, Liu Q, Cochran C, Bennett LM, Ding W, et al. A strong candidate for the breast and ovarian cancer susceptibility gene BRCA1. Science 1994;266:66–71.
2. Wooster R, Bignell G, Lancaster J, Swift S, Seal S, Mangion J, Collins N, Gregory S, Gumbs C, Micklem G. Identification of the breast cancer susceptibility gene BRCA2. Nature 1995;378:789–792.
3. Tavtigian SV, Simard J, Rommens J, Couch F, Shattuck-Eidens D, Neuhausen S, Merajver S, Thorlacius S, Offit K, Stoppa-Lyonnet D, Belanger C, Bell R, Berry S, Bogden R, Chen Q, Davis T, Dumont M, Frye C, Hattier T, Jammulapati S, Janecki T, Jiang P, Kehrer R, Leblanc JF, Goldgar DE, et al. The complete BRCA2 gene and mutations in chromosome 13q-linked kindreds. Nat Genet 1996;12:333–337.
4. Merajver SD, Frank TS, Xu J, Pham TM, Calzone KA, Bennett-Baker P, Chamberlain J, Boyd J, Garber JE, Collins FS et al. Germline BRCA1 mutations and loss of the wild-type allele in tumors from families with early onset breast and ovarian cancer. Clin Cancer Res. 1995;1:539–544.
5. Rosen EM, Fan S, Pestell RG, Goldberg ID. BRCA1 gene in breast cancer. J Cell Physiol. 2003;196:19–41.
6. Gudmundsdottir K, Ashworth A. The roles of BRCA1 and BRCA2 and associated proteins in the maintenance of genomic stability. Oncogene 2006;25:5864–5874 Review.
7. Tirkkonen M, Johannsson O, Agnarsson BA, Olsson H, Ingvarsson S, Karhu R, Tanner M, Isola J, Barkardottir RB, Borg A, Kallioniemi OP. Distinct somatic genetic changes associated with tumor progression in carriers of BRCA1 and BRCA2 germ-line mutations. Cancer Res. 1997;57:1222–1227.
8. Xu X, Weaver Z, Linke SP, Li C, Gotay J, Wang XW, Harris CC, Ried T, Deng CX. Centrosome amplification and a defective G2-M cell cycle checkpoint induce genetic instability in BRCA1 exon 11 isoform-deficient cells. Mol Cell. 1999;3:389–395.
9. Weaver Z, Montagna C, Xu X, Howard T, Gadina M, Brodie SG, Deng CX, Ried T. Mammary tumors in mice conditionally mutant for Brca1 exhibit gross genomic instability and centrosome amplification yet display a recurring distribution of genomic imbalances that is similar to human breast cancer. Oncogene 2002;21:5097–5107.
10. Thompson D, Easton DF Breast Cancer Linkage Consortium. Cancer Incidence in BRCA1 mutation carriers. J Natl Cancer Inst. 2002;94:1358–1365.

11. Elson DA, Riley RR, Lacey A, Thordarson G, Talamantes FJ, Arbeit JM. Sensitivity of the cervical transformation zone to estrogen-induced squamous carcinogenesis. Cancer Res. 2000;60:1267–1275.
12. Arbeit JM, Howley PM, Hanahan D. Chronic estrogen-induced cervical and vaginal squamous carcinogenesis in human papillomavirus type 16 transgenic mice. Proc Nat Acad Sci USA. 2003;93:2930–2935.
13. de Villiers EM. Relationship between steroid hormone contraceptives and HPV, cervical intraepithelial neoplasia and cervical carcinoma. Int J Cancer. 2003;103:705–758.
14. Liede A, Karlan BY, Narod SA. Cancer risks for male carriers of germline mutations in BRCA1 or BRCA2: a review of the literature. J Clin Oncol. 2004;22: 735–742.
15. Lubinski J, Phelan CM, Ghadirian P, Lynch HT, Garber J, Weber B, Tung N, Horsman D, Isaacs C, Monteiro AN, Sun P, Narod SA. Cancer variation associated with the position of the mutation in the BRCA2 gene. Familial Cancer. 2004;3:1–10.
16. Narod SA. Modifiers of risk of hereditary breast cancer. Oncogene 2006;25:5832–5836 Review.
17. Rosen EM, Fan S, Isaacs C. BRCA1 in hormonal carcinogenesis: basic and clinical research. Endocr Relat Cancer. 2005;12:533–548 Review.
18. Rebbeck TR, Lynch HT, Neuhausen SL, Narod SA, Van't Veer L, Garber JE, Evans G, Isaacs C, Daly MB, Matloff E, Olopade OI, Weber BL; Prevention and Observation of Surgical End Points Study Group. Prophylactic oophorectomy in carriers of BRCA1 or BRCA2 mutations. New Engl J Med 2002;346:1616–1622.
19. Kauff ND, Domchek SM, Friebel TM, Robson ME, Lee J, Garber JE, Isaacs C, Evans DG, Lynch H, Eeles RA, Neuhausen SL, Daly MB, Matloff E, Blum JL, Sabbatini P, Barakat RR, Hudis C, Norton L, Offit K, Rebbeck TR. Risk-reducing salpingo-oophorectomy for the prevention of BRCA1- and BRCA2-associated breast and gynecologic cancer: a multicenter, prospective study. J Clin Oncol 2008;26:1331–1337.
20. Monteiro AN, August A, Hanafusa H. Evidence for a transcription activation function of BRCA1 C-terminal region. Proc Nat Acad Sci USA 1996;93:13595–13599.
21. Hashizume R, Fukuda M, Maeda I, Nishikawa H, Oyake D, Yabuki Y, Ogata H, Ohta T. The RING heterodimer BRCA1–BARD1 is a ubiquitin ligase inactivated by a breast cancer-derived mutation. J Biol Chem. 2001;276:14537–14540.
22. Boulton SJ. BRCA1-mediated ubiquitylation. Cell Cycle. 2006;5:1481–1486.
23. Shakya R, Szabolcs M, McCarthy E, Ospina E, Basso K, Nandula S, Murty V, Baer R, Ludwig T. The basal-like mammary carcinomas induced by Brca1 or Bard1 inactivation implicate the BRCA1/BARD1 heterodimer in tumor suppression. Proc Nat Acad Sci USA 2008; Apr 28. [Epublished ahead of print].
24. Bork P, Hofmann K, Bucher P, Neuwald AF, Altschul SF, Koonin EV. A superfamily of conserved domains in DNA damage-responsive cell cycle checkpoint proteins. FASEB J. 1997;11:68–76.
25. Thakur S, Zhang HB, Peng Y, Le H, Carroll B, Ward T, Yao J, Farid LM, Couch FJ, Wilson RB, Weber BL. Localization of BRCA1 and a splice variant identifies the nuclear localization signal. Mol Cell Biol. 1997;17:444–452.
26. Rodriguez JA, Henderson BR. Identification of a functional nuclear export sequence in BRCA1. J Biol Chem. 2000;275: 38589–38596.
27. Rajan JV, Wang M, Marquis ST, Chodosh LA. Brca2 is coordinately regulated with Brca1 during proliferation and differentiation in mammalian epithelial cells. Proc Nat Acad Sci USA 1996;93:3078–3083.
28. Thomas JE, Smith M, Tonkinson JL, Rubinfeld B, Polakis P Induction of phosphorylation of BRCA1 during the cell cycle and after DNA damage. Cell Growth Differen. 1997;8:801–809.
29. Rosen EM, Fan S, Ma Y. BRCA1 regulation of transcription. Cancer Lett. 2006;236:175–185 Review.

30. Hu YF, Li R. JunB potentiates function of BRCA1 activation domain 1 (AD1) through a coiled-coil-mediated interaction. Genes Dev. 2002;16:1509–1517.
31. Fan S, Wang J, Yuan R, Ma Y, Meng Q, Erdos MR, Pestell RG, Yuan F, Auborn KJ, Goldberg ID, Rosen EM. BRCA1 inhibition of estrogen receptor signaling in transfected cells. Science 1999;284:1354–1356.
32. Zhang Y, Fan S, Meng Q, Ma Y, Katiyar P, Schlegel R, Rosen EM. BRCA1 interaction with human papillomavirus oncoproteins. J Biol Chem. 2005;280:33165–33177.
33. Fan S, Ma YX, Wang C, Yuan RQ, Meng Q, Wang JA, Erdos M, Goldberg ID, Webb P, Kushner PJ, Pestell RG, Rosen EM p300 Modulates the BRCA1 inhibition of estrogen receptor activity. Cancer Res. 2002;62:141–151.
34. Fan S, Ma YX, Wang C, Yuan RQ, Meng Q, Wang JA, Erdos M, Goldberg ID, Webb P, Kushner PJ, Pestell RG, Rosen EM. Role of direct interaction in BRCA1 inhibition of estrogen receptor activity. Oncogene 2001;20:77–87.
35. Fan S, Wang JA, Yuan RQ, Ma YX, Meng Q, Erdos MR, Brody LC, Goldberg ID, Rosen EM. BRCA1 as a potential human prostate tumor suppressor: modulation of proliferation, damage responses and expression of cell regulatory proteins. Oncogene 1998;16:3069–3082.
36. Fan S, Yuan R, Ma YX, Meng Q, Goldberg ID, Rosen EM Mutant BRCA1 genes antagonize phenotype of wild type BRCA1. Oncogene 2001;20:8215–8235.
37. Kawai H, Li H, Chun P, Avraham S, Avraham HK Direct interaction between BRCA1 and the estrogen receptor regulates vascular endothelial growth factor (VEGF) transcription and secretion in breast cancer cells. Oncogene 2002;21:7730–7739.
38. Ma YX, Tomita Y, Fan S, Wu K, Tong Y, Zhao Z, Song LN, Goldberg ID, Rosen EM. Structural determinants of the BRCA1: estrogen receptor interaction. Oncogene 2005;24:1831–1846.
39. Wu LC, Wang ZW, Tsan JT, Spillman MA, Phung A, Xu XL, Yang MC, Hwang LY, Bowcock AM, Baer R. Identification of a RING protein that can interact in vivo with the BRCA1 gene product. Nat Genet. 1996;14:430–440.
40. Ruffner H, Joazeiro CA, Hemmati D, Hunter T, Verma IM. Cancer-predisposing mutations within the RING domain of BRCA1: loss of ubiquitin protein ligase activity and protection from radiation hypersensitivity. Proc Nat Acad Sci USA. 2001;98:5134–5139.
41. Eakin CM, Maccoss MJ, Finney GL, Klevit RE. Estrogen receptor alpha is a putative substrate for the BRCA1 ubiquitin ligase. Proc Nat Acad Sci USA. 2007;104:5794–5799.
42. Pedram A, Razandi M, Levin ER. Nature of functional estrogen receptors at the plasma membrane. Mol Endocrinol. 2006;20:1996–2009.
43. Razandi M, Pedram A, Rosen EM, Levin ER. BRCA1 inhibits membrane estrogen and growth factor receptor signaling to cell proliferation in breast cancer. Mol Cell Biol. 2004;24:5900–5913.
44. Zheng L, Annab LA, Afshari CA, Lee WH, Boyer TG. BRCA1 mediates ligand-independent transcriptional repression of the estrogen receptor. Proc Nat Acad Sci USA. 2001;98:9587–9592.
45. Jones LP, Li M, Halama ED, Ma Y, Lubet R, Grubbs CJ, Deng C-X, Rosen EM, Furth PA. Promotion of mammary cancer development by tamoxifen in a mouse model of Brca1-mutation related breast cancer. Oncogene 2005;24:3554–3562.
46. Ma Y, Hu C, Riegel AT, Fan S, Rosen EM. Growth factor signaling pathways modulate BRCA1 repression of estrogen receptor-alpha activity. Mol Endocrinol. 2007;21:1905–1923.
47. Mosselman S, Polman J, Dijkema R. ER-beta: identification and characterization of a novel human estrogen receptor. FEBS Lett. 1996;392:49–53.
48. Pettersson K, Delaunay F, Gustafsson JA. Estrogen receptor beta acts as a dominant regulator of estrogen signaling. Oncogene 2000;19:4970–4978.
49. Weihua Z, Saji S, Makinen S, Cheng G, Jensen EV, Warner M, Gustafsson JA. Estrogen receptor (ER) beta, a modulator of ER alpha in the uterus. Proc Nat Acad Sci USA. 2000;97:5936–5941.

50. Jisa E, Jungbauer A. Kinetic analysis of estrogen receptor homo- and heterodimerization in vitro. J Steroid Biochem Mol Biol. 2003;84:141–148.
51. Hall JM, McDonnell DP. The estrogen receptor betaisoform (ERbeta) of the human estrogen receptor modulates ERalpha transcriptional activity and is a key regulator of the cellular response to estrogens and antiestrogens. Endocrinology 1999;140:5566–5578.
52. Hu Y, Ghosh S, Amleh A, Yue W, Lu Y, Katz A, Li R. Modulation of aromatase expression by BRCA1: a possible link to tissue-specific tumor suppression. Oncogene 2005;24:8343–8348.
53. Lu M, Chen D, Lin Z, Reierstad S, Trauernicht AM, Boyer TG, Bulun SE. BRCA1 negatively regulates the cancer-associated aromatase promoters I.3 and II in breast adipose fibroblasts and malignant epithelial cells. J Clin Endocrinol Metab. 2006;91:4514–4519.
54. Subbaramaiah K, Hudis C, Chang SH, Hla T, Dannenberg AJ. EP2 and EP4 receptors regulate aromatase expression in human adipocytes and breast cancer cells. Evidence of a BRCA1 and p300 exchange. J Biol Chem. 2008;283:3433–3444.
55. Ma Y, Katiyar P, Jones LP, Fan S, Zhang Y, Furth PA, Rosen EM. The breast cancer susceptibility gene BRCA1 regulates progesterone receptor signaling in mammary epithelial cells. Mol Endocrinol. 2006;20:14–34.
56. Poole AJ, Li Y, Kim Y, Lin SC, Lee WH, Lee EY. Prevention of Brca1-mediated mammary tumorigenesis in mice by a progesterone antagonist. Science 2006;314:1467–1470.
57. Henderson BE, Feigelson HS Hormonal carcinogenesis. Carcinogenesis 2000;21:427–433.
58. von Schoultz B. Androgens and the breast. Maturitas 2007;57:47–49 Review.
59. Park JJ, Irvine RA, Buchanan G, Koh SS, Park JM, Tilley WD, Stallcup MR, Press MF, Coetzee GA. Breast cancer susceptibility gene 1 (BRCA1) is a coactivator of the androgen receptor. Cancer Res. 2000;60:5946–5949.
60. Yeh S, Hu YC, Rahman M, Lin HK, Hsu CL, Ting HJ, Kang HY, Chang C. Increase of androgen induced cell death and androgen receptor transactivation by BRCA1 in prostate cancer cells. Proc Nat Acad Sci USA. 2000;97:11256–11261.
61. Ando S, De Amicis F, Rago V, Carpino A, Maggiolini M, Panno ML, Lanzino M. Breast cancer: from estrogen to androgen receptor. Mol Cell Endocrinol. 2002;193:121–128.
62. Ferro P, Catalano MG, Dell'Eva R, Fortunati N, Pfeffer U. The androgen receptor CAG repeat: a modifier of carcinogenesis? Mol Cell Endocrinol. 2002;193:109–120.
63. Hakem R, de la Pompa JL, Mak TW. Developmental studies of Brca1 and Brca2 knockout mice. J Mammary Gland Biol Neoplasia. 1998;3: 431–445 Review.
64. Hakem R, de la Pompa JL, Elia A, Potter J, Mak TW. Partial rescue of Brca1 (5–6) early embryonic lethality by p53 or p21 null mutation. Nat Genet. 1997;16:298–302.
65. Lane TF, Deng C, Elson A, Lyu MS, Kozak CA, Leder P. Expression of Brca1 is associated with terminal differentiation of ectodermally and mesodermally derived tissues in mice. Genes Dev. 1995;9:2712–2722.
66. Marquis ST, Rajan JV, Wynshaw-Boris A, Xu J, Yin GY, Abel KJ, Weber BL, Chodosh LA. The developmental pattern of Brca1 expression implies a role in differentiation of the breast and other tissues. Nat Genet. 1995;11:17–26.
67. Kubista M, Rosner M, Kubista E, Bernaschek G, Hengstschlager M. Brca1 regulates in vitro differentiation of mammary epithelial cells. Oncogene 2002;21:4747–4756.
68. Furuta S, Jiang X, Gu B, Cheng E, Chen PL, Lee WH. Depletion of BRCA1 impairs differentiation but enhances proliferation of mammary epithelial cells. Proc Nat Acad Sci USA. 2005;102:9176–9181.
69. Rajan JV, Marquis ST, Gardner HP, Chodosh LD. Developmental expression of Brca2 colocalizes with Brca1 and is associated with proliferation and differentiation in multiple tissues. Devel Biol. 1997;184:385–40.
70. Bennett LM, McAllister KA, Malphurs J, Ward T, Collins NK, Seely JC, Gowen LC, Koller BH, Davis BJ, Wiseman RW. Mice heterozygous for a Brca1 or Brca2 mutation display distinct mammary gland and ovarian phenotypes in response to diethylstilbestrol. Cancer Res. 2000;60:3461–3469.

71. Xu X, Wagner K-U, Larson D, Weaver Z, Li C, Ried T, Hennighausen L, Wynshaw-BorisA, Deng C-X Conditional mutation of Brca1 in mammary epithelial cells results in blunted ductal morphogenesis and tumour formation. Nat Genet. 1999;22: 37–43.
72. Phillips KA, Andrulis IL, Goodwin PJ Breast carcinomas arising in carriers of mutations in BRCA1 or BRCA2 are they prognostically different? J Clin Oncol. 1999;17:3653–3663.
73. Lakhani SR, Van De Vijver MJ, Jacquemier J, Anderson TJ, Osin PP, McGuffog L, Easton DF. The pathology of familial breast cancer predictive value of immunohistochemical markers estrogen receptor, progesterone receptor, HER-2, and p53 in patients with mutations in BRCA1 and BRCA2. J Clin Oncol. 2002;20:2310–2318.
74. Brodie SG, Xu X, Qiao W, Li WM, Cao L, Deng CX Multiple genetic changes are associated with mammary tumorigenesis in Brca1 conditional knockout mice. Oncogene 2001;20:17514–17523.
75. Deng CX Tumor formation in Brca1 conditional mutant mice. Environ Mol Mutagen. 2002;39:171–177.
76. Jones LP, Tilli MT, Assefnia S, Torre K, Halama ED, Parrish A, Rosen EM, Furth PA. Activation of estrogen signaling pathways collaborates with loss of Brca1 to promote development of ERalpha-negative and ERalpha-positive mammary preneoplasia and cancer. Oncogene 2008;27:794–802.
77. Bachelier R, Xu X, Li C, Qiao W, Furth PA, Lubet RA, Deng CX. Effect of bilateral oophorectomy on mammary tumor formation in BRCA1 mutant mice. Oncol Rep. 2005;14:1117–1120.
78. Holmes MD, Willett WC Does diet affect breast cancer risk? Breast Cancer Res. 2004;6:170–178.
79. Linos E, Willett WC. Diet and breast cancer risk reduction. J Natl Compr Canc Netw. 2007;5:711–718 Review.
80. Fan S, Meng Q, Gao B, Grossman J, Yadegari M, Goldberg ID, Rosen EM. Alcohol stimulates estrogen receptor signaling in human breast cancer cell lines. Cancer Res. 2000;60:5635–5639.
81. Rattenborg T, Gjermandsen I, Bonefeld-Jorgensen EC. Inhibition of E2-induced expression of BRCA1 by persistent organochlorines. Breast Cancer Res. 2007;4:R12.
82. Jeffy BD, Chirnomas RB, Chen EJ, Gudas JM, Romagnolo DF. Activation of the aromatic hydrocarbon receptor pathway is not sufficient for transcriptional repression of BRCA-1: requirements for metabolism of benzo[a]pyrene to 7r,8t-dihydroxy-9t,10-epoxy-7,8,9,10-tetrahydrobenzo[a]pyrene. Cancer Res. 2002;62:113–121.
83. Hockings JK, Thorne PA, Kemp MQ, Morgan SS, Selmin O, Romagnolo DF. The ligand status of the aromatic hydrocarbon receptor modulates transcriptional activation of BRCA-1 promoter by estrogen. Cancer Res. 2006;66:2224–2232.
84. Kang HJ, Kim HJ, Kim SK, Barouki R, Cho CH, Khanna KK, Rosen EM, Bae I. BRCA1 modulates xenobiotic stress-inducible gene expression by interacting with ARNT in human breast cancer cells. J Biol Chem. 2006;281: 14654–14662.
85. Shertzer HG, Senft AP. The micronutrient indole-3-carbinol: implications for disease and chemoprevention. Drug Metab Drug Interact. 2000;17:159–188.
86. Bradlow HL, Michnovich J, Telang NT, Osborne MP. Effects of dietary indole-3-carbinol on estradiol metabolism and spontaneous mammary tumors in mice. Carcinogenesis 1991;12:1571–1574.
87. Meng Q, Yuan F, Goldberg ID, Rosen EM, Auborn K, Fan S. Indole-3-carbinol is a negative regulator of estrogen receptor-alpha signaling in human tumor cells. J Nutr. 2000;130:2927–2931.
88. Meng Q, Qi M, Chen DZ, Yuan R, Goldberg ID, Rosen EM, Auborn K, Fan S. Suppression of breast cancer invasion and migration by indole-3-carbinol: associated

with up-regulation of BRCA1 and E-cadherin/catenin complexes. J Mol Med. 2000;78:155–165.

89. Carter TH, Liu K, Ralph W Jr, Chen D, Qi M, Fan S, Yuan F, Rosen EM, Auborn KJ Diindolylmethane alters gene expression in human keratinocytes in vitro. J Nutr. 2002;132:3314–3324.
90. Fan S, Meng Q, Auborn K, Carter T, Rosen EM BRCA1 and BRCA2 as molecular targets for phytochemicals indole-3-carbinol and genistein in breast and prostate cancer cells. Br J Cancer. 2006;94:407–426.
91. Cabanes A, Wang M, Olivo S, DeAssis S, Gustafsson JA, Khan G, Hilakivi-Clarke L. Prepubertal estradiol and genistein exposures up-regulate BRCA1 mRNA and reduce mammary tumorigenesis. Carcinogenesis 2004;25:741–748.
92. Barkhem T, Carlsson B, Nilsson Y, Enmark E, Gustafsson J, Nilsson S. Differential response of estrogen receptor alpha and estrogen receptor beta to partial estrogen agonists/antagonists. Mol Pharmacol. 1998;54:105–112.
93. Pike AC, Brzozowski AM, Hubbard RE, Bonn T, Thorsell AG, Engstrom O, Ljunggren J, Gustafsson JA, Carlquist M Structure of the ligand-binding domain of oestrogen receptor beta in the presence of a partial agonist and a full antagonist. EMBO J. 1999;18:4608–4618.
94. Yu B, Khan G, Foxworth A, Huang K, Hilakivi-Clarke L. Maternal dietary exposure to fiber during pregnancy and mammary tumorigenesis among rat offspring. Int J Cancer. 2006;119: 2279–2286.
95. Hilakivi-Clarke L, Olivo SE, Shajahan A, Khan G, Zhu Y, Zwart A, Cho E, Clarke R. Mechanisms mediating the effects of prepubertal (n-3) polyunsaturated fatty acid diet on breast cancer risk in rats. J Nutr. 2005;135(12 Suppl):2946S–2952S Review.
96. Verhoog LC, Brekelmans CT, Seynaeve C, van den Bosch LM, Dahmen G, van Geel AN, Tilanus-Linthorst MM, Bartels CC, Wagner A, van den Ouweland A, Devilee P, Meijers-Heijboer EJ, Klijn JG. Survival and tumour characteristics of breast-cancer patients with germline mutations of BRCA1. Lancet 1998;351:316–321.
97. Robson ME, Chappuis PO, Satagopan J, Wong N, Boyd J, Goffin JR, Hudis C, Roberge D, Norton L, Begin LR, Offit K, Foulkes WD. A combined analysis of outcome following breast cancer differences in survival based on BRCA1/BRCA2 mutation status and administration of adjuvant treatment. Breast Cancer Res. 2004;6:R8–R17.
98. Reis-Filho JS, Tutt AN. Triple negative tumours: a critical review. Histopathology 2008;52:108–118 Review.
99. Archey WB, McEachern KA, Robson M, Offit K, Vaziri SA, Casey G, Borg A, Arrick BA. Increased CpG methylation of the estrogen receptor gene in BRCA1-linked estrogen receptor-negative breast cancers. Oncogene 2002;21:7034–7041.
100. Hosey AM, Gorski JJ, Murray MM, Quinn JE, Chung WY, Stewart GE, James CR, Farragher SM, Mulligan JM, Scott AN, Dervan PA, Johnston PG, Couch FJ, Daly PA, Kay E, McCann A, Mullan PB, Harkin DP. Molecular basis for estrogen receptor alpha deficiency in BRCA1-linked breast cancer. J Natl Cancer Inst. 2007;99:1683–1694.
101. Ozcelik H, To MD, Couture J, Bull SB, Andrulis IL. Preferential allelic expression can lead to reduced expression of BRCA1 in sporadic breast cancers. Int J Cancer. 1998;77:1–6.
102. Taylor J, Lymboura M, Pace PE, A'hern RP, Desai AJ, Shousha S, Coombes RC, Ali S. An important role for BRCA1 in breast cancer progression is indicated by its loss in a large proportion of nonfamilial breast cancers. Int J Cancer. 1998;79:334–342.
103. Rio PG, Maurizis JC, Peffault de Latour M, Bignon YJ, Bernard-Gallon DJ. Quantification of BRCA1 protein in sporadic breast carcinoma with or without loss of heterozygosity of the BRCA1 gene. Int J Cancer. 1999;80:823–826.
104. Wilson CA, Ramos L, Villasenor MR, Anders KH, Press MF, Clarke K, Karlan B, Chen JJ, Scully R, Livingston D, Zuch RH, Kanter MH, Cohen S, Calzone FJ, Slamon

DJ. Localization of human BRCA1 and its loss in high-grade, non-inherited breast carcinomas. Nat Genet. 1999;21:236–240.
105. Rice JC, Massey-Brown KS, Futscher BW. Aberrant methylation of the BRCA1 CpG island promoter is associated with decreased BRCA1 mRNA in sporadic breast cancer cells. Oncogene 1998;17:1807–1812.
106. Esteller M, Silva JM, Dominguez G, Bonilla F, Matias-Guiu X, Lerma E, Bussaglia E, Prat J, Harkes IC, Repasky EA, Gabrielson E, Schutte M, Baylin SB, Herman JG. Promoter hypermethylation and BRCA1 inactivation in sporadic breast and ovarian tumors. J Natl Cancer Inst. 2000;92:564–569.
107. Staff S, Isola J, Tanner M Haplo-insufficiency of BRCA1 in sporadic breast cancer. Cancer Res. 2003;63:4978–4983.
108. Butcher DT, Rodenhiser DI. Epigenetic inactivation of BRCA1 is associated with aberrant expression of CTCF and DNA methyltransferase (DNMT3B) in some sporadic breast tumours. Eur J Cancer. 2007;43:210–219.
109. MacDonald G, Stramwasser M, Mueller CR. Characterization of a negative transcriptional element in the BRCA1 promoter. Breast Cancer Res. 2007;9:R49.
110. Wang C, Fan S, Li Z, Fu M, Rao M, Ma Y, Lisanti MP, Albanese C, Katzenellenbogen BS, Kushner PJ, Weber B, Rosen EM, Pestell RG. Cyclin D1 antagonizes BRCA1 repression of estrogen receptor alpha activity. Cancer Res. 2005;65:6557–6567.

Metastasis of Hormone Receptor Positive Breast Cancer

Monica M. Richert and Danny R. Welch

Background

Metastasis

Metastasis, or the movement of tumor cells away from the primary tumor to develop independent tumors at a secondary site, is the final step in tumor progression toward autonomy from the host [1–4]. In order to metastasize, tumor cells must invade surrounding tissues and enter the bloodstream or lymphatics through a process termed intravasation. The neovasculature within a primary tumor is permeable which allows the tumor cell access to the bloodstream [5]. Once in the bloodstream, the cell may remain as a single cell or form an embolus with other tumor cells or other cell types. The disseminated tumor cells must be capable of surviving the sheer forces it encounters while traveling through the vasculature. Once the tumor cell reaches its target organ it adheres either to the vascular or to the lymphatic endothelium or arrests due to the physical limitation of size within the capillary [6, 7]. The tumor cell will then either begin to proliferate within the vessel and eventually break through or leave the vessel through a process termed extravasation. If the tumor cells extravasate, they must invade the surrounding tissue and begin to proliferate to form a secondary mass. The formation of this secondary mass is necessary for metastasis.

The process of metastasis is highly inefficient with less than 0.001% of the $1–4\times10^6$ cells per gram of tumor per day that leave the primary tumor establishing secondary masses [8, 9]. While the inefficiency of this process is due to a number of factors including cell death caused by physical trauma, immune clearance, and anoikis, as many as 80% of the cells complete most steps of the metastatic cascade, but either die at the secondary site or never proliferate

D.R. Welch (✉)
Division of Molecular and Cellular Pathology, Department of Pathology, University of Alabama at Birmingham, Birmingham, AL 35294, USA
e-mail: danwelch@uab.edu

S.A.W. Fuqua (ed.), *Hormone Receptors in Breast Cancer*,
Cancer Treatment and Research 312, DOI 10.1007/978-0-387-09463-2_6,

[9–11]. A small portion of the cells will begin to proliferate and an even smaller percentage goes on to form macrometastases. If any step of this metastatic cascade cannot be completed, then metastases will not develop. Therefore, targeting any step of this process could aid in the control of metastatic disease.

Estrogen Receptor and Breast Cancer Metastasis

Several of the risk factors for breast cancer have indicated that steroid hormones play a role in development and progression of this disease. According to the American Cancer Society, women are at greater risk for breast cancer when they have an early age of menarche, late first full-term pregnancy, and late age of menopause. Therefore, it appears that the length of time the breast is exposed to steroid hormones, both in the overall and in the undifferentiated (pre-lactation) state, correlates with incidence of breast cancer. Several hormone receptors including estrogen receptor and progesterone receptor are critical for development and differentiation of the breast and have been shown to be expressed in some breast cancers. This chapter will focus specifically on estrogen receptor-positive breast cancers.

Estrogen receptor (ER) is a nuclear hormone receptor that binds to specific elements within the DNA after ligand binding to result in transcriptional regulation of several genes. There are two isoforms, ERα and ERβ [12–14], and it is believed that ERα plays a predominant role in breast cancer. Some studies have indicated that a change in expression from ERα to ERβ indicates that a tumor has become endocrine resistant [15]. Along with its effects in the nucleus, ER is capable of binding to and activating signaling pathways such as Src-PI3K-Akt [16] or Src-Ras-ERK [17], both of which have been shown to contribution to tumor progression.

Estrogen receptor expression in tumors is generally associated with decreased aggressiveness. Expression of ER is generally correlated with decreased rate of cell proliferation and histologically differentiated tumors [18]. ER-positive tumors tend to have a lower rate of recurrence in the first years after diagnosis, but there is a higher recurrence rate in later years. The presence of ER is thought to have a stimulatory role in cancer cell proliferation, but an inhibitory effect on invasion and metastasis [15, 19]. Estrogens can increase the growth of breast cancer cells by causing cells to enter the cell cycle. Anti-estrogens prevent this activity in breast cancer cells. The partial agonist/antagonist, Tamoxifen (Nolvadex), is capable of acting as an anti-estrogen against breast cancer cells while acting as a partial agonist against other tissues such as the uterus.

In spite of this ability of estrogens to promote a mitogenic response in breast tumors, expression of ER is most often associated with a more differentiated and less invasive phenotype along with a more favorable prognosis. Interestingly, ER-positive tumors are more likely to metastasize to the bone, and most bone metastases are ER positive [20, 21]. This is paradoxical as ER-positive tumors are less invasive and metastatic. When ERα-positive cells are implanted into nude mice, they only form tumors in the presence of supplemental estrogen and, compared to ERα-negative cell lines, are poorly metastatic [22]. Mechanistically, it has been determined that these effects on invasion and metastasis are due to transcriptional effects of ER and signaling events due to ER interaction with cytoplasmic proteins (reviewed in [18]). While ER-positive tumors are generally less likely to metastasize, they are still capable of forming distant tumors and therefore, treatments for hormone-responsive metastases are necessary.

It is also important to note that hormone-responsive tumors will eventually progress to a hormone-refractory state making them more aggressive and metastatic. Recent work to understand how tumors become hormone refractory has led to the understanding that expression of the epidermal growth factor receptor (EGFR) correlates with a lack of response to endocrine therapy [23, 24]. EGFR belongs to a family of receptor tyrosine kinases including ErbB2/HER2, ErbB3/HER3, and ErbB4/HER4. EGFR activation occurs by ligand binding and either homodimerization or heterodimerization with other family members followed by autophosphorylation [25]. Cross-activation of the receptors is common; homo- or heterodimerization determines the specificity of ligand binding; and several of the ligands are capable of activating more than one family member.

EGFR signaling promotes tumor cell proliferation, survival, migration, angiogenesis, and metastasis. Estrogen can upregulate TGFα and amphiregulin, ligands of EGFR, in an ER-dependent manner causing the formation of an autocrine loop [26, 27]. Studies are currently underway to determine whether combination of endocrine treatment with ZD1839 (Iressa), an EGFR inhibitor, can overcome the hormone-refractory state of most metastatic disease (reviewed in [28]). Since metastatic disease is the ultimate cause of cancer morbidity and death, it is therefore critical to address this final step of tumor progression in order to improve the survival rates of women with invasive breast cancer.

Effect of Metastatic Disease

It was estimated by the American Cancer Society that about 178,480 new cases of invasive breast cancer will be diagnosed in the United States in 2007. Breast cancer is the second leading cause of cancer death in women, with one in eight developing invasive breast cancer in their lifetime. Three percent of women will die from breast cancer. Localized disease is diagnosed in approximately 64% of patients. When tumor cells remain confined to the breast, long-term survival rates are very high at approximately 98%. Approximately 28% of patients are diagnosed after tumor cells have spread to regional lymph nodes. In these cases, the long-term survival rate decreases to 81%. This survival rate drops dramatically to only 27% once tumor cells have escaped the primary tumor and colonized secondary sites, which has already occurred in approximately 6% of cases at the time of diagnosis. The median survival for patients with metastatic disease is 2–4 years. This decreases to 4–13 months in patients with multiple visceral lesions.

In addition to decreased survival, the quality of life for patients with metastasis is far worse. Breast cancer cells predominantly metastasize to the lung, bone, and brain. Each site of metastasis has it own challenges. For example, bone metastases result in severe pain, fractures, hypercalcemia, spinal cord compression, and cachexia, while brain metastases are currently untreatable. The cost of metastastic disease is staggering with families spending up to 98% of their income on care of a breast cancer patient [29].

Current Therapies

The therapy chosen for treatment of metastatic breast cancer is very much dependent on each patient, with the extent of disease, general health, age, and hormone status taken into account. Endocrine therapy is generally the first line of treatment for hormone receptor-positive tumors, unless there are life-threatening visceral metastases which may cause organ failure. In this case, classical chemotherapy is used as the first therapy as a means of quickly shrinking tumor size.

Endocrine Therapy

Endocrine therapy consists of either selective estrogen receptor modulators (SERMs) or aromatase inhibitors. The best known SERM is Tamoxifen, a partial agonist/antagonist for ER. Tamoxifen is currently combined with total estrogen blockade by either oophorectomy or GnRH agonists to treat premenopausal women with ER-positive tumors. Once the disease becomes Tamoxifen resistant, aromatase inhibitors and the pure-anti-estrogen, fulvestrant (Faslodex), are used (reviewed in [30–35]).

For postmenopausal women, aromatase inhibitors such as letrozole (Femara), anastrozole (Arimidex), and exemestane (Aromasin) are the first line of treatment. It has been shown that these agents are more active than tamoxifen in terms of clinical benefit. When the disease progresses, tamoxifen and fulvestrant are turned to as second-line therapy. Fulvestrant has been shown to be a pure anti-estrogen with no partial agonist activity on the endometrium and vasculature as is found with tamoxifen. It is as active as tamoxifen or anastrozole in postmenopausal patients whose disease progresses during endocrine therapy.

The majority of hormone receptor-positive breast cancer will eventually progress to become refractory to endocrine treatment. Once this occurs, several options are available including standard chemotherapy and trastuzumab (Herceptin), as well as bisphosphonates and radiotherapy for bone metastases.

Standard Chemotherapy

Standard chemotherapy is generally comprised of anthracyclines, taxanes, or a combination therapy. Anthracyclines such as doxorubicin and epirubicin are limited by their dose-dependent cardiotoxicity. New formulations of anthracyclines including liposomal forms of these drugs are reducing cardiotoxicity, allowing higher cumulative doses of these drugs. Whether treatment is given singly or in combination is greatly dependent on the patient. Combination therapies are more effective, but are also more toxic to the patient and, therefore, less well tolerated. Single treatments or treatments given in succession rather than combined may be more readily tolerated by older or generally less healthy individuals. Due to these differences in tolerability, it must be decided between doctor and patient what the end point of chemotherapy will be (reviewed in [30, 31]).

Herceptin

Trastuzumab (Herceptin) is a monoclonal humanized antibody that recognizes the extracellular domain of HER2/Neu, a tyrosine kinase receptor. HER2 is overexpressed or amplified in approximately 25–30% of breast cancer. Breast cancers are classified as HER2 positive when they are scored as 3+ by immunohistochemistry or are positive for amplification by fluorescence in situ hybridization (FISH). It is important to note that gene amplification can occur without concomitant overexpression. Overexpression is associated with increased aggressiveness, rate of recurrence, and mortality in patients with regional lymph node involvement. Often HER2 expression is increased in tumors which are no longer hormone responsive. Trastuzumab has been shown to be effective against HER2-positive tumors with a greater effect on those that have amplification of HER2 versus overexpression. Metastasis of HER2-positive tumors has also been successfully treated using trastuzumab. The combination of trastuzumab with standard chemotherapy has been shown to be more effective than chemotherapy alone against HER2-positive tumors. One of the problems associated with use of this monoclonal antibody is that as lung metastases are cured using trastuzumab, there has been an increase in the incidence of brain metastases that cannot be treated using this antibody (reviewed in [30, 31]).

Bisphosphonates/Radiotherapy

Bone metastases result in immense pain, hypercalcemia, fractures, spinal cord compression, and cachexia. Radiotherapy has been used to prevent the continued growth of tumors within the skeletal system and is currently used in combination with chemotherapy for advanced disease. Bisphosphonates, which have been used as a treatment for osteoporosis, have been found to inhibit osteoclast recruitment and activation resulting in decreased bone loss. Bisphosphonates are also able to induce apoptosis of cancer cells and interfere with the attachment of cells to the bone matrix. All of these mechanisms aid in delaying the effects of bone metastasis. Zolendronic acid (Zometa) is now the standard bisphosphonate treatment for bone metastases (reviewed in [21, 30]).

Ongoing Research

While the above therapies can help to prolong life and have increased the quality of life for patients with metastatic disease, metastatic breast cancer is still currently essentially incurable. In order to begin to truly treat and control metastatic disease, we must increase our understanding of the molecular events involved in how a cell completes the metastatic cascade. As a tumor grows and progresses, it becomes more aggressive. This progression of the tumor toward metastasis is mediated by genetic instability and selection of subpopulations of cells within the tumor. Eventually, some of these populations will become competent to metastasize. The fraction of cells within a tumor that are capable of metastasis depends on several factors. If mutations allowing metastasis occur early in tumor development, a greater proportion of tumor cells will metastasize. Also, the size of a tumor can influence its ability to spread with larger tumors being more likely to metastasize [36, 37].

Cells within a tumor also interact with the surrounding environment. Each microenvironment can affect a tumor cell's ability to proliferate and invade the surrounding tissue. The tumor cell also affects the surrounding environment through the secretion of factors that can affect nearby stromal cells and extracellular matrix. These interactions can either promote or inhibit the ability of that tumor cell to form a mass at the secondary site. For example, a tumor cell can secrete cytokines and chemokines to recruit inflammatory cells, such as macrophages, neutrophils, and lymphocytes. These cells can then secrete proteases, cytokines, and cytotoxic mediators that can result in tumor cell killing or tissue remodeling, angiogenesis, and release of growth factors that cause the tumor cell to proliferate (reviewed in [38, 39]).

It is clear that the process of metastasis is complex. Each step of the cascade is regulated by several genes and in order for metastasis to be completed some of those genes must be misregulated or mutated. It is the understanding of these molecular interactions that will allow us to target therapies to kill tumor cells in the secondary site or prevent the outgrowth of established metastases to make this disease chronic rather than fatal.

Microarrays

Recent work using microarray technology to compare gene expression patterns between normal and tumor tissue as well as between tumor types has begun to identify gene signatures that indicate whether or not a tumor has the capacity to metastasize. It has been shown that breast tumors can be subclassified based on differences in their gene expression patterns. Five tumor subtypes have been defined [40]. Three are estrogen receptor negative, while two are estrogen receptor positive. These subtypes represent clinically distinct groups of patients that have different disease-free and overall survival. Furthermore, studies done by van't Veer and colleagues have identified a 70-gene expression profile that predicts the presence or absence of later metastatic disease in young patients [41–43]. This 70-gene profile has been used to develop a high-throughput diagnostic test that has been shown to be reproducible and reliable [44]. Liu et al. have demonstrated a significant correlation between a 186-gene invasiveness profile with both overall survival and metastasis-free survival [45]. Several of these microarray studies have been compared, and it has been found that the results were consistent in terms of the ability of these methods to classify tumors [46]. Recent work in mouse models indicates that these genetic profiles are found in normal tissues [47]. Mice with a range of metastatic efficiencies were tested for the latter profiles. The stratification of mice by profile correlated with their metastatic efficiency. This indicates that the genetic factors allowing metastasis may not be acquired features of a tumor, but rather the baseline genetic makeup of the person. Therefore, these gene profiles may be used clinically to determine which patients are most likely to develop metastases and the best treatment for the patient based on the tumor type, ultimately saving those who are unlikely to develop metastatic disease from undergoing toxic therapies that are unnecessary. In February 2007, the FDA approved the use of a 72-gene array (MammaPrint; Molecular Profiling Institute, Inc.) to classify breast cancers.

These microarray studies have also demonstrated that the expression patterns in primary tumors and metastases are similar, which has led to the conclusion that the genes that control tumor development also control metastasis and that genes specifically regulating metastasis do not exist [48]. In contrast to this conclusion, several labs have demonstrated that specific signatures exist that determine whether a tumor cell will metastasize to the lung [49], bone [50, 51], or regional lymph nodes [52]. For example, the Massague' and Guise laboratories have used microarray technology to identify a small subset of genes that control metastasis of breast cancer cells to bone [50]. MDA-MB-231 metastatic, ER-negative breast cancer cells were injected intracardially into mice. A subpopulation of cells that efficiently colonize bone was isolated and compared to the parental cell line using microarray. Several genes were identified that differed between the parental and the bone-colonizing populations. MMP-1, osteopontin, IL-11, CXCR4, and connective tissue-derived growth factor were found to be overexpressed. Individual transfection of these genes into the parental cell line modestly increased bone metastasis, while co-transfection of combinations of these genes resulted in bone metastasis as efficient as the bone-colonizing subpopulation. Some breast cancers produce osteoblastic bone metastases. The Guise laboratory has demonstrated that secretion of endothelin 1 from ZR75.1 breast cancer cells promotes osteoblastic bone metastases [53]. These metastases can be blocked by treatment with an orally active endothelin A receptor antagonist. These studies demonstrate that defined gene combinations can control metastasis and encourage the study of metastasis-controlling genes as potential therapeutic targets.

Metastasis-Promoting Genes

In order for metastasis to occur, there must be coordinated expression of multiple genes to allow the tumor cell to acquire the ability to complete each step of the metastatic cascade. Therefore, in studying metatasis-promoting genes, there is a high level of false-negative results. In spite of this, several genes have been identified that promote metastasis including Ras, MEK, and VEGF, while in breast cancer, osteopontin, NFκB, and Twist have been demonstrated to promote metastasis (reviewed in [54]).

Osteopontin

Osteopontin is a secreted acidic glycoprotein that interacts with a variety integrins to promote cell adhesion, migration, and invasion. It is variably phosphorylated on up to 28 sites that are distributed throughout the molecule. It can be cleaved by thrombin resulting in an enhancement of its function in promoting cell adhesion and migration [55].

There is a great deal of evidence for a role of osteopontin in tumor progression. Transfection of cells with osteopontin results in an increase in the malignant phenotype, while down-regulation causes a decrease in malignancy [56, 57]. Osteopontin knockout mice develop tumors at a slower rate compared to tumors in wild-type animals [58]. The interaction of osteopontin with $\alpha v\beta 3$ integrin has been implicated in its functions in cell adhesion, migration, and invasion [59–62]. Breast cancer cells that are more metastatic express higher levels of $\alpha v\beta 3$ integrin and are more sensitive to the effect of osteopontin [63]. It has also been demonstrated that osteopontin and $\alpha v\beta 3$ integrin are coordinately regulated in some tissues [64, 65]. Osteopontin is also capable of inducing extracellular matrix degradation and human breast epithelial cell invasion through induction of urokinase type plasminogen activator [63, 66]. This occurs through activation of PI3 kinase, Akt, and NFκB (reviewed in [67]). The activity of urokinase type plasminogen activator correlates with the metastatic ability of cells [68]. Finally, osteopontin has been shown to be differentially expressed during angiogenesis, indicating a possible role of this molecule in this process in tumor development and progression. Osteopontin can prevent apoptotic cell death of endothelial cells through activation of NFκB in a Ras- and Src-dependent manner [69].

Osteopontin expression in breast tumors has been correlated with increased aggressiveness (reviewed in [70]). It can be expressed either in the tumor cells themselves or in the associated macrophages, but it is unclear whether the location of osteopontin expression plays a role in its ability to promote metastasis. In a test of 154 women with lymph node-negative breast cancer, osteopontin expression was increased in tumor cells in 26% of the tumors [71]. A statistically significant association was identified between increased osteopontin expression and decreased disease-free and overall survival. Osteopontin can also be detected in the blood of patients with breast tumors (reviewed in [70]). It has been demonstrated that the median plasma level of osteopontin is almost tripled in patients with metastases, and modestly increased in patients with localized disease compared to healthy women. The level of plasma osteopontin also indirectly correlated with length of survival and was associated with the number of sites of metastatic disease. This indicates that plasma osteopontin levels may be a prognostic factor for women with metastatic disease.

NfκB

NFκB is a transcription factor involved in the control of expression of many genes involved in tumor progression including Twist [72], osteopontin [67, 70], matrix metalloproteinases [73–76], and urokinase type plasminogen activator [67]. During tumorigenesis, NFκB plays a role in protecting cells from apoptosis as inhibition of NFκB sensitizes tumor cells to chemotherapeutic-induced cell death [75, 76]. NFκB has recently been shown to induce and maintain epithelial-to-mesenchymal transition (EMT) in mammary epithelial cells [76]. Epithelial-to-mesenchymal transition involves the conversion of attached epithelial cells to more motile mesenchymal-like cells and has been most clearly described in embryogenesis. During tumor progression, EMT is hypothesized to be necessary for motility and invasion and the reverse process, MET, for cells to have an epithelial phenotype at the secondary site. Activation of NFκB promoted EMT, while inhibition prevented EMT in Ras-transformed cells and reversed EMT in mesenchymal cells [76]. Inhibition of NFκB activity significantly decreased metastasis of ras-transformed metastatic mammary epithelial cells after tail vein injection.

In the basal state, NFκB is inhibited by IκB. When cells are stimulated, IκB Kinase (IKK) complex phosphorylates IκB and relieves the inhibition of NFκB (reviewed in [77, 78]). Therefore, preventing phosphorylation of IκBα through inhibition of IKK or a repressor of IκBα would effectively inhibit NFκB activity. NFκB activity in breast cancer has recently been demonstrated to promote osteolytic bone metastases [79]. NFκB activity was found to be constitutive in the MDA-MB-231 breast cancer cell line which forms bone metastases after intracardiac injection. These cells were transduced with a specific NFκB inhibitor – super-repressor of IκBα (SR-IκBα) which is a non-degradable IκBα with substitutions at the IKK phosphorylation sites. Transduction with SR-IκBα resulted in inhibition, but not abrogation, of primary tumor growth, while incidence of bone metastasis and size of bone lesions after intracardiac injection were significantly decreased. Inhibitors of IKK2 were subsequently used to block NFκB activation and also showed a significant decrease in the size and number of osteolytic bone metastases. Primary tumor incidence was not affected, while growth was again inhibited. It was determined that the effect of NFκB on osteolytic bone metastases was due to its transcriptional control of granulocyte macrophage-colony-stimulating factor which mediates breast cancer bone metastasis by stimulating osteoclast development.

Twist

Twist is a transcription factor that regulates epithelial-to-mesenchymal transition and cell movement during embryogenesis (reviewed in [80]). Twist has been found to be highly expressed in invasive lobular carcinoma of the breast which is made up of epithelial cells that have lost the normal tissue structure found in less aggressive tumors [81]. Increased expression of Twist has been found to be associated with poor survival and metastatic disease in breast cancer patients. In a highly aggressive murine mammary carcinoma cell line, suppression of Twist resulted in inhibition of metastasis to the lung without affecting the formation of primary tumors [81]. It was determined that loss of Twist inhibited tumor cells from entering the bloodstream.

Twist has been shown to repress expression of E-cadherin, an epithelial expressed protein involved in cell/cell adhesion, and induce EMT in murine mammary carcinoma cells (reviewed in [80, 81]). Twist induces expression of the mesenchymal markers fibronectin and N-cadherin in human mammary epithelial cells. It is also capable of inhibiting Myc-induced apoptosis in some cell types [82, 83]. Each of these functions can contribute to the ability of Twist to promote metastasis. Twist has been demonstrated to be upregulated by NFκB, Wnt, and FGF pathways which are also implicated in breast tumor progression [84].

Metastasis Suppressors

Metastasis suppressors interfere with at least one step of the metastatic cascade resulting in suppression of metastasis without preventing primary tumor growth. These genes are distinct from tumor suppressor genes which prevent both tumorigenesis and metastasis. This makes metastasis suppressors distinct therapeutic targets. Currently, more than 20 metastasis suppressors have been identified. Three examples, Nm23, BRMS1, and KISS1, will be discussed here. Readers are referred to several excellent reviews for further details [85–88].

Nm23

Nm23 was the first metastasis suppressor identified. It was discovered using differential display of metastatic and non-metastatic murine melanoma cell lines [89]. It is located on chromosome 17q21 and encodes a 17 kDa nucleoside diphosphate kinase [90]. The kinase activity of Nm23 is not required for metastatic suppression, rather it is the histidine kinase activity that is responsible [91]. Nm23 forms a complex with a scaffold protein (KSR – kinase suppressor of ras) for the mitogen-activated protein kinases (MAPKs) resulting in phosphorylation of KSR within its 14-3-3-binding site [92]. This phosphorylation results in binding of KSR to 14-3-3, sequestration, and inhibition of MAPK activation. Transfection of Nm23 into MDA-MB-435 cells decreased both basal and stimulated MAPK phosphorylation indicating that Nm23 signals through the ERK/MAPK pathway [93, 94].

The Nm23 family has eight members, two of which (Nm23 H1 and H2) are metastasis suppressors [90]. Decreased expression of Nm23 correlates with metastatic potential in most tumor types, but expression in neuroblastomas correlates with an increase in aggressiveness suggesting that the function of Nm23 might be cell type specific (reviewed in [95]). Nm23 expression is decreased in late-stage metastatic breast, endometrial, ovarian, melanoma, and colon cancers; other studies have found no correlation with metastasis (reviewed in [96, 97]). Several studies have demonstrated an inverse correlation between Nm23 and EGFR and HER2 indicating a potential mechanism where Nm23 alters the responsiveness of a tumor cell to exogenous growth signals [98–103]. As with several metastasis suppressors, expression may be controlled by epigenetic mechanisms. It has been demonstrated that increased expression of Nm23 correlates with hypomethylation of the promoter [93].

BRMS1

BRMS1, or breast cancer metastasis suppressor 1, is located at 11q13.1–q13.2, a region that is frequently altered in metastatic breast cancer. BRMS1 was identified using differential display following microcell-mediated chromosomal transfer of chromosome 11 into a breast cancer cell line [104]. Enforced expression of BRMS1 suppresses metastasis of breast cancer, bladder carcinoma, ovarian cancer, and melanoma in vivo [104–109], but does not suppress in vivo or in vitro growth, adhesion to laminin, fibronectin, collagens I and IV, or Matrigel [105]. There is also no effect on expression of MMP-2 and -9 or heparanse as well as invasion in vitro [105]. Motility and growth in soft agar were modestly inhibited by expression of BRMS1 [105].

BRMS1 is a predominantly nuclear protein that contains a glutamate rich region, an imperfect leucine zipper, and two coiled-coil domains suggesting that BRMS1 may have a role in a transcriptional complex. Yeast 2-hybrid and co-immunoprecipitation studies have demonstrated that BRMS1 interacts with mSin3:HDAC complexes that may regulate gene expression including decreased NFκB activity [110]. This regulation is through deacetylation of the p65 subunit of NFκB by the BRMS1:HDAC complex resulting in decreased HDAC1 binding to p65 [111, 112]. Expression of BRMS1 in MDA-MB-435 breast cancer cells results in the restoration of gap junctional intercellular communication due in part to modification of connexin expression [105, 107]. Osteopontin transcription is decreased in the presence of BRMS1 expression through decreased NFκB activity [113]. BRMS1 has also been demonstrated to significantly decrease the levels of the phosphoinositide PI(4,5)P2 which is essential for PI3 kinase and Akt activation and downstream activation of NFκB [114, 115]. This indicates that BRMS1 modulates the response of tumor cells to external growth factors.

Clinical data concerning the role of BRMS1 in tumor progression and metastasis is conflicting [116–119]. Most studies have used RNA expression instead of protein. This is problematic in that BRMS1 RNA expression does not correlate with protein expression. It is also likely that the subcellular localization of BRMS1 is critical to its function. One study correlated BRMS1 immunohistochemistry with estrogen receptor, progesterone receptor, and HER2 status along with survival [119]. BRMS1 was lost in 25% of the tumors examined. Patients that were less than 50 years old at diagnosis and had tumors that were PR negative or HER2 positive were most likely to have lost BRMS1 expression. While there was no overall correlation between BRMS1 expression and disease-free survival, when stratified by loss of ER, PR, or overexpression of HER2, loss of BRMS1 expression significantly correlated with reduced disease-free survival.

KISS1

KISS1 was identified after microcell-mediated transfer of chromosome 6 into human melanoma cell lines followed by subtractive hybridization techniques [120, 121]. KISS1 maps to 1q32 and encodes a 15.4 kDa secreted protein [121]. It is a downstream effector of the metastasis suppressors TXNIP and CRSP-3 which are located on chromosome 6 [122]. Melanoma and breast cancer cell lines are suppressed for metastasis after enforced expression of KISS1, and there is an 80% correlation between KISS1 loss and melanoma metastatic progression as determined by in situ hybridization [123, 124]. Clinically, KISS1 has been shown to be inversely correlated with poor prognosis in a number of cancers including breast cancer (reviewed in [125]). Recent data demonstrates that KISS1 expression is regulated by the transcription factors AP2α and Sp1 [126, 127]. This provides a mechanism for loss of KISS1 in breast cancer where AP2α is frequently lost.

Metastin, a secreted 54-amino acid amidated fragment of KISS1, binds to GPR54, a G-protein-coupled receptor to induce activation of phospholipase C, hydrolysis of PIP_2 and calcium, and arachidonate release [128–132]. This signaling cascade results in affects on focal adhesion kinases suggesting a role for KISS1 in cell adhesion [129]. Activation of GPR54 by metastin resulted in a decrease in SDF-1-induced Akt activity and chemotaxis [133]. Treatment of GPR54-transfected B16BL6 melanoma cells with metastin-reduced metastasis and anchorage-independent growth, but it has not yet been demonstrated that the endogenous receptor is responsible for metastatic suppression of cancer cells [129]. GPR54 activity has been demonstrated to affect pubertal development and pregnancy in transgenic mice, but this does not indicate how KISS1 may be affecting metastasis. KISS1 is highly expressed in early placenta and molar pregnancies and is low in choriocarcinoma cells suggesting that KISS1 may play a role in the invasive and migratory properties of trophoblasts [134]. KISS1 can form a stable complex with pro-MMPs and MMP-2, -9, -14, -16 and -24 have been shown to cleave both KISS1 and metastasis [135]. Cleavage of metastin results in the formation of a decapeptide termed KP10 which can induce focal adhesion and stress fiber formation in cells expressing GPR54 [135]. Combination of KP10 and BB-94, an MMP inhibitor, treatment resulted in a significant block in HT1080 cell migration [135]. KP10 has also been shown to inhibit trophoblast migration and proteolytic activity without affecting proliferation [136]. Although these studies indicate that cleavage products of KISS1 may be important for metastatic suppression, it is not yet clear the exact mechanism of KISS1 action.

KISS1 inhibits metastasis in mouse models by inhibiting growth of tumor cells at the secondary site [D.R. Welch, personal communication]. It is not known whether this KISS1-induced dormancy is mediated through GPR54, but secretion of KISS1 is required in melanoma cells. As these cells express very little or no GPR54, it is likely that the tumor cell dormancy is induced through a paracrine mechanism or another unidentified receptor.

Potential Therapies

The discussion above gives a brief description of the types of research that are forwarding our understanding of the molecular controls of metastasis. It is clear that the identification of the molecular interactions occurring in each tumor will be critical in order to ultimately control metastatic disease. Several molecules have been identified which can predict the spread of primary tumors and may have therapeutic value. As more of these are identified, microarray technology can be employed to profile patient tumors. Based on these genetic profiles, the right combination of therapies can be determined for each patient [137, 138]. As we more clearly delineate the molecular interactions that allow tumor cell survival and metastasis, directed therapies can be developed to target specific molecules. Based on the molecules discussed above, several therapies could potentially be derived.

Inhibition of Signaling Molecules

Small molecule inhibitors of several signaling molecules have already been designed and tested in the laboratory and clinic. One of these, Iressa, an inhibitor of the epidermal growth factor receptor, as discussed above is being used in clinical trials to disrupt the signaling mechanisms that result in hormone-refractory breast cancer (reviewed in [28]). Likewise, inhibitors of molecules such as NFκB could be used to promote apoptosis of tumor cells and inhibit expression of molecules that promote invasion and metastasis such as the matrix metalloproteinases and urokinase type plasminogen activator. As described above, inhibitors of IKK which result in decreased activation of NFκB have been used in animal studies to decrease osteolytic bone metastases [79].

The effects of osteopontin in breast cancer cells occur predominantly through binding to the $\alpha v\beta 3$ integrin. Molecules targeting this integrin are being designed and tested [139]. Not only would they inhibit the effects of osteopontin on cell adhesion, migration, invasion, and potentially angiogenesis but also of other ligands that may work through the $\alpha v\beta 3$ integrin to promote tumor progression.

Treatment with Mimics of Secreted Inhibitory Molecules

KISS1 is secreted and cleaved to form a 10-amino acid fragment termed KP10. This fragment has been shown to inhibit migration and proteolytic activity of several cell types [135, 136]. The use of KP10 as a treatment to prevent the spread of metastasis or block the outgrowth of metastatic disease may be possible. Much work must be done to determine whether treatment must occur before cells begin to spread to the secondary site or whether KP10 interaction with tumor cells at the secondary site would be sufficient to render the metastatic cells dormant.

Epigenetic Modifications

Recently, much research has been focused on the epigenetic regulation of tumor-associated genes. Several of the metastasis suppressor genes have been shown to be regulated by epigenetic mechanisms including methylation of the promoter and acetylation of histones (reviewed in [85–88]). In these circumstances, it may be clinically possible to re-express these genes. This has been described for the metastasis suppressor Nm23. Treatment of metastatic breast cancer cell lines with either dexamethasone or medroxyprogesterone acetate results in increased Nm23 expression [140]. The same has been demonstrated with treatment with 5-azacytidine which results in hypomethylation of the Nm23 promoter and restoration of Nm23 expression

[93]. Treatment of mice with medroxyprogesterone acetate resulted in a significant decrease in the incidence and frequency of metastasis [141]. Histone deacetylase inhibitors, which can affect gene expression, are currently in clinical trials.

Perspectives

Throughout this chapter we have sought to critically evaluate the current state-of-the-art with regard to regulation of metastasis. Our charge was to assess metastasis in ER-positive breast cancer. Quite frankly, we can only report on associations rather than definitive cause and effect relationships. It is currently unclear whether a cause and effect relationship exits between estrogen receptor signaling and metastasis. While loss of ER correlates with decreased sensitivity to hormone treatment and increased likelihood of metastasis, the phenotypes have not been genetically linked. Emerging data on ER-dependent transcription and describing metastasis regulatory genes provides the possibility of defining a relationship. On an even more basic level, what determines the ER status of a tumor and its metastases? We know that tumors are more likely to develop in a breast that has been exposed to estrogen for longer periods of time. Do these tumors develop because of increased ER signaling or is ER expression simply correlative to tumor development? If hormone exposure is correlated with tumor development, it is surmised that ER signaling plays a role in the development of the tumor. Understanding how this happens will allow the development of more effective treatments for ER-positive breast cancer.

As the molecular basis of metastasis is unraveled, the inter-relationships of tumor cells with their microenvironments are increasingly appreciated. Cellular responses to steroid hormones, among other growth factors and growth inhibitors, clearly determines metastatic competency. Still, there remains much to be done to elucidate the cross-talk and determine which interactions are critical and which are ancillary associations. Several of the genes described above have functions that depend on the site of tumor cell growth indicating that they modulate the interpretation of extra-cellular signals. What signals differ between the site of primary tumor growth and metastases? What role does the microenvironment play in tumor cell dormancy? Also, some of the issues we have raised are paradoxical. For example, if ER-negative tumors are more aggressive and metastatic to visceral organs, why do ER-positive tumors preferentially metastasize to the bone? Understanding the molecular events that control the metastatic behavior of tumor cells including site-specific metastasis and tumor cell dormancy will provide critical information that will ultimately lead to more specific therapies to control metastasis making cancer a chronic rather than acute disease.

References

1. Lee K, Jessop H, Suswillo R, et al. Endocrinology: bone adaptation requires estrogen receptor-alpha. Nature 2003;424:389.
2. Steeg PS. Metastasis suppressors alter the signal transduction of cancer cells. Nature Rev Cancer. 2003;3:55–63.
3. Welch DR, Tomasovic SP. Implications of tumor progression on clinical oncology. Clin Exptl Metastasis. 1985;3:151–188.
4. Nowell P. The clonal evolution of tumor cell populations. Science 1976;194:23–28.
5. Jain RK, Munn LL, Fukumura D. Dissecting tumor pathophysiology using intravital microscopy. Nature Rev Cancer. 2002;2:266–276.
6. Chambers AF, Groom AC, MacDonald IC. Metastasis: dissemination and growth of cancer cells in metastatic sites. Nature Rev Cancer. 2002;2:563–572.
7. Chambers AF, MacDonald IC, Schmidt EE, et al. Steps in tumor metastasis: new concepts from intravital videomicroscopy. Cancer Metastasis Rev. 1995;14:279–301.
8. Weiss L. Concepts of metastasis. Cancer Metastasis Rev. 2000;19:219–234.
9. Weiss L. Metastatic inefficiency. Adv Cancer Res. 1990;54:159–211.
10. Fidler IJ. Selection of successive tumor lines for metastasis. Nature New Biol. 1973;242:148–149.
11. Chambers AF, Naumov GN, Vantyghem SA, et al. Molecular biology of breast cancer metastasis: clinical implications of experimental studies on metastatic inefficiency. Breast Cancer Res. 2000;2:400–407.
12. Korach KS. Insights from the study of animals lacking functional estrogen receptor. Science 1994;266:1524–1527.
13. Gustafsson JA. Estrogen receptor β – a new dimension in estrogen mechanism of action. J Endocrinol. 1999;163:379–383.
14. Dupont S, Krust A, Gansmuller A, et al. Effect of single and compound knockouts of estrogen receptors α (ERα) and β (ERβ) on mouse reproductive phenotypes. Development 2000;127:4277–4291.
15. Speirs V, Malone C, Walton DS, et al. Increased expression of estrogen receptor b mRNA in Tamoxifen-resistant breast cancer patients. Cancer Res. 1999;59:5421–5424.
16. Simoncini T, Hafezi-Moghadam A, Brazil DP, et al. Interaction of estrogen receptor with the regulatory subunit of phosphatidylinositol-3-OH kinase. Nature 2000;407: 538–541.
17. Kousteni S, Bellido T, Plotkin LI, et al. Nongenotropic, sex-nonspecific signaling through the estrogen and androgen receptors: dissociation from transcriptional activity. Cell 2001;104:719–730.
18. Platet N, Cathiard AM, Gleizes M, et al. Estrogens and their receptors in breast cancer progression: a dual role in cancer proliferation and invasion. Critical Rev Oncol. 2004;51:55–67.
19. Platet N, Prevostel C, Derocq D, et al. Breast cancer cell invasiveness: correlation with protein kinase C activity and differential regulation by phorbol ester in estrogen receptor-positive and -negative cells. Int J Cancer. 1998;75:750–756.
20. Coleman RE. Skeletal complications of malignancy. Cancer 1997;80:1588–1594.
21. Lipton A. Bisphosphonates and metastatic breast carcinoma. Cancer 2003;97:848–853.
22. Price JE, Polyzos A, Zhang RD, et al. Tumorigenicity and metastasis of human breast carcinoma cell lines in nude mice. Cancer Res. 1990;50:717–721.
23. Klijn JGM, Berns PMJJ, Schmitz PIM, et al. The clinical significance of epidermal growth factor receptor (EGF-R) in human breast cancer: a review on 5232 patients. Endocr Rev. 1992;13:3–17.
24. Nicholson RI, MeClelland RA, Gee JMW, et al. Epidermal growth factor receptor expression in breast cancer: association with response to endocrine therapy. Breast Cancer Res Treat. 1994;29:117–125.

25. Yarden Y, Sliwkowski MX. Untangling the ErbB signalling network. Nat Rev Mol Cell Biol. 2001;2:127–137.
26. Bates SE, Davidson NE, Valverius EM, et al. Expression of transforming growth factor-α and its messenger RNA in human breast cancer: its regulation by estrogen and its possible functional significance. Mol Endocrinol. 1988;2:543–555.
27. Martinez-Lacaci I, Secada M, Plowman G, et al. Estrogen and phorbol esters regulate amphiregulin expression by two separate mechanisms in human breast cancer cell lines. Endocrinology 1995;136:3983–3992.
28. Lichtner RB. Estrogen/EGF receptor interactions in breast cancer: rationale for new therapeutic combination strategies. Biomed Pharmacother. 2003;57:447–451.
29. Arozullah AM, Calhoun EA, Wolf M, et al. The financial burden of cancer: estimates from a study of insured women with breast cancer. J Support Oncol. 2004;2:271–278.
30. Guarneri V, Conte PF. The curability of breast cancer and the treatment of advanced disease. Eur J Nucl Med Mol Imaging. 2004;31:S149–S161.
31. Gralow JR. Optimizing the treatment of metastatic breast cancer. Breast Cancer Res Treat. 2005;89:S9–S15.
32. McKeage K, Curran MP, Plosker GL. Fulvestrant: a review of its use in hormone receptor-positive metastatic disease in postmenopausal women with disease progression following antiestrogen therapy. Drugs 2004;64:633–648.
33. Howell A, Robertson JFR, Vergote I. A review of the efficacy of anastrozole in post-menopausal women with advanced breast cancer with visceral metastases. Breast Cancer Res Treat. 2003;82:215–222.
34. Carlson RW, Henderson IC. Sequential hormonal therapy for metastatic breast cancer after adjuvant tamoxifen or anastrozole. Breast Cancer Res Treat. 2003;80:S19–S26.
35. Buzdar AU. Advances in endocrine treatments for postmenopausal women with metastatic and early breast cancer. Oncologist 2003;8:335–341.
36. Bernards R, Weinberg RA. Metastasis genes: a progression puzzle. Nature 2002;418:823.
37. Hahn WC, Weinberg RA. Rules for making human tumor cells. N Engl J Med. 2002;347:1593–1603.
38. Coussens LM, Werb Z. Inflammation and cancer. Nature 2002;420:860–867.
39. Egeblad M, Werb Z. New functions for the matrix metalloproteinases in cancer progression. Nature Rev Cancer. 2002;2:161–174.
40. Perou CM, Sorlie T, Eisen MB, et al. Molecular portraits of human breast tumours. Nature 2000;406:747–752.
41. Weigelt B, Hu Z, He X, et al. Molecular portraits and 70-gene prognosis signature are preserved throughout the metastatic process of breast cancer. Cancer Res. 2005;65:9155–9158.
42. Buyse M, Loi S, van't Veer L, et al. Validation and clinical utility of a 70-gene prognostic signature for women with node-negative breast cancer. JNCI 2006;98:1183–1192.
43. van de Vijver MJ, He YD, van't Veer L, et al. A gene-expression signature as a predictor of survival in breast cancer. N Engl J Med. 2002;347:1999–2009.
44. Glas AM, Floore A, Delahaye LJMJ, et al. Converting a breast cancer microarray signature a into high-throughput diagnostic test. BMC Genomics 2006;7:278–287.
45. Liu R, Wang X, Chen GY, et al. The prognostic role of a gene signature from tumorigenic breast-cancer cells. N Engl J Med. 2007;356:217–226.
46. Fan C, Oh D, Wessels L, et al. Concordance among gene-expression based predictors for breast cancer. N Engl J Med. 2006;355:560–569.
47. Yang H, Crawford N, Lukes L, et al. Metastasis predictive signature profiles pre-exist in normal tissues. Clin Exp Metastasis. 2005;22:593–603.
48. Ramaswamy S, Ross KN, Lander ES, et al. A molecular signature of metastasis in primary solid tumors. Nat Genet. 2003;33:49–54.
49. Minn AJ, Gupta GP, Siegel PM, et al. Genes that mediate breast cancer metastasis to lung. Nature 2005;436:518–524.

50. Kang Y, Siegel PM, Shu W, et al. A multigenic program mediating breast cancer metastasis to bone. Cancer Cell 2003;3:537–549.
51. Minn AJ, Kang Y, Serganova I, et al. Distinct organ-specific metastatic potential of individual breast cancer cells and primary tumors. J Clin Invest. 2005;115:44–55.
52. O'Donnell RK, Kupferman M, Wei SJ, et al. Gene expression signature predicts lymphatic metastasis in squamous cell carcinoma of the oral cavity. Oncogene 2005;24:1244–1251.
53. Yin JJ, Mohammad KS, Kakonen SM, et al. A causal role for endothelin-1 in the pathogenesis of osteoblastic bone metastases. Proc Natl Acad Sci USA 2003;100:10954–10959.
54. Debies MT, Welch DR. Genetic basis of human breast cancer metastasis. J Mam Biol Neo. 2001;6:441–451.
55. Senger DR, Perruzzi CA. Cell migration promoted by a potent GRGDS-containing thrombin-cleavage fragment of osteopontin. Biochim Biophys Acta. 1996;1314:13–24.
56. Wu Y, Denhardt DT, Rittling SR, Osteopontin is required for full expression of the transformed phenotype by the Ras oncogene. Br J Cancer. 2000;83:156–163.
57. Behrend EI, Craig AM, Wilson SM, et al. Expression of antisense osteopontin RNA in metastatic mouse fibroblasts is associated with reduced malignancy. Ann NY Acad Sci. 1995;760:299–301.
58. Denhardt DT, Guo X. Osteopontin: a protein with diverse functions. FASEB J. 1993;1475–1482.
59. Standal T, Borset M, Sundan A. Role of osteopontin in adhesion, migration, cell survival and bone remodeling. Exp Oncol. 2004;26:179–184.
60. Wai PY, Kuo PCJ. The role of osteopontin in tumor metastasis. Surg Res. 2004;121:228–241.
61. Philip S, Kundu GC. Osteopontin induces NF-kappa B mediated promatrix metalloproteinase-2 activation through IKK/IκBα signaling pathways and curcumin (diferulolylmethane) down regulates these pathways. J Biol Chem. 2003;278:14487–14497.
62. Das R, Mahabeleshwar GH, Kundu GC. Osteopontin induces AP-1-mediated secretion of urokinase type plasminogen activator through c-Src dependent EGF receptor transactivation in breast cancer cells. J Biol Chem. 2004;279:11051–11064.
63. Tuck AB, Arsenault DM, O'Malley FP, et al. Osteopontin induces invasiveness and plasminogen activator expression of human mammary epithelial cells. Oncogene 1999;18:4237–4246.
64. Liaw L, Lindner V, Schwartz SM, et al. Osteopontin and beta 3 integrin are coordinately expressed in regenerating endothelium in vivo and stimulate Arg-Gly-Asp-dependent endothelial migration in vitro. Circ Res. 1995;77:665–672.
65. Ellison JA, Velier JJ, Spera P, et al. Osteopontin and its integrin receptor alpha(v)beta3 are upregulated during formation of the glial scar after focal stroke. Stroke 1998;29:1698–1706.
66. Das R, Mahabeleshwar GH, Kundu GC. Osteopontin stimulates cell motility and nuclear factor kappy B-mediated secretion of urokinase plasminogen activator through phosphatidylinositol 3-kinase/Akt signaling pathways in breast cancer cells. J Biol Chem 2003;278:28593–28606.
67. Das R, Philip S, Ganapati H, et al. Osteopontin: It's role in regulation of cell motility and nuclear factor kB-mediated urokinase type plasminogen activator expression. IUBMB Life 2005;57:441–447.
68. MacDougall JR, Matrisian LM. Contributions of tumor and stromal matrix metalloproteinases to tumor progression, invasion and metastasis. Cancer Metastasis Rev. 1995;14:351–362.
69. Scatena M, Almeida M, Chaisson ML, et al. NF-kappa B mediates $\alpha v \beta 3$ integrin-induced endothelial cell survival. J Cell Biol. 1998;141:1083–1093.
70. Furger KA, Menon RK, Tuck AB, et al. The functional and clinical roles of osteopontin in cancer and metastasis. Curr Mol Med. 2001;1:621–632.

71. Tuck AB, O'Malley FP, Singhal H, et al. Osteopontin expression in a group of lymph node negative breast cancer patients. Int J Cancer. 1998;79:502–508.
72. Furlong EE, Andersen EC, Null B, et al. Patterns of gene expression during drosophila mesoderm development. Science 2001;293:1629–1633.
73. Fidler IJ. Critical determinants of metastasis. Semin Cancer Biol. 2002;12:89–96.
74. Chambers AF, Groom AC, MacDonald IC. Dissemination and growth of cancer cells in metastatic sites. Nat Rev Cancer. 2002;2:563–572.
75. Huang S, Pettaway CA, Uehara H, et al. Blockade of NF-κB activity in human prostate cancer cells is associated with suppression of angiogenesis, invasion, and metastasis. Oncogene 2001;20:4188–4197.
76. Huber MA, Azoitei N, Baumann B, et al. NF-κB is essential for epithelial-mesenchymal transition and metastasis in a model of breast cancer progression. J Clin Invest. 2004;114:568–581.
77. Ghosh S, May MJ, Kopp EB. NF-κB and Rel proteins: evolutionarily conserved mediators of immune responses. Ann Rev Immunol. 1998;16:225–260.
78. Karin M, Ben-Neriah Y. Phsophorylation meets ubiquitination: the control of NF-κB activity. Ann Rev Immunol. 2000;18:621–663.
79. Park BK, Zhang H, Zeng Q, et al. NF-κB in breast cancer cells promotes osteolytic bone metastasis by inducing osteoclastogenesis via GM-CSF. Nat Med. 2007;13:62–69.
80. Yang J, Mani SA, Weinberg RA. Exploring a new twist on tumor metastasis. Cancer Res. 2006;66:4549–4552.
81. Yang J, Mani SA, Donaher JL, et al. Twist, a master regulator of morphogenesis, plays an essential role in tumor metastasis. Cell 2004;117:927–939.
82. Maestro R, Dei Tos AP, Hamamori Y, et al. Twist is a potential oncogene that inhibits apoptosis. Genes Dev. 1999;13:2207–2217.
83. Valsesia-Wittmann S, Magdeleine M, Dupasquier S, et al. Oncogenic cooperation between H-Twist and N-Myc overrides failsafe programs in cancer cells. Cancer Cell 2004;6:625–630.
84. Meulemans D, Bronner-Fraser M. Gene-regulatory interactions in neural crest evolution and development. Dev Cell. 2004;7:291–299.
85. Steeg PS, Ouatas T, Halverson D, et al. Metastasis suppressor genes: basic biology and potential clinical use. Clin Breast Cancer. 2003;4:51–62.
86. Berger JC, Vander Griend DJ, Robinson VL, et al. Metastasis suppressor genes: from gene identification to protein function and regulation. Cancer Biol Ther. 2005;4: 805–812.
87. Berger JC, Vander Griend D, Stadler WM, et al. Metastasis suppressor genes: signal transduction, cross-talk and the potential for modulating the behavior of metastatic cells. Anticancer Drugs 2004;15:559–568.
88. Shevde LA, Welch DR. Metastasis suppressor pathways – an evolving paradigm. Cancer Lett. 2003;198:1–20.
89. Steeg PS, Bevilacqua G, Kopper L, et al. Evidence for a novel gene associated with low tumor metastatic potential. J Natl Cancer Inst. 1988;80:200–204.
90. Otsuki Y, Tanaka M, Yoshii S, et al. Tumor metastasis suppressor nm23H1 regulates Rac1 GTPase by interaction with Tiam1. Proc Natl Acad Sci USA. 2001;98: 4385–4390.
91. Wagner PD, Steeg PS, Vu ND. Two-component kinase-like activity of nm23 correlates with its motility-suppressing activity. Proc Natl Acad Sci USA. 1997;94:9000–9005.
92. Hartsough MT, Morrison DK, Salerno M, et al. NM23-H1 metastasis suppressor phosphorylation of kinase suppressor of ras via a histidine protein kinase pathway. J Biol Chem. 2002;277:32389–32399.
93. Hartsough MT, Clare SE, Mair M, et al. Elevation of breast carcinoma Nm23-H1 metastasis suppressor gene expression and reduced motility by DNA methylation inhibition. Cancer Res. 2001;61:2320–2327.

94. Steeg PS, Palmieri D, Ouatas T, et al. Histidine kinases and histidine phosphorylated proteins in mammalian cell biology, signal transduction and cancer. Cancer Lett. 2003;190:1–12.
95. Salerno M, Ouatas T, Palmieri D, et al. Inhibition of signal transduction by the nm23 metastasis suppressor: possible mechanisms. Clin Exptl Metastasis. 2003;20:3–10.
96. Freije JM, MacDonald NJ, Steeg PS. Nm23 and tumor metastasis: basic and translational advances. Biochem Soc Symp. 1998;63:261–271.
97. Lombardi D, Lacombe ML, Paggi MG. nm23: unraveling its biological function in cell differentiation. J Cell Physiol. 2000;182:144–149.
98. Scambia G, Ferrandina G, Marone M, et al. Nm23 in ovarian cancer: correlation with clinical outcome and other clinicopathologic and biochemical prognostic parameters. J Clin Oncol. 1996;14:334–342.
99. Yamashita H, Kobayashi S, Iwase H, et al. Analysis of oncogenes and tumor suppressors in human breast cancer. Jpn J Cancer Res. 1993;84:871–878.
100. Tommasi S, Fedele V, Crapolicchio A, et al. ErbB2 and the antimetastatic nm23/NDP kinase in regulating serum induced breast cancer invasion. Int J Mol Med. 2003;12:131–134.
101. Nakopoulou LL, Tsitsimelis D, Lazaris AC, et al. Nm-23, c-erbB-2, and progesterone receptor expression in invasive breast cancer: correlation with clinicopathological parameters. Cancer Detect Prev. 1999;23:297–308.
102. Ohba K, Miyata Y, Koga S, et al. Expression of nm23-H1 gene product in sarcomatous cancer cells of renal cell carcinoma: correlation with tumor stage and expression of matrix metalloproteinase-2, matrix metalloproteinase-9, sialyl Lewis X, and c-erbB-2. Urology 2005;65:1029–1034.
103. Suzuki E, Ota T, Tsukuda K, et al. Nm23-H1 reduces in vitro cell migration and the liver metastatic potential of colon cancer cells by regulating myosin light chain phosphorylation. Int J Cancer. 2004;108:207–211.
104. Seraj MJ, Samant RS, Verderame MF, et al. Functional evidence for a novel human breast carcinoma metastasis suppressor, *BRMS1*, encoded at chromosome 11q13. Cancer Res. 2000;60:2764–2779.
105. Samant RS, Seraj MJ, Saunders MM, et al. Analysis of mechanisms underlying *BRMS1* suppression of metastasis. Clin Exptl Metastasis. 2001;18:683–693.
106. Samant RS, Debies MT, Shevde LA, et al. Identification and characterization of muring ortholog (*Brms1*) of breast cancer metastasis suppressor 1 (*BRMS1*). Int J Cancer. 2002;97:15–20.
107. Saunders MM, Seraj MJ, Li ZY, et al. Breast cancer metastatic potential correlates with a breakdown in homospecific and heterospecific gap junctional intercellular communication. Cancer Res 2001;61:1765–1767.
108. Seraj MJ, Harding MA, Gildea JJ, et al. The relationship of *BRMS1* and *RhoGDI2* gene expression to metastatic potential in lineage related human bladder cancer cell lines. Clin Exptl Metastasis. 2001;18:519–525.
109. Shevde LA, Samant RS, Goldberg SF, et al. Suppression of human melanoma metastasis by the metastasis suppressor gene, BRMS1. Exp Cell Res. 2002;273: 229–239.
110. Meehan WJ, Samant RS, Hopper JE, et al. Breast cancer metastasis suppressor 1 (BRMS1) forms complexes with retinoblastoma-binding protein 1 (RBP1) and the mSin3 histone deacetylase complex and represses transcription. J Biol Chem. 2004;279:1562–1569.
111. Cicek M, Fukuyama R, Welch DR, et al. Breast cancer metastasis suppressor 1 inhibits gene expression by targeting nuclear factor-kappaB activity. Cancer Res. 2005;65: 3586–3595.
112. Liu Y, Smith PW, Jones DR. Breast cancer metastasis suppressor 1 functions as a corepressor by enhancing histone deacetylase1-mediated deacetylation of RelA/p65 and promoting apoptosis. Mol Cell Biol. 2006;26:8683–8696.

113. Samant RS, Clark DW, Fillmore RA, et al. Breast cancer metastasis suppressor 1 (BRMS1) inhibits osteopontin transcription by abrogating NF-kappaB activation. Mol Cancer. 2007;6:6–14.
114. DeWald DB, Torabinejad J, Samant RS, et al. Metastasis suppression by breast cancer metastasis suppressor 1 involves reduction of phosphoinositide signaling in MDA-MB-435 breast carcinoma cells. Cancer Res. 2005;65:713–717.
115. Ozes ON, Mayo LD, Gustin JA, et al. NF-kappaB activation by tumor necrosis factor requires the Akt serine-threonine kinase. Nature 1999;401:82–85.
116. Kelly LM, Buggy Y, Hill A, et al. Expression of the breast cancer metastasis suppressor gene, BRMS1, in human breast carcinoma: lack of correlation with metastasis to axillary lymph nodes. Tumor Biol. 2005;26:213–216.
117. Lombardi G, Di Cristofano C, Capodanno A, et al. High level of messenger RNA for BRMS1 in primary breast carcinomas is associated with poor prognosis. Int J Cancer. 2007;120:1169–1178.
118. Zhang Z, Yamashita H, Toyama T, et al. Reduced expression of the breast cancer metastasis suppressor 1 mRNA is correlated with poor progress in breast cancer. Clin Cancer Res. 2006;12:6410–6414.
119. Hicks DG, Yoder BJ, Short S, et al. Loss of breast cancer metastasis suppressor 1 protein expression predicts reduced disease-free survival in subsets of breast cancer patients. Clin Cancer Research. 2006;12:6702–6708.
120. Lee J-H, Welch DR. Identification of highly expressed genes in metastasis-suppressed chromosome 6/human malignant melanoma hybrid cells using subtractive hybridization and differential display. Int J Cancer. 1997;71:1035–1044.
121. Lee J-H, Miele ME, Hicks DJ, et al. *KiSS-1*, a novel human malignant melanoma metastasis-suppressor gene. J Natl Cancer Inst. 1999;88:1731–1737.
122. Goldberg SF, Miele ME, Hatta N, et al. Melanoma metastasis suppression by chromosome 6: Evidence for a pathway regulated by CRSP3 and TXNIP. Cancer Res. 2003;63: 432–440.
123. Lee J-H, Welch DR. Suppression of metastasis in human breast carcinoma MDA-MB-435 cells after transfection with the metastasis suppressor gene, KiSS-1. Cancer Res. 1997;57:2384–2387.
124. Shirasaki F, Takata M, Hatta, N, et al. Loss of expression of the metastasis suppressor gene KiSS1 during melanoma progression and its association with LOH of chromosome 6q16.3-q23. Cancer Res. 2001;61:7422–7425.
125. Nash KT, Welch DR. The KISS1 metastasis suppressor: mechanistic insights and clinical utility. Front Biosci. 2006;11:647–659.
126. Mitchell DC, Abdelrahim M, Weng J, et al. Regulation of KiSS-1 metastasis suppressor gene expression in breast cancer cells by direct interaction of transcription factors activator protein-2alpha and specificity protein-1. J Biol Chem. 2006;281:51–58.
127. Mitchell DC, Stafford LJ, Li D, et al. Transcriptional regulation of KiSS-1 gene expression in metastatic melanoma by specificity protein-1 and its coactivator DRIP-130. Oncogene 2006. doi: 10.1028/sj.onc.1209963, Epub September 11, 2006.
128. Kotani M, Detheux M, Vandenbogaerde A, et al. The metastasis suppressor gene KiSS-1 encodes kisspeptins, the natural ligands of the orphan G protein-coupled receptor GPR54. J Biol Chem. 2001;276:34631–34636.
129. Ohtaki T, Shintani Y, Honda S, et al. Metastasis suppressor gene KiSS1 encodes peptide ligand of a G-protein-coupled receptor. Nature 2001;411:613–617.
130. Ringel MD, Hardy E, Bernet VJ, et al. Metastin receptor is overexpressed in papillary thyroid cancer and activates MAP Kinase in thyroid cancer cells. J Clin Endocrin Metab. 2002;87:2399–2402.
131. Stafford LJ, Xia CZ, Ma WB, et al. Identification and characterization of mouse metastasis-suppressor KiSS1 and its G-protein-coupled receptor. Cancer Res. 2002;62: 5399–5404.

132. Muir AI, Chamberlain L, Elshourbagy NA, et al. AXOR12: A novel G protein-coupled receptor, activated by the peptide KiSS-1. J Biol Chem. 2001;276:28969–28975.
133. Navenot JM, Wang Z, Chopin M, et al. Kisspeptin-10-induced signaling of GPR54 negatively regulates chemotactic responses mediated by CXCR4: a potential mechanism for the metastasis suppressor activity of kisspeptins. Cancer Res. 2005;65:10450–10456.
134. Janneau JL, Maldonado-Estrada J, Tachdjian G, et al. Transcriptional expression of genes involved in cell invasion and migration by normal and tumoral trophoblast cells. J Clin Endocrin Metab. 2002;87:5336–5339.
135. Takino T, Koshikawa N, Miyamori H, et al. Cleavage of metastasis suppressor gene product KiSS-1 protein/metastin by matrix metalloproteinases. Oncogene 2003;22:4617–4626.
136. Bilban M, Ghaffari-Tabrizi N, Hintermann E, et al. Kisspeptin-10, a KiSS-1/metastin-derived decapeptide, is a physiological invasion inhibitor of primary human trophoblasts. J Cell Sci 2004;117:1319–1328.
137. Lymberis SC, Parhar PK, Katsoulakis E, et al. Pharmacogenomics and breast cancer. Pharmacogenomics 2005;5:31–55.
138. Bild AH, Yao G, Chang JT, et al. Oncogenic pathway signatures in human cancers as a guide to targeted therapies. Nature 2006;439:353–357.
139. Gutheil JC, Campbell TN, Pierce PR, et al. Targeted antiangiogenic therapy for cancer using Vitaxin: a humanized monoclonal antibody to the integrin alphavbeta3. Clin Cancer Res. 2000;6:3056–3061.
140. Ouatas T, Halverson D, Steeg PS. Dexamethasone and medroxyprogesterone acetate elevate Nm23-H1 metastasis suppressor expression in metastatic human breast carcinoma cells via glucocorticoid receptor-dependent, transcriptional and post-transcriptional mechanisms: New uses for old compounds. Clin Cancer Res. 2003;9:3763–3772.
141. Palmieri D, Halverson DO, Ouatas T, et al. Medroxyprogesterone acetate elevation of Nm23-H1 metastasis suppressor expression in hormone receptor-negative breast cancer. J Natl Cancer Inst. 2005;97:632–642.

Endocrine Therapy with Selective Estrogen Receptor Modulators (SERMs) and Aromatase Inhibitors in the Prevention and Adjuvant Therapy Settings

Shelly S. Lo, Kathleen I. Pritchard, Patricia Robinson, and Kathy S. Albain

Endocrine-Responsive Breast Cancer

Breast cancer is the most common malignancy in women worldwide. In 2007, approximately 178,480 invasive cases of breast cancer and 62,030 non-invasive cases were diagnosed in the United States [1]. Approximately 70–80% of female breast cancers will express receptors for estrogen and/or progesterone receptors [2].

Hormones have been linked to breast cancer since Beatson demonstrated in 1896 that oophorectomy in premenopausal women resulted in tumor regression [3]. For many years to follow, sequential surgical removal of the ovaries, adrenal glands, and pituitary gland to lower estrogen levels was the mainstay of breast cancer therapy. Supra-physiologic doses of estrogens and androgens were also used as treatments for advanced breast cancer.

The development of the selective estrogen receptor modulators (SERMs) in the 1970s, along with recognition of benefit only in estrogen receptor-positive disease, introduced the first targeted treatment for breast cancer. Currently, SERMs such as tamoxifen are mainstays in the prevention and treatment of breast cancer. Raloxifene has also demonstrated efficacy in the prevention setting [4]. In the 1990s, the aromatase inhibitors (AIs) demonstrated efficacy in the metastatic and adjuvant breast cancer, and trials are now underway regarding efficacy in prevention. This chapter will summarize findings from key clinical trials with these agents in both the prevention and the adjuvant settings.

S.S. Lo (✉)
Division of Hematology/Oncology, Department of Medicine, Loyola University Chicago Stritch School of Medicine, Cardinal Bernardin Cancer Center, Maywood, IL, USA
e-mail: shlo@lumc.edu

S.A.W. Fuqua (ed.), *Hormone Receptors in Breast Cancer*,
Cancer Treatment and Research 312, DOI 10.1007/978-0-387-09463-2_7,

Prevention

Selective Estrogen Receptor Modulators (SERMs)

Chemoprevention is the use of specific natural or synthetic chemical agents to reverse, suppress, or prevent the progression of premalignant lesions to invasive carcinoma [5]. Agents used as chemopreventives include SERMs, which are pharmacological agents that interact with the estrogen receptor (ER) and display either estrogen-agonistic or estrogen-antagonistic properties, depending on the specific tissue target and hormonal milieu. Tamoxifen, the best-studied SERM, is a synthetic non-steroidal agent that binds to the ER and acts as a competitive antagonist. Its use in the prevention setting is based on efficacy demonstrated in the adjuvant setting regarding reduction in second primary breast cancers, reviewed later in this chapter.

Acceptance of tamoxifen as a chemopreventive by both patients and physicians has been low, primarily due to toxicity concerns. Thus, the search for safer, more tolerable, but effective alternatives ensued [6–9]. Another SERM, raloxifene, demonstrated similar efficacy to tamoxifen in the STAR trial, with fewer side effects [4]. These agents are now reviewed in greater detail and are all summarized in Table 1.

Tamoxifen

The Breast Cancer Prevention Trial (BCPT)

The Breast Cancer Prevention Trial (BCPT) sponsored by the National Surgical Adjuvant Breast and Bowel Project (NSABP) randomized 13,388 North American women at high risk for the development of breast cancer to tamoxifen (20 mg/day) or placebo. Women who were more than 60 years in age, or had a history of lobular carcinoma in situ (LCIS), or had a 5-year predicted risk (Gail score) [10] for developing breast cancer of >1.66% were eligible. Tamoxifen reduced the risk of invasive breast cancer by 49% (two-sided P<0.00001) and of non-invasive breast cancer by 50% (two-sided P<0.002). ER-positive tumors decreased by 69%. There was no significant reduction in ER-negative breast cancer. Risk reduction was observed in women of all age groups, as well as women with a history of lobular carcinoma in situ or atypical hyperplasia. Tamoxifen did not alter the average annual rate of ischemic heart disease; although it did reduce the incidence of fractures of the hip, radius, and spine by 19%, which was almost statistically significant (RR = 0.81; 95% CI = 0.63–1.05). Specifically, hip fractures were decreased by 45% (RR = 0.55; 95% CI = 0.25–1.15) with tamoxifen. However, endometrial cancer was increased in the tamoxifen group (RR=2.53, 95% CI =1.35–4.97), as was the incidence of thromboembolism (RR =1.60 95% CI=0.91–2.86). Both endometrial cancer and thromboembolism were seen at an increased rate in women older than 50 years, but not in younger women [11].

Table 1 Summary of the completed Phase III prevention trials

Study	Number of patients	Menopausal status	Median F/U	Invasive breast cancer cases	Non-invasive cases	Invasive cases cumulative rate per 1,000 women	Non-invasive cases cumulative rate per 1,000 women	Relative risk reduction 95% CI
NSABP-P1 (tamoxifen vs placebo)	13,175	Pre- and postmenopausal	7 years	Tam: 145 Placebo: 250	Tam: 60 Placebo: 93	Tam: 24.8 Placebo: 42.5	Tam: 10.2 Placebo: 15.8	Invasive: 0.57 (0.46–0.70) Non-invasive: 0.63 (0.45–0.89)
IBIS-1 (tamoxifen vs placebo)	7,152	Pre- and postmenopausal	96 months	Tam: 124 Placebo: 168	Tam: 17 Placebo: 27	NA	NA	Invasive: 0.74 (0.58–0.94) Non-invasive: 0.63 (0.32–1.2)
STAR (tamoxifen vs raloxifene)	19,747	Postmenopausal only	3.9 years	Tam: 163 Ral: 168	Tam: 57 Ral: 80	Tam: 25.1 Ral: 24.8	Tam: 8.1 Ral: 11.6	Invasive: 1.02 (0.82–1.28) Non-invasive: 1.40 (0.98–2.0)
Royal Marsden	2,471	Pre- and postmenopausal	13 years, 2 months	Tam: 82 Placebo: 104	Tam: 14 Placebo: 9	Tam: 4.8 Placebo: 6.1	Tam: 0.8 Placebo: 0.5	Invasive: 0.7% (0.58–1.04)
Italian Tamoxifen Prevention Study	5,408	Pre- and postmenopausal	11 years	Tam: 62 Placebo: 74	Tam: 6 Placebo: 9	Annual rates breast cancer Tam: 2.07 per 1,000 Placebo: 2.48 per 1,000	N/A	Invasive: 0.84 Non-invasive: N/A

An update after 7 years of follow-up confirmed the reduction in the number of invasive breast cancers (RR=0.57, 95% CI=0.46–0.70) and non-invasive breast cancers (RR=0.63, 95% CI=0.45–0.89) in the tamoxifen group [12]. The incidence of side effects including thromboembolic events, strokes, and cataracts were similar to those initially reported.

Royal Marsden Hospital Chemoprevention Trial

The RMH Chemoprevention Trial was a pilot trial for the subsequent IBIS-I trial. The aim of this randomized placebo-controlled trial was to assess whether tamoxifen would prevent breast cancer in healthy women at increased risk of breast cancer based on family history. Each participant had at least one first-degree relative younger than 50 years with breast cancer, one first-degree relative with bilateral breast cancer, or one affected first-degree relative of any age and another affected first- or second-degree relative. Women were allowed to use hormone replacement therapy (HRT) during the study. Between 1986 and 1996, 2,494 women of age 30–70 years were randomized to receive tamoxifen (20 mg/day) or placebo for up to 8 years. The primary end point was the occurrence of breast cancer [13].

After 20 years of blinded follow-up (median follow-up 13 years), the trial reported a statistically significant decrease in ER-positive tumors. One hundred and eighty-six cancers were diagnosed, and 139 were ER positive. Of those cancers diagnosed, 53 occurred in the tamoxifen-treated arm, while 86 occurred in the placebo-treated arm (P=0.005). The risk of developing an ER-positive breast cancer was not lower in the tamoxifen-treated group compared to placebo during the 8-year treatment period, but was significantly lower in the post-treatment period (23 cases versus 47 cases, HR= 0.48, P=0.004) [14]. Therefore, tamoxifen was associated with an overall risk reduction in ER-positive cancers to a similar magnitude with the other prevention studies.

IBIS-I

The IBIS-I multi-national study randomized 7,152 women to tamoxifen (20 mg/day) or placebo for 5 years. Eligible women had risk factors for developing breast cancer based on family history, LCIS, atypical hyperplasia, nulliparity, and prior breast biopsy stratified by age. After a median follow-up of 50 months, breast cancer developed in 69 of the 3,578 participants in the tamoxifen group compared to 101 of the 3,566 women in the placebo group (P=0.013). A 32% (95% CI= 8–50) risk reduction of invasive and non-invasive breast cancer was noted in the tamoxifen arm. The risk reduction in ER-positive invasive tumors with tamoxifen was 31% [15]. As observed in the NSABP study, there was no risk reduction in ER-negative tumors.

The results of IBIS-I were updated after a median follow-up of 96 months. A 27% risk reduction overall was confirmed, with a 33% risk reduction in the ER-positive subgroup. The benefits of tamoxifen extended well beyond the treatment phase up to 10 years. The side effects of tamoxifen, namely, thrombosis and endometrial cancer were increased during the treatment phase only and did not persist once tamoxifen was discontinued [16]. The lower degree of risk reduction in this study compared to the NSABP P1 study may be due to the enrollment of patients who were allowed to take hormone replacement treatment while on study.

The Italian Tamoxifen Prevention Study

The Italian Tamoxifen Prevention Study evaluated tamoxifen in 5,408 healthy women of ages 35–70 years who had previously undergone a hysterectomy. Women were randomized to receive tamoxifen (20 mg/day) or placebo for 5 years. Among the 5,378 women with complete data, 48.3% had also undergone a prior bilateral oophorectomy and 18.2% had at least one first-degree relative or an aunt with breast cancer. As in IBIS-I, women were allowed to take HRT during the study. The primary end points were reduction in the frequency of and the mortality rate from breast cancer [17].

After 11 years of follow-up, 136 women (74 placebo and 62 tamoxifen) developed breast cancer (RR =0.84, 95% CI = 0.60–1.17). In the group defined as "high risk" with at least one functioning ovary, there was a 77% reduction in the incidence of breast cancer (HR=0.24, 95% CI = 0.10–0.59) [18].

Raloxifene

To compare the efficacy and safety of raloxifene and tamoxifen, the NSABP conducted the Study of Tamoxifen and Raloxifene (STAR) trial, a prospective, double-blind, randomized clinical trial. Patients were 19,747 postmenopausal women of mean age 58.5 years with increased 5-year breast cancer risk (mean risk, 4.03 ± 2.17%) as estimated by the Gail model. Participants were randomly assigned to receive either tamoxifen (20 mg/day) or raloxifene (60 mg/day) over 5 years. The results of the NSABP P-2 STAR trial after 47-month median follow-up showed that raloxifene was as effective as tamoxifen in decreasing the incidence of invasive breast cancer, but inferior to tamoxifen in reducing non-invasive breast cancer. Raloxifene was associated with fewer side effects including a lower cumulative incidence of endometrial carcinoma (RR = 0.62, P = 0.07), thromboembolic disease (RR = 0.70, P = 0.01), and cataracts (RR = 0.79, P = 0.002) [4]. The results of this large randomized study demonstrate that the SERM raloxifene is also an effective alternative for breast cancer risk reduction.

Aromatase Inhibitors (AIs)

Improvement in disease-free survival (DFS) in the adjuvant setting by aromatase inhibitors (AIs) compared to tamoxifen [19, 20] plus observed reductions

Table 2 Ongoing/proposed phase III prevention trials addressing the role of aromatase inhibitor

Study	Randomization
IBIS 2	Anastrozole vs placebo
APRES	Exemestane vs placebo in BRCA carriers
MAP 3	Exemestane vs placebo

in second primary breast cancers led to the study of aromatase inhibitors in the prevention setting, summarized in Table 2. Current trials include the National Cancer Institute Canada (NCIC) MAP 3 study, which randomizes postmenopausal women to exemestane or placebo, and the IBIS 2-trial, which is randomizing postmenopausal women to anastrozole versus placebo. To date, there are no active trials that compare an AI to a SERM as chemoprevention. The APRES study will enroll only BRCA 1 or 2 mutation carriers and randomize them to exemestane or placebo.

Prevention Summary

As summarized in Table 1, the development of invasive estrogen receptor-positive breast cancer can be delayed or prevented with the use of SERMs such as tamoxifen or raloxifene. Tamoxifen is superior compared to raloxifene in preventing non-invasive breast cancer. The role of the AIs in the prevention of breast cancer awaits completion of ongoing international trials. Overall, a significant reduction in annual rates of breast cancer could be achieved by widespread use of the SERMs in appropriately screened high-risk populations.

Adjuvant Therapy of Early Breast Cancer

Tamoxifen

After demonstrating efficacy in the metastatic setting versus medroxyprogesterone, oophorectomy, and diethylstilbestrol [21–24], tamoxifen became the first targeted therapy for cancer approved by the US Food and Drug Administration (US FDA) and was thus subsequently studied in the early breast cancer (adjuvant) setting.

Tamoxifen is a true targeted agent, since patients with ER- and PR-negative tumors do not respond to treatment [25]. In the 2000 update published in 2005, the Early Breast Cancer Trialists' Collaborative Group demonstrated that 5 years of adjuvant tamoxifen reduced the annual breast cancer death rate by 31% in women with ER-positive disease, irrespective of age, use of adjuvant chemotherapy, PR status, nodal status, or other tumor characteristics and that 5 years of use was more effective than 1–2 years of use [26]. However, tamoxifen was associated with a non-significant increase in pulmonary embolism and uterine cancer. The 2005 Oxford Overview confirmed efficacy in the ER-positive subset, irrespective of PR status for recurrence, and found an absolute survival benefit of 9.3% after 15 years of follow-up in the ER-positive subgroup ($p = 0.00001$) [27].

Carry-Over Benefit of Tamoxifen

Several studies in the literature have reported a carry-over benefit in which 5 years of tamoxifen in both the preventive and the adjuvant therapy settings produce a substantial protective effect not only while it is being taken but also during the follow-up period. This in particular has been striking in the Oxford Overview of tamoxifen benefit [26], as well as individual adjuvant and prevention trials.

For example, the NSABP P1 prevention trial demonstrated an early benefit to tamoxifen therapy with a 49% risk reduction of invasive breast cancer at 47.7 months (RR=0.51, 95% CI= 0.39–0.66, $p<.00001$). During that same time period, there was a 50% risk reduction of non-invasive breast cancers [11]. After 7 years of follow-up, the risk reduction was similar to the initial report at 43%. In other words, the benefit carried over as did the degree of benefit. The incidence of invasive breast cancer (RR = 0.57, 95% CI = 0.46–0.70) and non-invasive breast cancer (RR = 0.63, 95% CI = 0.45–0.89) was lower in the tamoxifen arm relative to the placebo arm [12].

The Royal Marsden prevention trial failed to demonstrate a beneficial effect of tamoxifen for the early risk reduction of invasive breast cancer during the first interim analysis (RR=1.06 [95% CI = 0.7–1.7]). There was equal distribution of invasive and non-invasive breast cancers [13]. However, long-term results with a median follow-up time of 13 years reported a reduction in risk of breast cancers in the tamoxifen arm (HR=0.84, 95% CI=0.64–1.10; P=0.2) [14].

The IBIS-I trial reported a 31% risk reduction for invasive and non-invasive breast cancers in the tamoxifen arm compared to the placebo arm during active therapy (OR=0.68, 95% CI= 0.50–0.92, P=0.013). The 96 month median follow-up reported fewer breast cancer incidents in the tamoxifen arm versus the placebo arm. The incidence of invasive and non-invasive breast cancers in the tamoxifen group were 27% lower than the placebo group in the early setting (years 0–4) and 44% lower in the long-term follow-up (years 5 and beyond). The absolute risk reduction of breast cancer increased from 1.1% at 5 years to 1.7% at 10 years. The absolute risk reduction of ER-positive breast cancer increased from 1.4% at 5 years to 1.7% at 10 years [16].

The Italian prevention trial also initially reported a null effect of tamoxifen in reducing the risk of invasive breast cancer (P=0.63) [17]. At 11 years of follow-up, the study demonstrated a statistically significant reduction of ER-positive breast tumors among women in the tamoxifen group relative to the placebo group (HR=0.84, [95%CI = 0.60–1.17] P=.30). There were fewer incidences of non-invasive breast cancer in the tamoxifen arm as compared to placebo [6 (81%) versus 9(14.5%), respectively] [18].

Thus, the data from the Oxford Overview in the adjuvant setting together with emerging benefits with longer follow-up in several prevention trials support the concept that the efficacy of tamoxifen is durable, may emerge late, and may even grow (or "carry over") in the long-term follow-up period.

Specific Adjuvant Tamoxfen Trials

As previously indicated, tamoxifen is a SERM that inhibits the growth of breast cancer cells by competitively antagonizing estrogen at the estrogen receptor. Tamoxifen has partial estrogen agonist activity that can be both beneficial (increasing bone mineral density) and detrimental (increased risk of uterine cancer and thromboembolic events). A number of large adjuvant tamoxifen trials informed the EBCTCG Overview because of efficacy compared to no systemic treatment in early breast cancer.

The Nolvadex Adjuvant Trial Organization (NATO) study showed a benefit for tamoxifen versus placebo that was independent of menopausal status, stage, grade, and ER status [28]. The NSABP B-14 study randomized predominantly lymph node-negative women with resected early-stage breast cancer to tamoxifen versus placebo. The tamoxifen-treated group experienced an improvement in DFS at 4 years versus placebo (83 versus 77%, $p<0.00001$). Tamoxifen also reduced local and distant recurrences, as well as contralateral breast cancers. Updated results through 10 years of follow-up showed a survival benefit (80% versus 76%, $p= 0.02$) in favor of the tamoxifen arm [29].

Four studies addressed the optimal duration of adjuvant tamoxifen for early breast cancer: NSABP B-14, the Scottish study, ECOG 4181/E5181, and ATLAS (Adjuvant Tamoxifen: Longer Against Shorter). NSABP B14 reported that greater than 5 years of tamoxifen use was no better than 5 years of tamoxifen use (overall survival 91% versus 94%, respectively, $P=0.07$) [29]. A Scottish study of 1,312 lymph node-negative patients also showed benefit from tamoxifen in the adjuvant setting [30]. Updated results 5 years after study closure showed prolonged DFS in premenopausal women and postmenopausal women [31]. A second randomization of the treatment arm to an additional 5 years of tamoxifen versus placebo showed that at after a median follow-up of 6 years, additional benefit from tamoxifen was unlikely. Event-free survival analysis showed a trend in favor of discontinuing tamoxifen that did not meet statistical significance (HR=1.27). Endometrial carcinoma was also non-statistically elevated in the group continuing tamoxifen [32]. Evidence from this study led the authors to conclude that tamoxifen use for greater than 5 years was not beneficial.

ECOG 4181/5181 examined duration of tamoxifen in patients with lymph node-positive breast cancer. All patients received adjuvant chemotherapy and tamoxifen for 5 years at the time of randomization. There was no difference in overall survival, time to relapse, toxic side effects, or second cancers in the tamoxifen arm versus placebo. In an exploratory subset analysis, the time to recurrence in patients with ER-positive tumors was significantly in favor of those receiving tamoxifen. The authors concluded, however, that the data did not support use of tamoxifen longer than 5 years though continued evaluation of tamoxifen use beyond 5 years was reasonable in the LN-positive, ER-positive subset [33].

Results from the ATLAS trial demonstrated that after a mean duration of 4.2 years from randomization between continuation of tamoxifen during years 5–10 and discontinuation of tamoxifen following completion of 5 years of therapy, there was a reduction in recurrence in the arm allocated to longer duration tamoxifen therapy. In this preliminary analysis presented at the 2007 San Antonio Breast Cancer Symposium, no significant difference in breast cancer survival or overall survival was reported [34]. Details regarding risk of endometrial cancer and other toxicities are awaited.

Based on the results of the published studies plus the EBCTCG update, 5 years of adjuvant tamoxifen remains the standard duration of adjuvant hormonal therapy. It is hoped that further follow-up of the ATLAS trial and results of the Adjuvant Tamoxifen Treatment – offer more Trial (aTTom) study will help clarify the optimal duration of adjuvant tamoxifen therapy. Since the NSABP B-14 and the Scottish study enrolled predominantly lymph node-negative patients, perhaps patients at higher risk of relapse, such as those with involved lymph nodes, will benefit from a longer duration of endocrine therapy.

Timing of Tamoxifen in Relation to Other Therapies

Starting adjuvant tamoxifen after completion of the systemic chemotherapy, when given, has become the standard approach after an intergroup study (INT0100) showed greater benefit in the arm receiving sequential chemotherapy followed by tamoxifen versus the concurrent chemotherapy plus tamoxifen group [35]. Retrospective case series of concurrent tamoxifen use with radiation appear to have equivalent outcomes compared to concurrent treatment [36–38]. Timing of hormonal therapy with radiation therapy may be examined in a proposed prospective adjuvant NCIC study.

Adjuvant Endocrine Therapy in Premenopausal Women

The EBCTCG overview confirmed a significant reduction in risk of recurrence and death for premenopausal women with ER-positive breast cancer treated with adjuvant tamoxifen [39]. This was true for studies of tamoxifen versus nil as well as for those of chemotherapy plus tamoxifen versus chemotherapy alone. There is also evidence that ovarian function suppression (OFS) with or without added tamoxifen is equivalent to adjuvant cytoxan, methotrexate, 5-fluorouracil (CMF) chemotherapy in premenopausal patients with endocrine responsive disease [40–43].

There may be additive benefit when OFS is given after chemotherapy. The IBCSG Trial VIII randomized 1,063 premenopausal women with node-negative breast cancer to adjuvant CMF chemotherapy plus goserelin or either modality alone. As expected, in patients with ER-negative disease, 5-year DFS was better for those who received chemotherapy compared to goserelin alone. In contrast, in ER-positive disease overall, chemotherapy-alone and goserelin-alone arms provided similar outcomes. For those who received sequential treatment, there was a non-significant trend toward improved DFS. However, an unplanned subset analysis showed a marked advantage to CMF followed by goserelin in the cohort of women $\leq$39, providing provocative information on a potentially useful treatment strategy in younger patients [44].

INT-0101 was a study of 1,504 premenopausal, node-positive women that compared oral cyclophosphamide, doxorubicin (Adriamycin), and 5-fluorouracil (CAF), CAF plus goserelin, and CAF plus goserelin and tamoxifen. After a median follow-up of 9.6 years, there was an improvement in DFS with the combination of CAF plus goserelin and tamoxifen compared to CAF plus goserelin alone. There was no advantage with the addition of goserelin to CAF versus CAF alone. Exploratory, retrospective subset analyses suggested that women under age 40 years had the most benefit from the addition of goserelin to CAF, possibly due to incomplete cessation of menses after chemotherapy alone [45]. Unfortunately, this study lacked an informative fourth arm of chemotherapy followed by tamoxifen treatment, which would have allowed this study to answer the question whether OFS is required in addition to treatment with a SERM after adjuvant chemotherapy in premenopausal women. A meta-analysis of 16 trials, which included 11,906 premenopausal women with early breast cancer, showed that the addition of luteinizing hormone-releasing hormone (LHRH) agonists to tamoxifen, chemotherapy, or both reduced recurrence by 13% ($P=0.02$) and death after recurrence by 15% ($P=0.03$) [46].

Currently, there are two ongoing clinical trials that prospectively address critical questions regarding the optimal adjuvant endocrine therapy in premenopausal women. For premenopausal women with hormone receptor-positive tumors who maintain ovarian function after adjuvant chemotherapy or do not receive adjuvant chemotherapy, the Suppression of Ovarian Function Trial (SOFT) compares the use of tamoxifen alone versus ovarian function suppression (OFS) plus tamoxifen versus OFS plus an aromatase inhibitor (exemestane). For premenopausal, hormone receptor-positive patients who are prescribed ovarian suppression (with or without chemotherapy), the Tamoxifen and Exemestane Trial (TEXT) evaluate OFS and tamoxifen versus OFS plus exemestane.

Adjuvant Endocrine Therapy in Postmenopausal Women

Aromatase Inhibitors

The third-generation aromatase inhibitors (AIs) include two non-steroidal agents (anastrozole and letrozole) and one steroidal agent (exemestane). The AIs are only effective in postmenopausal women in whom the majority of estrogen production is the result of bio-conversion from androgens in the peripheral tissues. Aromatase inhibitors inhibit the aromatase enzyme, which is involved in the last step of the bio-conversion of androgens to estrogens. In premenopausal women, AIs are ineffective, as an intact hypothalamic–pituitary–ovarian axis will sense a decrease in circulating estrogen, thereby increasing ovarian estrogen production. The major, completed phase III adjuvant hormonal studies that include AIs are summarized in Table 3.

Aromatase Inhibitors as Upfront Hormonal Therapy

Arimidex, Tamoxifen Alone or in Combination (ATAC) Study

The ATAC (Anastrozole Tamoxifen Alone or in Combination) study was conducted in 9,366 postmenopausal women with early breast cancer, node-positive or -negative, hormone receptor positive or unknown who were randomized to tamoxifen or anastrozole or both between 1996 and 2000. The primary end points of this study included disease-free survival (DFS) and safety/tolerability. Study reports at 33, 47, and 68 months of follow-up showed an improvement in DFS, time to recurrence, and a reduction in the incidence of contralateral breast cancer in favor of the anastrozole-alone treatment arm compared to tamoxifen. The concurrent AT arm was not significantly different from tamoxifen alone (RR = 0.02, P = 0.8) [19, 47, 48]. In the latest update, after a median follow-up of 100 months, anastrozole significantly prolonged DFS (HR = 0.85, P=0.003), time to recurrence (HR = 0.76, P=0.0001), reduced distant metastases (HR 0.84, P = 0.022), as well as contralateral breast cancers (HR 0.60, P = 0.004) in the hormone receptor-positive patients (ATAC Trialists' Group, 2007). There was no difference noted in overall survival. (HR = 0.97, P = 0.7) [49].

The ATAC trial also demonstrated a carry-over benefit, similar to that described in long-term follow-up of the tamoxifen trials (reviewed above). The absolute differences in the time to recurrence increased from 2.8% (anastrozole 9.7% versus tamoxifen 12.5%) at 5 years to 4.8% at 9 years (anastrozole 17% versus 21.8%) (HR=0.76, [95%CI = 0.67–0.87] P = 0.0001). Other treatment outcomes including distant metastases (HR = 0.84, [95%CI = 0.72–0.97], P=0.022) and contralateral breast cancers (HR = .60, [95%CI = 0.42–0.85], P=0.004) also demonstrated a carry over effect with a greater long-term magnitude of benefit by the use of anastrozole in comparison to tamoxifen. There was no difference in deaths following recurrence or overall survival between the

Table 3 Summary of the adjuvant aromatase inhibitor studies

	ATAC	BIG 1-98	MA-17	ARNO 95	ABCSG 8	ITA	IES
AI vs comparator	Anastrozole vs tamoxifen	Letrozole vs tamoxifen	Letrozole vs placebo	Anastrozole vs tamoxifen	Anastrozole vs tamoxifen	Anastrozole vs tamoxifen	Exemestane vs tamoxifen
Setting	Initial adjuvant	Initial adjuvant	Extended adjuvant	Sequential adjuvant	Sequential adjuvant	Sequential adjuvant	Sequential adjuvant
Median follow-up (months)	100	25.8	54	30.1	31.1 following switch	64	58
DFS, HR, p value	ITT:0.86 p=0.022 HR + : 0.84 p=0.022	0.81 p=0.003	ITT: 0.64 p=0.00003	0.66 p=0.049	0.61 p=0.01	0.57 p=0.005	ITT: 0.76 p=0.0001 ER + /?: 0.75 p=0.0001
OS, HR, p value	0.97 p=0.7	0.86 p=0.16	ITT:1.0 p=0.99	0.53 p=0.045	No difference	0.56 p=0.1	ITT: 0.85 (p=0.08) ER+/?: 0.83 (p=0.05)
Contralateral breast cancer	HR 0.6, p=0.004	Not reported	HR 0.61 p=0.037	Not reported	No difference	No difference	ITT:0.56 p=0.04 ER + /?: 0.55 p=0.03
Ischemic cardiovascular disease	No difference	2.1 vs 1.1% in favor of tamoxifen p<0.0001	Not reported	Not reported	No difference	No difference	No statistically significatn difference in MI, angina, or CVA observed

Table 3 (continued)

	ATAC	BIG 1-98	MA-17	ARNO 95	ABCSG 8	ITA	IES
Subgroup analysis		Letrozole more effective in ER+/ PR+ subgroup	Survival benefit seen in ER+ disease. Longer duration of letrozole use associated with greater benefit. Postunblinding: Improved DFS, DDFS, OS, CBC	Survival benefit seen in meta-analysis of ARNO/ ABCSG/ ITA: HR 0.71; p=0.038.	Survival benefit seen in meta-analysis of ARNO/ ABCSG/ ITA: HR 0.71; p=0.038.	Survival benefit seen in meta-analysis of ARNO/ ABCSG/ ITA: HR 0.71; p=0.038.	Survival benefit seen in ER+ /unknown subset.

two arms. Analysis for the combination arm was discontinued due to no outcomes differences at the first interim analysis [49].

Anastrozole was associated with statistically significantly fewer hot flashes, less vaginal bleeding/discharge and endometrial cancer, as well as fewer ischemic cerebrovascular events, and venous thromboembolic events compared with tamoxifen. There continues to be no difference in ischemic cardiovascular disease between anastrozole and tamoxifen at the 9-year follow-up. There was a statistically significant increase in joint symptoms and fractures in the anastrozole arm [49].

Bone loss is a known consequence of AI use. In the ATAC bone sub-protocol, patients assigned to anastrozole had a decrease in bone mineral density (BMD) at the lumbar spine and hip from baseline, whereas patients randomized to tamoxifen had an increase in BMD. Although half of the patients randomized to anastrozole with normal bone mineral density at baseline became osteopenic at 5 years, no patients in this group became osteoporotic. In the patients with baseline osteopenia receiving anastrozole, very few became osteoporotic [50]. These data are somewhat reassuring and suggest that patients with normal BMD at baseline may not need yearly bone density measurements. Also reassuring are data from the 100-month follow-up. The incidence of fractures decreased after completion of 5 years of anastrozole, and the fracture rate in the two groups was equivalent at 9 years [49].

Breast International Group (BIG) 1-98 Study

This phase III, four arm randomized multi-national study involved 8,028 postmenopausal women with hormone receptor-positive, node-positive or -negative disease who were randomized between 1998 and 2003 to tamoxifen for 5 years (arm A), letrozole for 5 years (arm B), tamoxifen for 2 years followed by letrozole for 3 years (arm C), or letrozole for 2 years followed by tamoxifen for 3 years (arm D). After a median follow-up of 25.8 months, the upfront letrozole arms (B and D) were compared to the upfront tamoxifen arms (A and C). The 5-year DFS was 84% versus 81.4% in favor of the letrozole arms ($HR = 0.81$, $P = 0.003$). There was no difference in relative benefit between women whose tumors were ER/PR positive and those whose tumors were ER positive/PR negative in this study.

Fractures were more common in the letrozole group (5.7% versus 4.0%, $P<0.001$). Letrozole was associated with statistically fewer thromboembolic events, vaginal bleeding, fewer endometrial biopsies, and endometrial cancers. Arthralgias were more common in the letrozole arm (any grade 20.3%) than in the tamoxifen arm (any grade 12.3%), $p<0.001$. There was, however, an increased incidence of grade 3, 4, or 5 cardiac events in the letrozole group compared to the tamoxifen group (2.1% versus 1.1%, $P<0.001$) [18, 51]. The authors speculated that this may be due in part to the protective effect of tamoxifen on arteries, but concluded that there was insufficient information to fully determine the effect of AIs on cardiovascular disease. Longer follow-up of this study will provide additional follow-up on efficacy and toxicity, as well as assess the optimal role of sequential endocrine agents compared with endocrine monotherapy. This is the only study that examines 2–3 years of an aromatase inhibitor followed by a switch to a SERM (arm D).

Tamoxifen for 2–3 Years Prior to Switching to Aromatase Inhibitors

There have been four studies that have examined the role of aromatase inhibitors after 2–3 years of tamoxifen. Three studies used anastrozole after tamoxifen (Italian Tamoxifen-Arimidex Trial [ITA], the Austrian Breast and Colorectal Cancer Study Group trial 8 [ABCSG8], and the Arimidex-Nolvadex 95 study [ARNO95]) [52–58]. One study utilized exemestane after 2–3 years of tamoxifen (Intergroup Exemestane Study [IES]) [59, 60].

The rationale for switching from a SERM to an AI is based on several concepts. First, tamoxifen use is associated with rare though potentially adverse life-threatening events including thromboembolic events. Limiting the duration of tamoxifen use may decrease the overall number of adverse events. Second, primary tamoxifen resistance in hormone receptor-positive tumors has been described, in addition to secondary tamoxifen resistance and tamoxifen-induced tumor growth [61]. These reasons may explain why longer durations of tamoxifen use have not been beneficial [62]. Therefore, switching from tamoxifen to another endocrine-based therapy may improve long-term outcome with fewer complications.

Italian Tamoxifen–Arimidex Trial (ITA)

The ITA study was an open label, prospective study of 448 women with hormone receptor-positive, lymph node-positive disease who were randomized if free of recurrence *after* completion of 2–3 years of tamoxifen to continue on tamoxifen or switch to anastrozole. After a median follow-up of 36 months from randomization, the anastrozole group experienced an improvement in recurrence-free survival (HR = 0.35, P = 0.0002). Overall, more adverse events were recorded in the anastrozole arm (203 versus 150, P = 0.04), though there was fewer life-threatening events or events that required hospitalization (33 of 150 events versus 28 of 203 events) [53].

Updated results after 64 months of median follow-up continue to show improvement in DFS (HR 0.57, P = 0.005) in favor of the anastrozole arm. There was no difference in cardiovascular events, although significantly more patients who switched to anastrozole had an increase in cholesterol levels (1.4% versus 8.1%, P = 0.01) [54].

Austrian Breast and Colorectal Cancer Study Group Trial 8 (ABCSG8) and the Arimidex-Nolvadex 95 Study (ARNO95)

A combined analysis of two prospective, multi-center, randomized trials (ABCSG trial 8 and ARNO 95) demonstrated efficacy in favor of anastrozole over tamoxifen. Both studies involved postmenopausal women with hormone receptor-positive breast cancer who had completed 2 years of adjuvant tamoxifen followed by 3 years of anastrozole versus tamoxifen for 5 years. Two thirds of patients were lymph node negative. After a median follow-up of 28 months, a 40% decrease in the risk for an event was seen in the anastrozole group compared to the tamoxifen group (HR = 0.60, P = 0.0009). No difference in overall survival was reported at the 2005 publication between the two groups. The side effects noted in this study were similar to the other anastrozole versus tamoxifen studies demonstrating a statistically significant increase in fractures (P = 0.015) and fewer thromboses (P = 0.034) in favor of the anastrozole arm [55].

The first report of an improvement in overall survival with the aromatase inhibitors came from a meta-analysis of the three trials switching to anastrozole (ARNO 95, ABCSG 8, and ITA), which included 3,500 patients. As reported with each individual trial, there was a statistically significant improvement in DFS in the meta-analysis (HR = 0.59, P<0.0001). With an increased number of patients in the meta-analysis, an improvement in overall survival for the first time was reported with the use of AIs. A 29% improvement in overall survival (HR = 0.71, P = 0.0377) was seen in the switching arm compared to the tamoxifen arm [57].

Individual updates of the ARNO 95 and ABCSG 8 trials were also recently reported. The ABCSG trial 8 randomized patients *after* surgery to 5 years of tamoxifen or tamoxifen for 2 years followed by anastrozole for 3 years. This was the only study that randomized patients to switch *prior* to starting any hormonal therapy. The primary end point of this study is event free survival. After a median follow-up of 31.1 months following the switch, event-free survival was associated with a HR of 0.61 (P = 0.01). The number of events in the first 2 years (prior to the switch) was non-statistically in favor of the group randomized to tamoxifen with 24 versus 29 events in the tamoxifen followed by anastrozole arm. After the switch, statistically significantly more events occurred in the tamoxifen arm (HR = 0.63, P = 0.010). Overall, 5-year analysis of ABCSG Trial 8 showed the event-free survival to be superior, though diluted due to the events in the first 2 years, in the switching arm with a HR of 0.68, P = 0.02 [56]. An improvement in OS has not yet been seen in this study.

In contrast to ABCSG Trial 8, the ARNO95 Trial randomized 979 patients after they had received 2 years of adjuvant tamoxifen to continued tamoxifen for an additional 3 years or switch to anastrozole. Interim analysis at 30.1 months median follow-up demonstrated statistically significant improvements in DFS and for the first time in overall survival (HR = 0.53, P = 0.045) [58].

Intergroup Exemestane Study (IES)

This international study randomized 4,742 postmenopausal women with ER+/unknown, node-positive or -negative breast cancer who remained disease free after 2–3 years of tamoxifen to either continue tamoxifen for a total of 5 years or switch to exemestane to complete a total of 5 years of treatment. A 32% reduction in breast cancer recurrence was seen at 3 years (HR 0.68, $P<0.001$) [52]. Thromboembolic events were statistically increased in the tamoxifen group. The incidence of cardiac deaths was similar in both groups.

When updated at 58 months of median follow-up, an analysis excluding 2.5% of patients ultimately found to have ER-negative disease after enrollment was performed. A statistically significant improvement in OS was seen in the ER-positive/unknown group (HR 0.83, $P=0.05$) compared to the intention to treat analysis group (HR 0.85, $P=0.08$). Patients who switched to exemestane had a higher incidence of myocardial infarction than patients who remained on tamoxifen (1.3% versus 0.8), which did not meet statistical significance ($P=0.08$) [59]. In this study, patients were not stratified according to cardiovascular risk factors. There was no difference in quality of life in regards to hot flashes, night sweats, weight gain, loss of libido, or diarrhea. There was a statistical difference in the incidence of vaginal discharge in favor of exemestane ($P=0.002$) [60].

Extended Adjuvant Hormonal Therapy

The risk of breast cancer recurrence continues for an indefinite period after primary surgical, radiotherapy, and systemic adjuvant therapy in hormone receptor-positive disease [63]. Over half of all recurrences and deaths occur 5 years after breast cancer diagnosis [26]. In the early 1990s, extended tamoxifen was felt to be no better than 5 years of use and was associated with increased side effects [29]. Data from the ECOG studies demonstrated that recurrences in ER-positive patients were most frequently seen in the first 3 years after diagnosis, but continued through year 12 [64]. Breast cancer growth requires estrogen, so suppression of estrogen production by extension of adjuvant therapy with subsequent aromatase inhibitors was postulated to lower risk of recurrence without the adverse side effects associated with extended tamoxifen.

Two studies were designed to examine the use of aromatase inhibitors after 5 years of initial tamoxifen use. Due to the robustness of the data favoring letrozole use, MA-17 was unblinded in 2003. As a result, the other extended AI study, NSABP B-33 that looked at exemestane use after 5 years of tamoxifen, was also unblinded and patients receiving placebo were allowed to switch to exemestane.

MA-17 Extended Adjuvant Study

This phase III study randomized women who had completed approximately 5 years of adjuvant tamoxifen therapy to letrozole or placebo for 5 years. The study was stopped early in 2003 after its primary end point of improved disease-free survival had been met. Four-year disease-free survival was 93% versus 87% ($P \leq 0.001$) in favor of the group receiving letrozole. The side-effect profile of letrozole was similar to the other aromatase inhibitor studies. The incidence of osteoporosis was not statistically different, and the rates of fracture were similar between the two groups [65]. Updated results at 48 months showed an improvement in overall survival in the lymph node-positive subset (HR = 0.61, P = 0.04) [66].

In an intent to treat (ITT) analysis, the hazard ratios for events in DFS and distant disease-free survival (DDFS) progressively decreased over time favoring letrozole with the trend being statistically significant ($P<0.0001$ and $P=0.0013$, respectively) up to 48 months. The DFS hazard ratio progressively decreased in favor of letrozole (HR = 0.52 at 12 months to HR = 0.19 at 48 months, $P<0.0001$) indicating a greater letrozole benefit over the time period examined. In addition, in the node-positive subset, a trend toward improved overall survival ($P=0.038$) was seen [67, 68]. In the node-negative subset, an improved trend was seen only in DFS but not in DDFS or overall survival [66].

An intent to treat (ITT) analysis after 54 months median follow-up continued to show a decreasing hazard radio in DFS in favor of letrozole (HR = 0.64; $P=0.00003$) as well as DDFS (HR = 0.76; $P=0.045$) despite the fact that 73% of patients switched to letrozole at the time the study was unblinded [68]

After 2003, the patients who had completed 5 years of tamoxifen and who had initially been randomized to the placebo arm were offered letrozole. Over 1,600 women accepted letrozole treatment. The women who switched from placebo to letrozole tended to be younger, had more advanced disease, a worse performance status, and were more likely to have received adjuvant chemotherapy. Results from this analysis showed that patients who were off adjuvant hormonal therapy from 1 to 7 years prior to unblinding derived a benefit from switching to letrozole even though there was the hiatus in adjuvant therapy. At a median follow-up of 5.3 years from initial randomization, an improvement in DFS (HR = 0.39; $P<0.0001$), DDFS (HR = 0.37; $P=0.0008$), OS (HR = 0.32; $P<0.0001$), and contralateral breast cancer (HR = 0.21; $P=0.012$) was seen in favor of patients who crossed over to letrozole [66]. Patients who received letrozole following a “prolonged delay” after completing tamoxifen therapy had improved outcomes associated with letrozole administration. Therefore, consideration should be given to re-starting adjuvant hormonal therapy with an AI in patients who have been off endocrine therapy with tamoxifen from 1 to 5 years. It is still unclear which subsets are more likely to benefit from re-starting treatment and whether the duration off tamoxifen or LN positivity have any impact.

Another unanswered question is the optimal total duration of adjuvant endocrine therapy in general, and specifically, the optimal duration of the AI. As previously noted, it appears that extending adjuvant therapy with letrozole beyond 5 years of tamoxifen confers greater benefit with a statistically significant trend in DFS and DDFS hazard ratios out to 48 months [65]. Longer treatment duration, therefore, appears to be beneficial in this scenario. Whether 5 years of tamoxifen followed by 5 years of an AI is to be preferred over a switching strategy of tamoxifen to an AI (total therapy of 5 years) or a "few" years of tamoxifen then 5 years of an AI remains unsettled.

An extension of MA-17 is being conducted in which women receiving 5 years of letrozole are re-randomized again to stop or continue the drug for 5 more years. In addition, NSABP B42 will investigate the role of letrozole in the extended adjuvant setting. Postmenopausal patients will be randomized to letrozole or placebo after completing 5 years of adjuvant hormonal therapy.

NSABP B-33

This study was designed as a phase III placebo-controlled study of postmenopausal women who had completed 5 years of tamoxifen, randomized to continue hormonal therapy with exemestane or placebo. B-33 was prematurely stopped in 2003 after 1,598 women had been randomized due to the unblinding of MA-17. Of the 1,598 patients randomized, 52% had lymph node-negative disease and 49% were under the age of 60. After unblinding, 560 of the 783 patients remained on exemestane, while 344 patients originally randomized to placebo switched to exemestane. After a median follow-up of 30 months, a trend toward improvement in DFS (RR = 0.68, p = 0.07), RFS (96% versus 94%; RR = 0.44; p = 0.004) was seen in favor of the original exemestane arm. No improvement in OS was seen (RR = 1.2, P = 0.63) [70]. Despite early termination of this study, and crossover to exemestane, original exemestane assignment was associated with improved DFS and RFS in a magnitude similar to that seen in MA-17.

Other Adjuvant Hormonal Studies

The results from a number of studies of drug choice, duration, and/or sequence are not yet mature. They address direct upfront AI comparisons, extended treatment with AIs, and re-treatment with AIs after a prolonged treatment break.

MA.27

Postmenopausal women with hormone receptor-positive disease are randomized to anastrozole versus exemestane for 5 years. This study was activated in 2003 and has completed accrual.

FACE Trial

This adjuvant upfront AI study randomized women with node-positive disease to letrozole versus anastrozole for 5 years. The study was activated in 2005 and completed accrual in early 2008.

NSABP B-42

This study activated in 2006 has an accrual goal of 3,840 postmenopausal patients who will be randomized to letrozole or placebo after completing 5 years of adjuvant hormonal therapy. Patients completing 5 years of an aromatase inhibitor or 2–3 years of tamoxifen followed by an AI will be eligible for this study.

US Oncology Study

In an upcoming study to be sponsored by US Oncology, women who have completed tamoxifen who are currently not on hormonal treatment will be given an AI versus placebo. This study will serve to validate the MA-17 finding of benefit from an AI after a prolonged hiatus of hormonal treatment.

TEAM

The TEAM trial is a multi-national, phase III trial being conducted in approximately 4,400 postmenopausal women with ER-positive and/or PR-positive early breast cancer. Patients are randomized to receive exemestane or tamoxifen as upfront adjuvant monotherapy for 5 years. The primary end point is DFS, with secondary end points of OS, contralateral breast cancer, and safety. Due to the results of the IES study, this study was amended to allow patients who had received 2–3 years of tamoxifen to be switched to exemestane.

SOLE Trial

The SOLE trial is an international study randomizing women who have completed tamoxifen and are not currently on any hormonal treatment to be given letrozole versus placebo in an attempt to further elucidate the use of an AI after intervals of no treatment following tamoxifen [71].

Weighing Options for Adjuvant Hormonal Therapy

What is the optimal sequence of hormonal therapy in a postmenopausal woman? Should women start off with an aromatase inhibitor, switch after 2–3 years of tamoxifen treatment, or switch after 5 years of tamoxifen? At this point, there is no clear answer based on evidence from prospective clinical trials. Guidelines have been published to assist medical oncologists on this aspect of adjuvant hormonal treatment.

Guidelines and Panel Recommendations

American Society of Clinical Oncology (ASCO) Guidelines

The ASCO updated guidelines published in 2005 concluded that optimal adjuvant hormonal therapy for a postmenopausal woman with hormone receptor-positive breast cancer includes an aromatase inhibitor as either initial therapy or after treatment with tamoxifen. Whether the initial tamoxifen duration should be a few years or 5 years remains uncertain as is whether there might be a benefit to the specific sequencing of the therapies. This technology assessment acknowledges our limited knowledge of long-term side effects of AI use [72].

NCCN Guidelines

The National Cancer Center Network (NCCN) guidelines [73] have incorporated the ASCO guidelines by including aromatase inhibitors into the treatment of postmenopausal women with early-stage breast cancer. Premenopausal women are offered tamoxifen for 2–3 years, and menopausal status is re-assessed. Those who remain premenopausal complete 5 years of tamoxifen when reassessment of menopausal status is again performed. Those who remain premenopausal receive no additional therapy. Those who become postmenopausal after 5 years of tamoxifen can be offered letrozole for 5 years. Women who become postmenopausal after 2–3 years may be offered a switch to exemestane or anastrozole to complete a total of 5 years of therapy or may complete a total of 5 years of tamoxifen prior to switching to letrozole for 5 years. Postmenopausal women may be treated with upfront anastrozole or letrozole, or started on tamoxifen for 2–3 years before switching to exemestane or anastrozole to complete a total of 5 years. Alternatively, tamoxifen may be used for 4.5–6 years and then switched to letrozole [72]. It is controversial whether the duration of the AI after a few years of tamoxifen should be that required to complete a total of 5 years of therapy with all agents, or a total of 5 additional years of the AI. Tamoxifen for 5 years is an option only for women with a contraindication or who decline aromatase inhibitors.

St. Gallen Guidelines

The 2005 St. Gallen expert consensus meeting highlighted breast cancer endocrine responsiveness [74]. Three categories (endocrine responsive, endocrine non-responsive, and tumors of uncertain endocrine responsiveness) were acknowledged. These categories were further divided according to menopausal status and level of risk. The panel recommended adjuvant chemotherapy for endocrine non-responsive patients.

For the premenopausal, low-risk endocrine responsive/uncertain groups, tamoxifen, ovarian function suppression, or no treatment were suggested.

Options for the low-risk postmenopausal women included tamoxifen, an AI or no treatment. For premenopausal, intermediate-risk patients in the endocrine responsive/uncertain group, tamoxifen or chemotherapy followed by tamoxifen with or without OFS, or OFS alone were suggested options. In the postmenopausal, intermediate-risk endocrine responsive/uncertain group, either tamoxifen, an AI or chemotherapy followed by tamoxifen or an AI were reasonable options, along with switching at 2–3 years to anastrozole or exemestane or after 5 years to letrozole.

The premenopausal, high-risk women were encouraged to have chemotherapy followed by tamoxifen with or without OFS, or chemotherapy followed by OFS plus an AI if there is a medical contraindication to tamoxifen use. In postmenopausal high-risk women with endocrine-responsive/uncertain disease, chemotherapy followed by tamoxifen, an AI, or sequential hormonal treatment with tamoxifen for 2–3 years followed by a switch to anastrozole or exemestane were options. Switching to letrozole after 5 years of tamoxifen was also a reasonable choice.

The St. Gallen 2007 conference echoed similar opinions as in 2005. In addition, panelists concluded that adjuvant endocrine treatment for patients with hormone-responsive breast cancer is mandatory and is not a matter of controversy. The agent of choice, timing, duration, and combination continues to be a matter of debate [75].

Decision-Making Models

Two decision-making models have been proposed to assist in the adjuvant endocrine therapy choice. To determine benefit of sequential versus upfront AI use, the first model suggested that sequential tamoxifen followed by a crossover to an AI at 2.5 years provided a modest improvement in DFS compared to either drug alone or crossing over after 5 years of tamoxifen [76]. This result contradicts the United Kingdom's model that used time to recurrence as the end point rather than DFS. In that model, upfront AI use was deemed more favorable than sequential AI use [77]. Fortunately, prospective results from the four-arm BIG 1-98 study will shed some light on the optimal sequencing of hormonal agents.

Theoretical Considerations

Proponents of using an aromatase inhibitor upfront state that the use of the better agent upfront will minimize the risk of early relapse. If tamoxifen is chosen as the upfront regimen, patients may be at increased risk of relapse in the first 3 years prior to the switch. Upfront AI also avoids the potentially life-threatening side effects with tamoxifen such as thromboembolic events, ischemic cerebrovascular events, and endometrial cancer which are not associated with the AIs. Proponents of the switch (from tamoxifen to an AI) approach note, however, that side effects will be minimized due to differing side-effect profiles of the SERMs and AIs and that the short-term losses will be compensated by the long-term gains. Patients who have not relapsed after 2 years of tamoxifen may be less likely to develop tamoxifen resistance if they are switched to an aromatase inhibitor at year 2–3.

Overall Survival Data from Clinical Trials

Thus far, improvements in overall survival have been seen only in the switching studies. Survival benefit has not been demonstrated in the upfront aromatase inhibitor studies despite long-term follow-up. Updates from two switching studies (IES and ARNO) have reported OS benefits as did the extended hormonal trial (MA-17) involving a switch after 5 years of tamoxifen. The lack of survival benefit for the overall group seen in some of these trials, such as MA.17 and B-33, probably relates to the fact that these studies were closed early because of results on disease-free survival, which crossed O'Brian–Fleming boundaries for early termination of the studies. Following this, women on the placebo arms were given the active drug, thereby greatly reducing any chance of survival benefit eventually being seen.

Proponents of upfront AI use point out that it required greater than 10 years of follow-up to demonstrate a survival benefit in the tamoxifen versus placebo studies. Further follow-up is required for all of these studies to better define optimal adjuvant endocrine therapy.

Impact of Drug Metabolism Phenotype on Adjuvant Hormonal Choice

Endoxifen, a metabolite of tamoxifen, is thought to play an important role in the anti-cancer effect of tamoxifen. The CYP2D6 enzyme plays an important role in the conversion of tamoxifen to endoxifen. Patients who have a genetic variation associated with the CYP2D6 poor metabolizer phenotype (CYP2D6*4/*4) and therefore lack functional CYP2D6 have a higher risk of relapse while on tamoxifen [78]. Compared to intermediate metabolizers or extensive metabolizers, poor metabolizers of CYP2D6 or those on medications causing CYP2D6 inhibition, had a significantly worse time to recurrence and disease-free survival [79]. Therefore, patients that are poor metabolizers of CYP2D6 perhaps should not receive tamoxifen. Patients on tamoxifen should not also be on medications (fluoxetine, paroxetine, sertraline, cimetidine, and amiodarone) that inhibit CYP2D6. There are also data emerging on the pharmacogenetics of AIs, so that trials are being planned to select optimal first-line agent (tamoxifen or AI) based on drug metabolism phenotypes.

Toxicity Considerations and Choice of Agent

Both tamoxifen and the aromatase inhibitors may increase the incidence of hot flashes. They differ in many other respects. SERMs have estrogenic effects on bones, by increasing bone mineral density and reducing bone fractures. Their estrogenic effect on the uterine lining increases the risk for the development of endometrial cancer. SERMs are also associated with an increased incidence of thromboembolic events compared to the AIs.

All AIs are associated with a decrease in bone mineral density and an increased incidence of musculoskeletal complaints (5–10%, ranging from mild to severe) when compared to tamoxifen. Unlike tamoxifen, AIs are not associated with an increased risk of endometrial cancer or thromboembolism.

An important concern regarding the use of aromatase inhibitors in postmenopausal women is the incidence of cardiovascular disease. Although the numbers are small, BIG 1-98 showed a statistically significant increase in grade 3, 4, or 5 cardiac events (2.1% versus 1.1%, $P<0.0001$) [20]. It is possible that tamoxifen's cholesterol-lowering effect may have resulted in a cardioprotective effect in the tamoxifen-treated group. Hypercholesterolemia was reported in 43.6% of patients treated with letrozole versus 19.2% of patients treated with tamoxifen [20]. The IES study also demonstrated an increased incidence of cardiac events, which did not meet statistical significance in the exemestane treatment arm [52].

Further follow-up of all AI studies is needed to fully elucidate the long-term effects of this class of medications.

Summary and Unanswered Questions

Both the tamoxifen and the aromatase inhibitors have an established role in the adjuvant treatment of breast cancer. How to best utilize them is still unclear. An improvement in DFS is seen in the upfront and sequential treatment from the AIs. However, OS has been described only in the sequential studies and is not yet seen in the upfront AI studies. Although there are now hints of a carry-over benefit to the AIs, this is established for tamoxifen 5–10 years after therapy has stopped and must be considered in the equation of treatment choice as well.

What is the optimal duration and sequence of aromatase inhibitor therapy in relation to tamoxifen, or with no tamoxifen at all? Are all the aromatase inhibitors equally efficacious as upfront adjuvant treatment or as sequential treatment after tamoxifen? What is the best AI to use upfront? What are the long-term side effects of continued AI use? Is there an optimal patient subset that can be identified that can predict who will benefit from AI use versus tamoxifen use? In premenopausal women rendered postmenopausal with the use of LHRH agonists, are AIs efficacious? These are among the many questions that remain unanswered. A better understanding of the biology of SERM and AI resistance and how to counteract it will impact on our use of these agents in the future.

Given the heterogeneity of hormone receptor-positive breast cancer, one strategy is unlikely to fit all tumors and patients. More information from clinical trials with biomarker correlates, currently underway, will assist in the appropriate tailoring of adjuvant hormonal treatment. For now, it is not unreasonable to tailor adjuvant hormonal treatment based on the individual's co-morbidities and anticipated side effects from the drug while bearing well in mind long-term survival outcomes reported to date.

References

1. Retrieved June 16, 2008, from American Cancer Society Website: http://www.cancer.org,
2. Osborne CK. Adjuvant Endocrine Therapy in Diseases of the Breast, 3rd ed. Lippincott Philadelphia, 2004. Chapter 53. p 870.
3. Beatson GW. On the treatment of inoperable carcinoma of the mamma: suggestions for a new method of treatment with illustrative cases. Lancet 1896;2:104.
4. Vogel VG, Costantino JP, Wickerham DL, et al. Effects of tamoxifen vs raloxifene on the risk of developing invasive breast cancer and other disease outcomes. The NSABP study of tamoxifen and raloxifene (STAR) P-2 Trial. JAMA 2006;295:2727–2741.
5. Vogel VG. Chemoprevention: reducing breast cancer risk. In Vogel VG (ed) *Management of patients at high risk for breast cancer*. Malden, MA: Blackwell Science Inc., 2001, pp 201–227.
6. Port ER, Montgomery LL, Heerdt AS, et al. Patient reluctance toward tamoxifen use for breast cancer primary prevention. Ann Surg Oncol. 2001;8:580–585.
7. Melnikow J, Paterniti D, Azart R, et al. Preferences of women evaluating risks of tamoxifen (POWER) study of preferences for tamoxifen for breast cancer risk reduction. Cancer 2005;103:1996–2005.
8. Tchou J, Hou N, Rademaker A, et al. Acceptance of tamoxifen chemoprevention by physicians and women at risk. Cancer 2004:100:1800–1806.
9. Taylor R, Taguchi K. Tamoxifen for breast cancer chemoprevention: low uptake by high-risk women after evaluation of a breast lump. Ann Fam Med. 2005:3:242–247.
10. Gail MH, Brinton LA, Byar DP, Corle DK. Projecting individualized probabilities of developing breast cancer for white females who are being examined annually. *J Natl Cancer Inst*. 1989;81:1879–1886.
11. Fisher B, Costantino JP, Wickerham DL, Redmond CK. Tamoxifen for prevention of breast cancer: report of the national surgical adjuvant breast and bowel project P-1 study. *J Natl Cancer Inst*. 1998;90:1371–1388.
12. Fisher B, Costantino JP, Wickerham DL, et al. Tamoxifen for the prevention of breast cancer: current status of the national surgical adjuvant breast and bowel project P-1 study. JNCI 2005;97:1652–1662.
13. Powles T, Eeles R, Ashley S, Easton D, Chang J, Dowsett M, Tidy, A, Viggers, J, Davey J. Interim analysis of the incidence of breast cancer in the Royal Marsden Hospital tamoxifen randomized chemoprevention trial. The Lancet 1998;352:98–101

14. Powles TJ, Ashley S, Tidy A, Smith IE, Dowsett M. Twenty-year follow-up of the Royal Marsden randomized, double-blinded tamoxifen breast cancer prevention trial, JNCI 2007;99:283–290.
15. Cuzick J, Forbes J, Edwards R, Baum M. First results form the International Breast Cancer Intervention Study (IBIS-1): a randomized prevention trial. *The Lancet* 2002;360:817–824.
16. Cuzick J, Forbes JF, Sestak I, Cawthorn S, Hamed H, Holli K, Howell A. International Breast Cancer Intervention Study I investigators. Long-term results of tamoxifen prophylaxis for breast cancer-96-month follow-up of the randomized IBIS-I trial. JNCI 2007;99:272–282.
17. Veronesi U, Maisonneuve P, Costa A, Sacchini V, Maltoni C, Robertson C, Rotmensz N, Boyle P. Prevention of breast cancer with tamoxifen: preliminary findings from the Italian randomized trial among hysterectomized women. The Lancet 1998:352–93
18. Veronesi, U, Maisonneuve P, Rotmensz N, Bonanni B, Boyle P, Viale G, Costa A, Sacchini V, Travaglini R, D'Aiuto G, Oliviero P, Lovison F, Gucciardo G, del Turco MR, Muraca MG, Pizzichetta MA, Conforti S, Decensi A. Italian tamoxifen study group tamoxifen for the prevention of breast cancer: late results of the Italian randomized tamoxifen prevention trial among women with hysterectomy. JNCI 2007;99:727–737.
19. The ATAC Trialists'Group. Anastrozole alone or in combination with tamoxifen versus tamoxifen alone for adjuvant treatment of postmenopausal women with early breast cancer: first results of the ATAC randomized trial. Lancet 2002;359:2131–2139.
20. The Breast International Group (BIG) 1-98 Collaborative Group. A Comparison of Letrozole and Tamoxifen in Postmenopausal Women with Early Breast Cancer. NEJM 2005;353:2747–57.
21. Muss HB, Case LD, Atkins JN, Bearden JD III, Cooper MR, Cruz JM, Jackson DV Jr., O'Rourke MA, Pavy MD, Powell BL. Tamoxifen versus high-dose oral medroxyprogesterone acetate as initial endocrine therapy for patients with metastatic breast cancer: a Piedmont Oncology Association study. JCO 1994;12:1630–1638.
22. Ingle JN; Krook JE; Green SJ, et al. Randomized trial of bilateral oophorectomy versus tamoxifen in premenopausal women with metastatic breast cancer. J Clin Oncol. 1986;Feb;4(2):178–185.
23. Ingle JN, Ahmann DL, Green SJ, et al. Randomized clinical trial of diethylstilbestrol versus tamoxifen in postmenopausal women with advanced breast cancer. N Engl J Med. 1981;Jan 1;304(1):16–21.
24. Sawka CA, Pritchard KI, Shelley W, et al. A randomized crossover trial of tamoxifen versus ovarian ablation for metastatic breast cancer in premenopausal women: a report of the National Cancer Institute of Canada Clinical Trials Group (NCIC CTG) trial MA.1. Breast Cancer Res Treat. 1997;Jul;44(3):211–215.
25. Fisher B, Costantino J, Redmond C. A randomized clinical trial evaluating tamoxifen in the treatment of patients with node negative breast cancer who have estrogen-receptor-positive tumors. NEJM 1989;320:479–484.
26. Early Breast Cancer Trialists' Collaborative Group (EBCTCG). Effects of chemotherapy and hormonal therapy for early breast cancer on recurrence and 15-year survival: an overview of the randomized trials. Lancet 2005;365:1687–1717.
27. Peto Richard for the Early Breast Cancer Trialists' Collaborative Group (EBCTG). The worldwide overview: Updated (2005–6) meta-analyses of trial results. Presented at the San Antonio Breast Cancer Symposium, 2007.
28. Controlled trial of tamoxifen as a single adjuvant agent in the management of early breast cancer. "Nolvadex" Adjuvant Trial Organisation. Br. J Cancer. 1988;57:608–611.
29. Fisher B, Dignam J, Bryant J, DeCillis A, Wickerham DL, Wolmark N, Costantinio J, Redmond C, Fisher ER, Bowman DM, Deschenes L, Dimitrov NV, Margolese RG, Robidoux A, Shibata H, Terz J, Paterson AH, Feldman MI, Farrar W, Evans J, Lickley Hl. Five versus more than five years of tamoxifen therapy for breast cancer patients with negative lymph nodes and estrogen receptor-positive tumors. JNCI 2001;93:684–690.

30. Adjuvant tamoxifen in the management of operable breast cancer: the Scottish Trial. Report from the Breast Cancer Trials Committee, Scottish Cancer Trials Office (MRC), Edinburgh. Lancet 1987;2:171–175.
31. Stewart HJ for the Scottish Cancer Trials Breast Group. The Scottish Trial of Adjuvant Tamoxifen in Node-Negative Breast Cancer. JNCI 1992;11:117–120.
32. Stewart HJ, Forrest AP, Everington D, et al. Randomised comparison of 5 years of adjuvant tamoxifen with continuous therapy for operable breast cancer. The Scottish Cancer Trials Breast Group. Br J Cancer. 1996;74:297–299.
33. Tormey DC, Gray R, Falkson HC. Postchemotherapy adjuvant tamoxifen therapy beyond five years in patients with lymph node-positive breast cancer. JNCI 1996;88:1828–1833.
34. Peto R, Davies C, on Behalf of the ATLAS Collaboration. ATLAS (Adjuvant Tamoxifen, Longer Against Shorter): international randomized trial of 10 versus 5 years of adjuvant tamoxifen among 11500 women – preliminary results. SABCS 2007, abstract 48.
35. Albain KS, Barlow W, O'Malley F, et al. Concurrent (CAFT) versus sequential (CAF-T) chemohormonal therapy (cyclophosphamide, doxorubicin, 5-fluorouracil, tamoxifen) versus T alone for postmenopausal, node-positive, estrogen (ER) and/or progesterone (PgR) receptor-positive breast cancer: mature outcomes and new biologic correlates on phase III intergroup trial 0100 (SWOG-8814). SABCS 2004, abstract #37.
36. Harris EE, Christensen VJ, Hwang WT, et al. Impact of concurrent versus sequential tamoxifen with radiation therapy in early-stage breast cancer patients undergoing breast conservation treatment. JCO 2005;23:11–16.
37. Ahn PH, Vu HT, Lannin D, et al. Sequence of radiotherapy with tamoxifen in conservatively managed breast cancer does not affect local relapse rates. JCO 2005;23:17–23.
38. Pierce LJ, Hutchins LF, Green SR, et al. Sequencing of tamoxifen and radiotherapy after breast-conserving surgery in early-stage breast cancer. JCO 2005;23:24–29.
39. Early Breast Cancer Trialists' Collaborative Group (2005) Effects of chemotherapy and hormonal therapy on recurrence and 15-year survival: an overview of the randomized trials. Lancet 365:1687–1717
40. Scottish Cancer Trials Breast Group and ICRF, Breast Unit, Guy's Hospital, London. Adjuvant ovarian ablation versus CMF chemotherapy in premenopausal women with pathological stage II breast carcinoma: the Scottish Trial. Lancet 1993:341:1293–1298.
41. Boccardo F, Robagotti A, Amoroso D, Mesiti M, Romeo D, Sismondi P, Giai M, Genta F, Pacini P, Distante V, Bolognesi A, Aldrighetti D, Farris A. Cyclophosphamide, methotrexate, and fluorouracil versus tamoxifen plus ovarian suppression as adjuvant treatment of estrogen receptor-positive pre-/perimenopausal breast cancer patients: results of the Italian Breast Cancer Adjuvant Study Group 02 randomized trial. J Clin Oncol. 2000;18:2718–2727.
42. Jakesz R, Hausmaninger H, Kubista E, Gnant M, Menzel C, Bauernhofer T, Seifert M, Haider K, Mlineritsch B, Steindorfer P, Kwasny W, Fridrik M, Steger G, Wette V, Samonigg H. Randomized adjuvant trial of tamoxifen and goserelin versus cyclophosphamide, methotrexate, and fluorouracil: evidence for the superiority of treatment with endocrine blockade in premenopausal patients with hormone-responsive breast cancer – Austrian Breast and Colorectal Cancer Study Group Trial 5. J Clin Oncol. 2002;20:4621–4627.
43. Jonat W, Kaufmann M, Sauerbrei W, Blamey R, Cuzick J, Namer M, Fogelman I, de Haes JC, de Matteis A, Stewart A, Eiermann W, Szakolczai I, Malmer M, Schumacher M, Geberth M, Lisboa B. Goserelin versus cyclophosphamide, methotrexate, and fluorouracil as adjuvant therapy in premenopausal patients with node-positive breast cancer: the Zoladex Early Breast Cancer Research Association Study. J Clin Oncol. 2002;20:4628–4635
44. International Breast Cancer Study Group .Adjuvant chemotherapy followed by goserelin versus either modality alone for premenopausal lymph node-negative breast cancer: a randomized trial. J Natl Cancer Inst. 2003;95:1833–1846

45. Davidson N, O'Neill A, Vukov A, Osborne CK, Martino S, White D, Abeloff MD. Chemohormonal therapy in premenopausal, node-positive, receptor positive breast cancer: an Eastern Cooperative Oncology Group Phase III Intergroup Trial (E5188, INT-0101). Proc Am Soc Clin Oncol. 2003;22:15a
46. LHRH-agonists in Early Breast Cancer Overview group. Lancet 2007;369:1711–1723.
47. The ATAC Trialists' Group. Anastrozole alone or in combination with tamoxifen versus tamoxifen alone for adjuvant treatment of postmenopausal women with early breast cancer. Results of the ATAC (Arimidex, Tamoxifen, Alone or in Combination) trial efficacy and safety update analyses. Cancer 2003;98:1802–1810.
48. The ATAC Trialists' Group. Results of the ATAC (Arimidex, Tamoxifen, Alone or in Combination) trial after completion of 5 years' adjuvant treatment for breast cancer. Lancet 2005;365:60–62.
49. The ATAC Trialists' Group. Effect of anastrozole and tamoxifen as adjuvant treatment for early-stage breast cancer: 100 month analysis of the ATAC trial. Lancet, published on-line 1/08.
50. Coleman RE, on behalf of the ATAC Trialists' Group. Effect of anastrozole on bone mineral density: 5-year results from the 'Arimidex', Tamoxifen, Alone or in Combination (ATAC) trial. J Clin Oncol. 2006 ASCO Annual Meeting Proceedings Part I. Vol 24, No. 18S (June 20 Supplement), 2006: 511.
51. Ingle JN, Tu D, Pater JL, et al. Duration of letrozole treatment and outcomes in the placebo-controlled NCIC CTG MA.17 extended adjuvant therapy trial. Breast Cancer Res Treat. 2006;99:295–300.
52. Coombes RC, Hall E, Gibson LJ, et al. A randomized trial of exemestane after two to three years of tamoxifen therapy in postmenopausal women with primary breast cancer. NEJM 2004;350:1081–1092.
53. Boccardo F, Rubagotti A, Puntoni M, et al. Switching to anastrozole versus continued tamoxifen treatment of early breast cancer: preliminary results of the Italian tamoxifen anastrozole trial. JCO 2005;22:5138–5147.
54. Boccardo F, Fubagotti A, Guglielmini P, et al. Switching to anastrozole versus continued tamoxifen treatment of early breast cancer: updated results of the Italian tamoxifen anastrozole (ITA) trial. Ann Oncol. 2006;17:supplement 7:vii10–vii14.
55. Jakesz R, Jonat W, Gnant M, et al. Switching of postmenopausal women with endocrine-responsive early breast cancer to anastrozole after 2 years' adjuvant tamoxifen: combined results of ABCSG trial 8 and ARNO 95 trial. Lancet 2005;366:455–462.
56. Jakesz R, Gnant M, Greil R, et al. The benefits of sequencing adjuvant tamoxifen and anastrozole in postmenopausal women with hormone-responsive early breast cancer: 5 year-analysis of ABCSG Trial 8. SABCS 2005 abstract #13.
57. Jonat W, Gnant M, Boccardo F, et al. Switching from adjuvant tamoxifen to anastrozole in postmenopausal women with hormone-responsive early breast cancer: a meta-analysis of the ARNO 95 trial, ABCSG Trial 8, and the ITA trial. SABCS 2005 abstract #18.
58. Kaufmann M, Jonat WW, Hilfrich J, et al. Survival benefit of switching to anatrozole after 2 years' treatment with tamoxifen versus continued tamoxifen therapy: the ARNO 95 study. ASCO 2006, abstract #547.
59. Coombes RC, Paridaens R, Jassem J, et al. First mature analysis of the Intergroup Exemestane Study. ASCO 2006, abstract #LBA527.
60. Fallowfield LJ, Bliss JM, Porter LS, et al. Quality of life in the Intergroup Exemestane Study: a randomized trial of exemestane versus continued tamoxifen after 2 to 3 years of tamoxifen in postmenopausal women with primary breast cancer. JCO 2006;20:910–7.
61. Clarke R, Leonessa F, Welch NJ, et al. Cellular and molecular pharmacology of anti-estrogen action and resistance. Pharmacol Rev. 2001;53:25–71.
62. Gottardis MM, Jordan VC. Development of tamoxifen stimulated growth of MCF-7 tumors in athymic mice after long-term antiestrogen administration. Cancer Res. 1988;48:5183–5187.

63. Early Breast Cancer Trialists' Collaborative Group. Systemic treatment of early breast cancer by hormonal, cytotoxic, or immune therapy: 133 randomised trials involving 31000 recurrences and 24000 deaths among 75000 women. Lancet 1992;339:71–85.
64. Saphner T, Tormey DC, Gray R. Annual hazard rates of recurrence for breast cancer after primary therapy. JCO 1996;14:2738–2746.
65. Goss PE, Ingle JN, Martino S, et al. A randomized trial of letrozole in postmenopausal women after five years of tamoxifen therapy for early-stage breast cancer. NEJM 2003;349:1793–1802.
66. Goss PE, Ingle JN, Martino S, et al. Randomized trial of letrozole following tamoxifen as extended adjuvant therapy in receptor-positive breast cancer: updated findings from NCIC CTG MA.17. J Natl Cancer Inst. 2005;97:1262–1271.
67. Ingle JN, Goss PE, Tu D. Analysis of duration of letrozole extended adjuvant therapy as measured by hazard ratios of disease recurrence over time for patients on NCIC CTG MA.17. SABCS 2005, abstract #17.
68. Ingle J, Tu D, Shepherd L, et al. NCIC CTG MA. 17: Intent to treat analysis (ITT) of randomized patients after a median follow-up of 54 months. J Clin Oncol. 2006 ASCO Annual Meeting Proceedings Part I. Vol 24, No. 18S (June 20 Supplement), 2006:549.
69. Goss PE, Ingle JN, Pater JL, et al. Late extended adjuvant treatment with letrozole improves outcome in women with early-stage breast cancer who complete 5 years of tamoxifen. JCO 2008;26;1949–1955.
70. Mamounas E, Jeong JH, Wickerham L, et al. Benefit from exemestane as extended adjuvant therapy after 5 years of adjuvant tamoxifen: intention-to-treat analysis of the national surgical adjuvant breast and bowel project B-33 trial. JCO 2008;26:1965–1971.
71. John Forbes, personal communication, 2008
72. Winer EP, Hudis C, Burstein HJ, et al. American Society of Clinical Oncology Technology assessment on the use of aromatase inhibitors as adjuvant therapy for postmenopausal women with hormone receptor-positive breast cancer: status report 2004. JCO 2005;23:619–629.
73. Retrieved June 16, 2008, from National Cancer Center Network Website: http://www.NCCN.org,
74. Goldhirsch A, Glick JH, Gelber RD, et al. Meeting highlights: international expert consensus on the primary therapy of early breast cancer 2005. Ann Oncol. 2005;16:1569–1583.
75. Rabaglio M, Aebi S, Castiglione-Gertsch M. Controversies of adjuvant endocrine treatment for breast cancer an recommendations of the 2007 St Gallen conference. Lancet Oncol. 2007;8:940–949.
76. Punglia RS, Kuntz KM, Winer EP, et al. Optimizing adjuvant endocrine therapy in postmenopausal women with early-stage breast cancer: a decision analysis. JCO 2005;23:5178–5187.
77. Cuzick J, Sasieni P, Howell A. Should aromatase inhibitors be used as initial adjuvant treatment or sequenced after tamoxifen? Br J Cancer. 2006;94:460–464.
78. Goetz MP, Rae JM, Suman VJ, et al. Pharmacogenetics of tamoxifen biotransformation is associated with clinical outcomes of efficacy and hot flashes. JCO 2005;23:9312–9318.
79. Knox SK, Ingle JN, Suman VJ, et al. Cytochrome P450 2D6 status predicts breast cancer relapse in women receiving adjuvant tamoxifen. ASCO 2006, abstract #504.

Biomarkers in Neoadjuvant Trials

Regina M. Fearmonti, Khandan Keyomarsi, and Kelly K. Hunt

Introduction

Neoadjuvant chemotherapy trials have consistently reported lower response rates in patients with hormone receptor-positive (HR+) breast cancers when compared with hormone receptor-negative (HR–) tumors. There are now many pharmacologic agents on the market for both the treatment and the prevention of breast cancer, while even more agents are being studied in the setting of clinical trials. Endocrine therapy is delivered in the neoadjuvant or adjuvant settings and in cases of advanced or metastatic disease. No available agent is free of adverse effects, however, and a mechanism by which to determine which patients will achieve the most benefit with the fewest side effects is needed. Biomarkers allow tumor characterization at the molecular level, providing additional information beyond grade and stage that assists the clinician with patient selection and in determining prognosis. A risk-benefit profile can thus be developed for each patient based on tumor-specific information, allowing the most effective therapeutic approach possible with the least possible morbidity.

Neoadjuvant studies provide a valuable setting in which to identify promising potential therapies without the large numbers of patients that are needed to assess benefit in adjuvant trials. The neoadjuvant approach also allows the clinician to assess response in an individual patient as well as identify those tumors that are resistant to therapy. They serve as a venue to obtain preliminary data on which to build the most promising agents to be moved to the adjuvant setting. Therapies targeted against tumor biological properties are an essential part of the individualized treatment of breast cancer. Characterization of reliable biomarkers is essential for the clinical translation of potential anti-cancer therapies, for in clinical trials these surrogate markers are essential for

K.K. Hunt (✉)
Department of Surgical Oncology, The University of Texas M. D. Anderson Cancer Center, 1515 Holcombe Boulevard, Unit 444, Houston, TX 77030, USA
e-mail: khunt@mdanderson.org

S.A.W. Fuqua (ed.), *Hormone Receptors in Breast Cancer*,
Cancer Treatment and Research 312, DOI 10.1007/978-0-387-09463-2_8,

determining whether a new drug has "hit its target" by providing some indication of therapeutic response and prognosis aside from interpreting complicated cell-signaling data. A review of completed trials and those trials currently underway is essential for understanding what has been gained from studying tumor biomarkers and what we can hope to gain in the next decade as other trials approach fruition. This chapter will review the role of hormones in breast tumorigenesis, agents available for targeting the hormone receptors, agents used in the adjuvant and neoadjuvant setting, and the role of biomarkers in assessing response to endocrine therapies.

Role of Hormones in Oncogenesis

Estrogen and its metabolites, progesterone, and other steroid hormones play a key role in breast tumorigenesis. This is best demonstrated by the association of hormone replacement therapy (HRT) with increased breast cancer risk. HRT is often used in postmenopausal patients to treat symptoms of estrogen withdrawal, notably vasomotor and urogenital symptoms and decreased libido. Its harmful effects have been evidenced in two large recent studies, and clinicians now consider that risk-benefit considerations do not favor the use of HRT for prevention of cardiovascular disease, bone fractures, or even short-term use to treat vasomotor symptoms. For over two decades the precise role of HRT—estrogen alone or estrogen plus progestin—on breast cancer was not known, as there was no evidence backed by a randomized prospective clinical trial on the effect of HRT on healthy postmenopausal women. The initial report from the Women's Health Initiative (WHI), a randomized, double-blind prospective trial encompassing 40 centers, compared an estrogen–progestin combination (conjugated equine estrogens [CEE] plus medroxyprogesterone acetate [MPA]) to placebo in otherwise healthy postmenopausal women. The trial was stopped early when potential benefits were exceeded by observed risks, which included increases in coronary heart disease and thromboembolic events as well as an increased frequency of abnormal mammograms and invasive breast cancers, with those cancers diagnosed at a more advanced stage. They observed approximately a 4% increase in abnormal mammograms after only 1 year of estrogen plus progestin use, and women who remained in the study for the 5.6-year median average duration had about a 10% chance of having an abnormal mammogram [1]. The doses and formulations of CEE and MPA used in the WHI, though standard clinical doses used in the United States at that time, gave rise to questions regarding the timing of initiation of therapy, dosage and formulations, and their relationship to breast cancer risk. The follow-up analysis of the WHI demonstrated that the breast cancers found in women taking estrogen plus progestin, compared with those in women taking the placebo, were comparable in grade, receptor status, and histology, but were significantly larger and associated more often with positive lymph nodes. These findings directly challenged the concept that cancers resulting from the use of estrogen plus progestin were early stage, had a more favorable prognosis, and were more easily treated [2].

The Million Women Study from the United Kingdom concluded that use of HRT was associated with an increased incidence of fatal breast cancers, with the combined effect of estrogen plus progesterone greater than the effect of estrogen monotherapy. The risk of breast cancer increased the longer a woman used HRT. Oral, transdermal, and implanted hormones also were associated with increased breast cancers. For the estrogen plus progestin combinations, similar effects were seen regardless of progestin constituent and regimen. Confirming the larger size and advanced stage reported for breast cancers seen with hormone use in the WHI, the British investigators reported, for the first time, an increased risk of breast cancer mortality associated with HRT [3].

More recent experimental and clinical studies have indicated that the adverse effects of HRT may largely depend on the estrogen and progesterone/progestin formulation, dosage, mode of administration, patient age, associated diseases, and duration of treatment. Cardiovascular events and increased risk of invasive breast cancers are higher with oral estrogen than with transdermal estradiol, as well as with many progestin compounds than with micronized progesterone. Similarly, recent observational studies suggest that long-term (>5 years) HRT, especially with an estrogen–progestin combination, is associated with increased breast cancer risk.

Taken together, the WHI trial and the Million Women Study provide compelling evidence regarding HRT use and the increased risk of developing potentially life-threatening breast cancer.

Rationale for Hormone-Targeted Therapy

Approximately 75% of all breast cancers express estrogen receptors (ER), progesterone receptors (PgR), or both. Likewise, tumors positive for ER or PgR demonstrate a response rate to endocrine therapies approaching 50%, compared to response rates of <10% observed in ER- and PgR-negative tumors. This provides the rationale for treating only patients with HR-positive tumors with endocrine therapy, since this subgroup receives the most benefit in terms of reduction in risk of recurrence and odds of death due to breast cancer.

Benefits of Neoadjuvant Endocrine Therapy for Breast Cancer

Neoadjuvant, or preoperative, therapy is administered before surgical intervention with the intact tumor remaining in the breast and/or regional nodes. Historically, most neoadjuvant therapy has been limited to chemotherapy, and most often it has been administered to patients with large, locally advanced tumors. The goal of this treatment is to shrink the primary tumor and regional nodal disease in order to convert patients with inoperable to operable disease and to decrease the extent of surgical resection required to control the local-regional disease. The use of endocrine therapy in the adjuvant, or postoperative, setting has been well established for patients with hormone-sensitive disease. Neoadjuvant endocrine therapy has largely been utilized in patients with hormone-sensitive disease who are not felt to be good candidates for chemotherapy, or even surgical intervention, due to advanced age or significant medical co-morbidities. Increased experience with neoadjuvant endocrine therapies has demonstrated that endocrine agents can also downsize locally advanced and large operable breast cancers and allow for breast conservation strategies in women who would have required mastectomy if surgery was performed as the initial intervention. In addition, neoadjuvant chemotherapy trials have begun to report that patients with HR-rich tumors are less likely to experience a complete pathologic response or even a significant partial response with chemotherapy. These patients are likely better candidates for neoadjuvant endocrine therapies if tumor downsizing is desired.

Experiences with neoadjuvant endocrine therapy are now being reported with increasing frequency. The strategy of initiating primary therapy with tamoxifen alone has been practiced in the United Kingdom and some European centers [4]. The 2007 St. Gallen Consensus panel guidelines stress the importance of determining endocrine responsiveness of a particular tumor prior to selecting systemic therapy, yet the clinical practice of prescribing neoadjuvant endocrine therapy is not routine [5]. Possible reasons rest in the finding that tamoxifen, for example, can take up to 5 weeks to achieve steady-state plasma levels, thus limiting its usefulness as a single neoadjuvant agent. A retrospective study published in 2002 by Mauriac et al. analyzed 199 women $\geq$50 years of age with HR-positive breast cancer who were treated with neoadjuvant tamoxifen. They reported rates of breast-conserving surgery for operable breast tumors of approximately 54%, concluding that successes observed with neoadjuvant tamoxifen therapy in elderly women could be applied to younger women [6]. Similarly, Dixon et al. reported their results comparing neoadjuvant tamoxifen with AIs, citing at least a 50% reduction in tumor volume on ultrasound following neoadjuvant tamoxifen and reductions of 88 and 78% with neoadjuvant letrozole and anastrozole, respectively [7].

Patient selection is important to optimize neoadjuvant endocrine therapy: only patients with HR-positive breast cancers are candidates, and as preliminary studies dictate, postmenopausal women are likely to benefit the most. Such patients can expect a high probability of responses over a 3-month treatment period. Response to therapy can be monitored by clinical examination as well as by ultrasound, mammography, or other imaging procedures. There is some evidence to suggest that the nature of the tumor response is different for preoperative endocrine therapy compared with chemotherapy. In the case of neoadjuvant chemotherapy, partial or even complete responses can be realized within one to two cycles of chemotherapy. With neoadjuvant endocrine therapy, response time is much slower and may not be fully realized until 3–4 months of therapy has been completed. Investigators have reported a higher rate of complete tumor excisions with breast-conserving surgery following neoadjuvant endocrine treatment without the need for as many re-excisions to achieve negative margins. There also appears to be a low rate of subsequent local recurrence in patients undergoing breast-conserving therapy following neoadjuvant endocrine therapy.

While tamoxifen has been the workhorse of endocrine therapy for many years, third-generation aromatase inhibitors (letrozole, anastrozole, and exemestane) have recently been shown to be more effective than tamoxifen in postmenopausal women with hormone-sensitive breast cancer. In a large randomized trial of neoadjuvant endocrine therapy in postmenopausal women, letrozole achieved significantly higher response rates than tamoxifen, and a correspondingly higher rate of breast-conserving surgery was possible in the letrozole-treated patients [8].

Neoadjuvant endocrine therapy provides a useful model system by which to identify mechanisms associated with de novo resistance and signs of early acquired resistance. Clinical trials examining neoadjuvant endocrine therapy are underway and promise to identify and validate surrogate markers for therapeutic responsiveness, resistance, and prognosis.

Available Hormonal Agents for Neoadjuvant Treatment

Estrogen effects in breast tissue can be manipulated by interfering with its interaction at the receptor level or by altering its downstream-signaling pathways. Available hormonal agents that have been used in breast cancer treatment include selective estrogen receptor modulators (SERMs), aromatase inhibitors (AIs), progestins, androgens, and luteinizing hormone-releasing hormone (LHRH) agonists. All classes of agents employ distinct approaches to the treatment of estrogen-dependent breast cancer. As their differing efficacies, tolerabilities, and toxicities stem from these biological differences, an understanding of their mechanisms of action is essential.

Selective Estrogen Receptor Modulators

Selective estrogen receptor modulators, or SERMS, include a group of synthetic non-steroidal compounds that interact with intracellular estrogen receptors in target organs as estrogen receptor agonists and antagonists. These drugs have been intensively studied over the past decade and have proven to be a highly versatile group for the treatment of different conditions associated with aging, including hormone-responsive cancer and osteoporosis. This class of agents includes tamoxifen, raloxifene, and newer agents currently under evaluation. Tamoxifen complexes to the ER and blocks estrogen action in addition to conferring altered gene regulatory properties. These alterations are collectively referred to as selective estrogen receptor modulation, which defines this class of agents. The complex pharmacology of SERMs has resulted in a growing interest in the development of even more selective agents for other members of this nuclear receptor superfamily to allow an even more individualized treatment approach.

Tamoxifen

Tamoxifen is the most commonly utilized endocrine agent in the treatment of ER-positive breast cancer. Beginning as the failed postcoital contraceptive ICI 46474, tamoxifen quickly rose to become the first targeted anti-estrogenic therapy for the prevention and treatment of breast cancer [9]. It is an anti-estrogen that competes with estrogen for binding to the ER. Tamoxifen binds to the ER with high affinity and activates ER dimerization and DNA binding. In normal tissues, tamoxifen acts as an estrogen receptor agonist, and like HRT agents, tamoxifen-bound ER promotes bone mineralization and endometrial proliferation. As a consequence, risks associated with tamoxifen use mimic those seen with estrogen-replacement therapy, notably deep venous thrombosis, pulmonary embolism, stroke, and endometrial cancer, in addition to cataract formation [10, 11]. All risks are more pronounced in women $\geq$50 years of age, especially the risk of endometrial cancer, with an observed almost fourfold increase. A meta-analysis of 32 published randomized controlled trials demonstrated that tamoxifen was associated with significantly increased risks of endometrial cancer (relative risk [RR] 2.70; 95% CI, 1.94–3.75) as well as gastrointestinal cancers (RR 1.31; 95% CI, 1.01–1.69), strokes (RR 1.49; 95% CI, 1.16–1.90), and pulmonary emboli (RR 1.88; 95% CI, 1.77–3.01), with postmenopausal women having the greatest increases in neoplastic outcomes [12]. Consideration of tamoxifen use requires balance of potential benefits and risks.

In vivo, tamoxifen is transformed by polymorphic and inducible enzymes of the cytochrome P450 family, mainly via N-desmethylation, into over 12 characterized metabolites, each with varying biological activity [13]. It is these metabolites that modulate estrogen action at distinct target sites. Coactivators are the principal players that assemble a complex of functional proteins around the ligand ER complex to initiate transcription of a target gene at its promoter site. Tamoxifen thus demonstrates a variable treatment response with as many as 33% of patients not benefiting from treatment [14]. Debate still ensues regarding which metabolites are responsible for tamoxifen's anti-tumoral effects, yet the metabolites 4-hydroxytamoxifen and *N*-desmethyl-4-hydroxytamoxifen demonstrate strong anti-proliferative activity and likely play key roles [15]. For many years, a 5-year course of treatment with tamoxifen was the gold standard of adjuvant treatment. Tamoxifen has demonstrated efficacy in both premenopausal and postmenopausal women and across all age groups.

Raloxifene

Like tamoxifen, raloxifene belongs to the family of SERMs, yet it is a pure estrogen antagonist. It exerts its effects in breast and endometrial tissue as well as bone. Raloxifene remains the only SERM approved worldwide for the prevention and treatment of postmenopausal osteoporosis and vertebral fractures. Raloxifene maintains bone density (estrogen-like effect) in postmenopausal osteoporotic women, but at the same time reduces the incidence of breast cancer in both high-risk and low-risk postmenopausal women. Unlike tamoxifen, raloxifene does not increase the incidence of endometrial cancer.

Newer Agents

Search for the ideal SERM that exerts favorable estrogenic effects on bone and serum lipids, minimal effects on the endometrium, and anti-estrogenic effects on breast tissue is currently underway and has led to the development of newer agents. Toremifene, like tamoxifen, is currently used to treat advanced breast cancer and also has beneficial effects on bone mineral density and serum lipids in postmenopausal women. Ospemifene, lasofoxifene, bazedoxifene, and arzoxifene are new SERM molecules with potentially greater efficacy and potency than previous SERMs. Investigations are currently underway examining these agents for use in the treatment and prevention of osteoporosis. These drugs have been shown to be comparably effective to conventional HRT in animal models of osteoporosis with potentially improved safety profiles. Clinical efficacy data from ongoing phase III trials will lend insight into their full therapeutic potentials.

Aromatase Inhibitors

Unlike tamoxifen, aromatase inhibitors (AIs) do not exhibit intrinsic hormonal properties, but rather effect ER function indirectly. They exert their effects in the peripheral (i.e., non-ovarian) tissues, inhibiting the aromatization of androgens to estrogens and thus decreasing circulating estrogen levels [16]. For this reason, AIs are only effective in postmenopausal women. The two categories of AIs, type I and II, mimic the endogenous substrates androstenedione and testosterone, competing with them for binding to the enzyme aromatase. This halts aromatization which normally leads to the conversion of androgens to estrogens in peripheral tissues. When deprived of estrogens, ERs cannot bind to DNA and are thus not capable of engaging signaling pathways. Consequentially, the side effects of AIs stem from estrogen deprivation, namely bone loss and atrophic vaginitis. Likewise, the estrogen agonist effects observed with tamoxifen are avoided.

AIs have been applied in both neoadjuvant and adjuvant settings with excellent results, as AIs, unlike tamoxifen, are capable of achieving therapeutic concentrations within a matter of days [17].

The third-generation AIs, anastrozole, letrozole, and exemestane, appear to result in better overall response rates and improved DFS compared to tamoxifen in postmenopausal women with hormone receptor-positive breast cancer. They are associated with fewer gynecologic and thromboembolic side effects, which is advantageous in this older, high-risk patient population. The finding that AIs are more effective than tamoxifen for HR-positive breast cancer in both the neoadjuvant and the adjuvant settings has set the stage for the development of newer agents under investigation in clinical trials.

Steroidal (Type I) Aromatase Inhibitors

Type I agents, also referred to as suicidal inhibitors or steroidals, include exemestane and formestane. These type I inhibitors bind their active sites and initiate a chain of enzymatic reactions, ultimately leading to hydroxylation and an irreversible inhibitor-enzyme covalent bond. Enzyme activity is thus permanently halted until new enzyme synthesis ensues.

Non-steroidal (Type II) Aromatase Inhibitors

Anastrozole, letrozole, and fadrozole are type II aromatase inhibitors, differing from the type I subset in that their binding to the active site of aromatase is reversible. Their effectiveness is thus dependent on their relative concentrations and binding affinities in relation to endogenous substrate. Anastrozole and letrozole are the subject of numerous trials that will be discussed later in this chapter. Fadrozole, a second-generation non-steroidal AI, has been shown to be equivalent to tamoxifen [18] but inferior to letrozole in the neoadjuvant treatment of advanced breast cancer [19]. To date, its approval is restricted to Japan.

Predictors of Response to Hormonal Therapy Patient Characteristics

Menopausal Status

Postmenopausal women rely on the peripheral aromatization of adrenal androgens to estrogen, which results in overall lower serum estrogen levels as compared to premenopausal women with ovarian estrogen production. Postmenopausal women with ER-positive tumors that receive treatment with AIs experience increased response rates, longer times to disease progression, and fewer side effects compared to treatment with tamoxifen. In contrast, premenopausal women with ER-positive cancers achieve greater benefit from treatment with tamoxifen or LHRH agonists. Menopausal status is thus key in patient selection.

BRCA Mutations

Familial breast cancer represents 5–10% of all breast tumors. Mutations in the two known major breast cancer susceptibility genes, BRCA1 and BRCA2, account for a minority of familial breast cancer, whereas families without mutations in these genes (BRCAX group) account for 70% of familial breast cancer cases. Phenotypic and genotypic heterogeneities are the rule with hereditary breast cancers and thus dictate a spectrum of treatment approaches. BRCA1 mutation-positive breast cancers are frequently ER negative in contrast to BRCA2 mutation-positive cancers, which are more frequently ER positive. Therefore, significant differences exist with respect to anti-estrogen therapy which will be more amenable to BRCA2 versus BRCA1 mutation carriers manifesting breast cancer. Tumors that are negative for ER, PR, and Her2-neu, or "triple negative" tumors, may also harbor a unique basal-like gene expression profile and are characterized by poor prognosis wherein endocrine and/or Her2-neu-targeted therapies are not effective treatment options. As we learn more about the biology and the molecular aspects of hereditary forms of breast cancer, it will be crucial for the treating clinician to integrate this knowledge with pharmacologic, radiologic, and surgical treatment options for these high-risk patients [20].

Tumor Markers

Breast cancer is a heterogeneous disease, and there has been significant interest in identifying markers that will aid in predicting prognosis and response to therapy. To date, relatively few markers have established prognostic power, as experience with endocrine therapy has shown that targeted therapies require the target to be not merely expressed in the cancer phenotype, but important in regulating growth of cancer cells. The estrogen receptor (ER) is probably the most powerful predictive marker in breast cancer management, both in determining prognosis and in predicting response to hormone therapies. The progesterone receptor (PgR) is also a widely used marker, although its value is less well established. HER-2 status has also been established as a powerful prognostic and predictive factor in breast cancer. Given the importance of these biological markers in patient management, it is essential that assays are quality controlled and that interpretation is standardized. Furthermore, it is important to be aware of the limitations in their predictive power and how this may be refined through addition of further biological markers. The list of biomarkers for breast cancer currently undergoing investigation is quite exhaustive; for the present discussion we will focus on those biomarkers that are being analyzed in the context of neoadjuvant endocrine therapy trials.

IHC Technique and Scoring

More sophisticated techniques for measuring the amount of receptor expression in the primary tumor have evolved from what was once a tedious process of performing Southern blots for DNA determination, Northern blots at the transcript mRNA level, and reverse transcriptase PCR (RT-PCR), eventually evolving into FISH and chromogenic in situ hybridization (CISH). Immunohistochemical staining has become the preferred method for quantitating hormone receptor expression due to its ease of performance even in community laboratories. It has a steep learning curve and does not require fresh or fresh-frozen tissue samples. Enzyme-based IHC was introduced in the 1970s, and a series of advancements in technology in the 1980s and 1990s led to the development of antigen retrieval techniques to make IHC possible on nearly all archival tissue. This, coupled with sensitive detection systems and better antibodies has made this technique routine in evaluating receptor expression.

Hormone receptor status can be determined from a cell block obtained from fine-needle aspiration or core needle biopsy with good correlation to corresponding surgical specimens, giving it a role in receptor assessment for patients planned for neoadjuvant treatment. Immunohistochemistry can also be performed on tissue biopsies obtained during the course of treatment to assess treatment response, ER or PgR status, or markers of proliferation in tumor tissue.

IHC employs an antibody that targets an extracellular or intramembranous domain of the receptor. The bound antibody is then visualized by attaching a color-emitting molecule that detects the antigen–antibody reaction, and scoring is performed under a light microscope.

A variety of IHC antibodies and testing protocols exist. For most currently used IHC antibodies, a score ranging from 0 to 3+ reflecting the intensity of staining of the cell membrane in more than 10% of the cells is applied, but different cutoffs have been established to reflect specific hormone receptor status. In 1999, the College of American Pathology (CAP) approved the use of IHC for assessing ER and PgR in routine clinical practice yet did not provide guidelines as to how the testing should be performed [21]. Thereafter, the American Society of Clinical Oncology and expert panels of pathologists, oncologists, and surgeons have published general guidelines for assessing and applying tumor biomarkers [22]. Discrepancies still arise in cases related to weak-positive staining or with values close to the respective cutoffs. Most pathologists initially employ IHC to screen, relying on FISH as a confirmatory technique and in intermediate cases.

In an effort to overcome the interobserver and intraobserver differences in scoring that results in borderline or weakly staining cases and to make ER quantification more objective, a variety of automated scoring systems have been proposed. The ChromaVision Automated Cellular Imaging System and the Applied Imaging Ariol SL-50 quantify the color intensity of the immunoreactive product. Studies comparing these systems to the traditional manual scoring have demonstrated significant agreement between systems and only mild discrepancies when compared with manual scoring, with discrepant results more frequently seen when analyzing tumors with low levels (0–20%) of ER-positive cells [23].

Estrogen Receptor

The estrogen receptor (ER) belongs to a superfamily of nuclear hormone receptors which includes the progesterone receptor (PgR) as well as the thyroid hormone receptor, vitamin D receptor, and retinoic acid receptors that share in their ability to function as transcription factors when bound to their respective ligands. Since cloning of ER cDNA in 1986 by Green and colleagues, much has been learned about its structure and role in breast cancer [24].

The ER has two structurally and functionally distinct isoforms, ERα and ERβ. It has been demonstrated that ERβ is coexpressed with ERα in over 76% of breast tumors [25]. In general, patients whose tumors have the highest ER level derive a statistically significant greater reduction in tumor volume with neoadjuvant treatment [26]. The concentration of receptor isoforms, however, varies in a tissue-specific manner as do the functions of the receptor ligand. The ERα and ERβ isoforms have contradictory functions, with ERα having a growth-promoting action and ERβ having a growth-inhibitory action in certain tissues [27]. The tissue-selective ratio of ERα to ERβ translates into tissue-specific functions. The ER is the switch that initiates estrogen action in its target tissues, which include the uterus, vagina, and pituitary gland. The subsequent identification of the ER in some breast cancers and not others has created a mechanistic link to explain the observed heterogeneity of hormonal dependence.

Endocrine therapies, such as tamoxifen, are commonly given to most patients with ERα-positive breast carcinoma but are not indicated for ERα-negative cancers. The factors responsible for response to tamoxifen in 5–10% of patients with ERα-negative tumors are not clear. There is also controversy among studies examining ERß, with most studies associating it with better prognosis, increased DFS survival, and predictive of favorable response to tamoxifen [28–31], though a few studies cite the contrary [32]. The utility of ERß as an independent marker for prognosis and tamoxifen responsiveness is thus limited [33].

Endocrine responsiveness is a continuous variable dependent on levels of ER, and to a lesser extent, PgR. Because tumors with even a small amount of measurable protein (3–10 fmol/mg) have response rates to endocrine therapy in the 20–30% range, stringently low cutoff points should be adopted to avoid denying patients the benefits of neoadjuvant endocrine therapy. A range for ER negativity of <3 fmol/mg of cytosolic protein and $\geq 1\%$ of positively stained cells by IHC best separates who will and will not derive benefit from neoadjuvant therapy [34].

Progesterone Receptor

Large clinical trials have demonstrated that tumors expressing progesterone receptor (PgR) in addition to ER have a higher response rate to tamoxifen and other endocrine therapies, and increasing PgR levels are associated with better prognosis, longer time to treatment failure, and longer survival [35, 36]. Like the ER, the progesterone receptor also has two described isoforms, PR-A and PR-B. It is known that the two isoforms may mediate different effects of progesterone, possibly by varying in response to different PgR modulators. PgR modulators are a research interest, as they may be designed to be PgR isoform and cellular pathway selective to achieve targeted breast cancer therapy [37]. PgR scoring is similar to that for ER, as are the potential pitfalls.

Ki67

Ki67 is a cell cycle marker that is an assessment of proliferation. Ki67 has been applied in the assessment of prognosis in breast cancer patients and the efficacy of neoadjuvant endocrine therapy [38]. It can be measured in a surgical specimen and used to objectively assess tumor sensitivity to the prescribed treatment. Ki67 has been studied in numerous trials, as well as in the letrozole P024 trial and in a 2007 update from the IMPACT trialists group. In the P024 trial, the post-treatment reduction in Ki67 was significantly greater with letrozole (87%) than tamoxifen (75%; analysis of covariance $P = 0.0009$).

Similar studies have found that by integrating the prognostic value of the Ki67 level at baseline with the changes in Ki67 level associated with treatment benefit, Ki67 has served as useful marker for predicting recurrence-free survival in neoadjuvant endocrine treatment [39–41]. The results of these trials and others will be discussed in more detail in the sections that follow.

HER1 (EGFR) and HER2 (ErbB2)

HER1 (epidermal growth factor receptor) and HER2 (ErbB2 or neu) are members of the HER (erb-b) family of transmembrane receptor tyrosine kinases. HER1, like other members of this superfamily, depends on HER2 to act as the signal amplifier for the HER network. Increased levels of HER2 are causally associated with malignant transformation of mammary epithelial cells, with approximately 25% of invasive cancers exhibiting HER2 amplification [42, 43]. HER2 also confers shorter survival in breast cancer patients, and hence has been extensively evaluated in the context of neoadjuvant endocrine therapy trials.

The letrozole P024 study analyzed pre- and post-treatment specimens for Ki67, ER, PgR, as well as HER1 and HER2 (ErbB2 or neu) by IHC. The treatment-induced differences in the average Ki67 reduction observed in the letrozole arm were particularly marked for ER-positive tumors that overexpressed HER1 and/or HER2 (88 versus 45%, respectively; $P = 0.0018$). Of those tumors in both arms that demonstrated a paradoxical increase in Ki67 with treatment, the majority of the cases were HER1/2 negative. The findings that letrozole inhibited tumor proliferation to a greater extent than tamoxifen were shown to have a molecular basis. Specifically, possible tamoxifen agonist effects on the cell cycle in both HER1/2-positive and HER1/2-negative tumors were proposed [44]. In an era of personalized targeted therapy, HER1/2 expression and their coexpressive patterns with other EGFR family members could be an important determinant for appropriate agent selection in neoadjuvant endocrine breast cancer therapy.

Trials of Neoadjuvant Endocrine Therapy

Tamoxifen

Early trials examining neoadjuvant therapy with tamoxifen were conducted on patients that were not pre-screened for ER and PgR status to determine those most likely to respond. Rather, participants were elderly women with locally advanced breast cancer [45]. Since then, numerous phase III randomized trials have been conducted to address the effectiveness of tamoxifen as sole therapy versus as part of a combined therapeutic approach.

Bates et al. (1991) randomized 381 postmenopausal women ≥70 years old with operable breast cancer to receive tamoxifen (40 mg daily) alone versus tamoxifen and immediate surgery in the Cancer Research Campaign (CRC) trial. At a median follow-up of 34 months there was no statistically significant difference in overall survival (OS), yet more patients treated with tamoxifen alone went on to receive subsequent surgery for local treatment failure [46]. Van Dalsen et al. (1995) performed a retrospective review of 210 postmenopausal breast cancer patients that had received tamoxifen as primary treatment versus tamoxifen with surgery. With a mean follow-up of 41 months, they noted local progressive disease in 27% of those patients treated with tamoxifen ($P < 0.005$) that resulted in the need for further surgery. There was no difference between the two groups in terms of OS or incidence of metastases. They concluded that treatment of breast cancer in postmenopausal women with reasonable life expectancy should include surgery rather than tamoxifen alone [47].

Tan et al. (2001) conducted a prospective randomized phase III study out of Nottingham examining tamoxifen alone versus multimodal treatment, the latter of which consisted of neoadjuvant chemotherapy and surgery followed by postoperative radiation, then adjuvant tamoxifen. This study enrolled 108 premenopausal patients with locally advanced breast cancer and followed them for a mean of 52 months. There were no statistically significant differences noted in terms of OS or disease-free survival (DFS) between the two groups, yet the time to initial locoregional failure was noted to be significantly shorter in the group receiving tamoxifen alone [48].

Gazet and colleagues (1994) conducted a prospective randomized trial enrolling 200 elderly (≥70 years old), postmenopausal patients with surgically resectable breast cancer, allocating them to receive tamoxifen alone (20 mg daily) or primary surgery. At a median follow-up of 72 months they noted no statistically significant differences in the rates of DFS between the two treatment arms [49]. In 2003 Mustacchi et al. published the long-term follow-up results of the Group for Research on Endocrine Therapy in the Elderly study, known as the GRETA trial, which was designed to evaluate the efficacy of tamoxifen as primary treatment in women with operable breast cancer and ≥70 years of age in terms of OS and DFS. This randomized trial assigned 235 patients to receive tamoxifen alone (160 mg on day 1, then 20 mg daily) for a 5-year course and 239 patients to undergo surgery plus tamoxifen (20 mg daily) for 5 years total. After a mean follow-up of 80 months, no statistically significant differences were noted between the two arms with regard to OS and DFS. Similar to the conclusions drawn from preceding studies, they recommended surgery when medically feasible with tamoxifen due to the high rate of local disease progression observed with tamoxifen alone [50]. Nonetheless, both studies again demonstrated the time to first locoregional recurrence to be significantly shorter in the tamoxifen alone arms.

The EORTC 10851 trial sought to further examine tamoxifen in the treatment of early breast cancer in older women. A randomized trial comparing modified radical mastectomy to tamoxifen as the sole initial therapy in 164 women aged ≥70 years with operable breast cancer, survival curves were estimated and end points included survival, time to first relapse, locoregional progression, time to distant progression, and progression-free survival. After a median follow-up of approximately 10 years, there were significantly decreased times to progression and shorter times to local progression in the tamoxifen arm, though OS was similar between the two groups [51].

Table 1 further characterizes the key randomized prospective trials of neoadjuvant tamoxifen.

Letrozole (Femara)

In 2001, Dixon et al. reported the first experience of using neoadjuvant letrozole in the treatment of locally advanced and large operable breast carcinomas. In this phase I study, 24 postmenopausal women with ER-positive breast cancer were treated with either 2.5 or 10 mg of letrozole for 3 months. The study reported that only one patient treated with the 2.5 mg dose demonstrated a clinical and pathological complete response (CR), yet 15 patients planned for mastectomy appreciated such significant reduction in tumor volume that they were able to undergo breast-conserving surgery [52]. The small sample size and short-term follow-up in this study prohibited analysis of OS and DFS, yet its results inspired numerous other studies.

Paepke and colleagues (2003) sought to examine whether longer treatment with letrozole would increase clinical and pathological response rates. A trial was conducted enrolling 33 postmenopausal women that received letrozole (2.5 mg daily) for a period spanning from 4 to ≤8 months preceding surgery. Longer treatment resulted in a statistically significant decrease in tumor

Table 1 Prospective randomized trials of neoadjuvant therapy with tamoxifen

Study (number of patients)	Patient characteristics	Regimen	Duration of treatment (months)	Median follow-up (months)	Time to progression	ORR	OS/DFS
The Elderly Breast Cancer Working Party (n=381) [98]	≥70 years old, operable breast cancer	TAM 40 mg vs TAM + SURG	Until PD	34	NA	TAM 25% at 6 months	NS/NS
Gazet et al. (n=210) [99]	≥70 years old, operable breast cancer	TAM 20 mg vs SURG	Until PD	72	NA	NA	NA/NS
Nottingham (n=108) [100]	Pre + Post, LABC	TAM 20 mg vs Multi	Until PD	52	Shorter with TAM (P = 0.001)	TAM 36.5% vs Multi 55.4%	NS/NS
GRETA (n=474) [101]	≥70 years old, operable breast cancer	TAM (160 then 20 mg) + SURG + TAM 20 mg	60	80	NA	41.6%	NS/NS
EORTC 10851 (n=164) [102]	≥70 years old, operable breast cancer	TAM 20 mg vs MRM	Until PD	120	Shorter with TAM alone only (P<0.0001)	TAM 41.7%	NS/NA

TAM, tamoxifen; SURG, surgery; Pre, premenopausal; Post, postmenopausal; LABC, locally advanced breast cancer; Multi, multimodal treatment (neoadjuvant chemotherapy + surgery then postoperative radiation + TAM); MRM, modified radical mastectomy; ORR, overall response rate (CR + PR); PD, progression of disease; LR, local recurrence; OS, overall survival; DFS, disease-free survival; NS, not significant; NA, not analyzed.

volume, and 90% of the patients that received neoadjuvant letrozole for ≥4 months had a measurable response compared to 57% of the patients who were treated <4 months [53].

In a similar study, Renshaw et al. (2004) assessed response to neoadjuvant letrozole therapy after 3 months, directing non-responders and new breast conservation candidates to surgery while continuing neoadjuvant letrozole on the other patients for up to 12 months. At 3, 6, and 12 months, they observed complete response rates of 95, 29, and 36%, respectively [54].

Both studies suggested that the neoadjuvant treatment effects of letrozole are in some capacity duration dependent.

In a 2006 study by Miller et al., 63 postmenopausal women with large primary breast cancers were treated with neoadjuvant letrozole (2.5 mg daily) for 3 months and both pre- and post-treatment (at 10–14 days and 3 months) tumor samples were analyzed. Immunohistochemical staining for Ki67, ER, and PgR was performed and characterized in terms of clinical response and pathological response after 3 months of treatment. A clinical response was observed in 76.2% of cases and pathologic response in 75.8% of cases, although the degree of response was not specified. A statistically significant decrease in Ki67 was observed in all tumor subgroups at 10–14 days ($P<0.005$), and at 3 months, decreases from pre-treatment Ki67 scores were highly significant in all tumor subgroups irrespective of response status. Treatment also significantly reduced PgR expression at 14 days and 3 months (both $P<0.0001$), but the level of change did not correlate with pathologic response. They thus concluded that letrozole produces rapid and profound decreases in expression of Ki67 and PgR irrespective of clinical and pathological response rates [55].

Letrozole Versus Tamoxifen

Additional trials emerged comparing neoadjuvant tamoxifen with AIs to assess overall response rates and disease progression. The results of a 2001 randomized trial comparing neoadjuvant letrozole and tamoxifen in postmenopausal women with hormone receptor-positive disease demonstrated that letrozole produced higher clinical and mammographic response rates and incidence of conversion to breast-conserving surgery than tamoxifen. Supporting the findings from the 2002 ATAC trial of adjuvant endocrine therapy, Eiermann and colleagues demonstrated that a third-generation AI is more effective than tamoxifen in the treatment of breast cancer in the neoadjuvant setting as well [56]. In a further analysis of trial outcomes, HER1 and HER2 surfaced as possible biomarkers for drug effectiveness, that is, differences in the observed effects of letrozole and tamoxifen were more pronounced in tumors co-expressing HER1 and/or HER2 with ER [57].

Letrozole was compared to tamoxifen in a phase III randomized trial from the International Letrozole Breast Cancer Group known as the Femara Study

P025. Nine hundred and seven patients with positive or unknown hormone receptor status were enrolled. Letrozole therapy was found to be superior to tamoxifen, with a median time to progression of 41 versus 26 weeks. In addition, the median time to treatment failure (40 versus 25 weeks), overall response rate (30 versus 20%, $P = 0.0006$), and clinical benefit rate (49 versus 38%, $P = 0.001$) were significantly better in the patients treated with letrozole versus tamoxifen [58]. A 2003 update after a median follow-up of 32 months confirmed the superiority of letrozole over tamoxifen in terms of time to progression (median 9.4 versus 6.0 months, respectively, $P < 0.0001$), time to treatment failure (median 9 versus 5.7 months, respectively, $P < 0.0001$), overall objective response rates, and clinical benefit. Of note, the total duration of endocrine therapy was significantly longer for first-line letrozole than first-line tamoxifen (median 16 versus 9 months, respectively, $P = 0.005$), while the time to worsening Karnofsky performance index was significantly delayed in the letrozole group [59]. This suggested possible palliative benefits of a first-line AI approach.

Miller et al. further analyzed the effects of neoadjuvant AIs at differing doses and subsequent effects on tumor volume reduction and pathology. Postmenopausal women with large primary ER-positive breast cancers were randomized to receive neoadjuvant treatment with either letrozole (2.5 or 10 mg daily) or anastrozole (1 or 10 mg daily), and results of both arms were compared to those observed in a non-randomized group of patients treated with tamoxifen (40 mg daily) over the same time course. Tumors were analyzed pathologically before treatment and after 3 months of treatment. Clinical response to treatment was assessed by sequential measurements of tumor volume based on caliper assessment, ultrasound, and mammography. Following 3 months of treatment, the groups treated with AIs experienced more tumor shrinkage (88 and 77% reduction in volumes for letrozole and anastrozole, respectively) than the tamoxifen-treated group (46% volume reduction), a difference that was statistically significant ($P<0.0001$). In addition, pathological responses, defined as a decrease in tumor cellularity or increased fibrosis, were observed in 32 cases (68%). There was a decrease in immunohistochemical staining for Ki67 in all tumors treated with AIs, irrespective of clinical and pathological responses. Staining for PgR was also reduced in all 21 PgR-positive cancers treated with letrozole and in 16 out of 17 positive cancers treated with anastrozole [60]. These observations on IHC staining provided some objective measurement of the biological differences between AIs and tamoxifen. As the PgR is regarded as a marker of a functioning estrogen-signaling pathway, the reduction in PgR staining corresponds to the described estrogen-deprivation mechanism of action of AIs.

Miller et al. later analyzed further pathological changes associated with neoadjuvant letrozole treatment in two further studies. In 2003, they examined morphological characteristics, grading features, proliferation marker MIB1, apoptosis Bcl-2 expression, and ER and PgR status in ER-positive breast cancers before and after 3 months of neoadjuvant therapy with either letrozole

(2.5 or 10 mg daily) or tamoxifen (20 mg daily). Letrozole treatment was associated with a pathologic PR in 71% of patients, manifesting as a decrease in mitosis and reduction in the expression of MIB1. While only small changes were observed in ER expression following letrozole therapy, PgR reactivity was reduced in 20 of 21 evaluable cases which were initially PgR positive, becoming undetectable in 16 patients. Tamoxifen treatment was associated with a pathological PR in 63% of tumors. In contrast to letrozole, the dominant change in grading feature was an increase in tubule formation, reduction in ER score, and increased PgR expression. Following treatment with either tamoxifen or letrozole, variable effects were observed in the apoptotic index and expression of Bcl-2. These results indicated that both letrozole and tamoxifen have marked influences on the pathological features of breast cancer during neoadjuvant therapy, though effects on clinical and pathologic responses were frequently discordant [61].

Ellis and colleagues published preliminary results of a randomized, double-blind, multicenter, and multinational phase III trial comparing the antitumoral activity of neoadjuvant tamoxifen with AIs. This study, known as the letrozole P024 trial, included 337 postmenopausal women with ER-positive and/or PgR-positive primary breast cancers from 55 centers in 16 countries [62]. Overall response rates (clinical CR and PR) by clinical and radiographic measurements were better in patients that received letrozole, who demonstrated overall response rates of 60% versus 41% in the taxoxifen arm. Though not statistically significant, more women in the letrozole group were able to undergo successful post-treatment breast conservation therapy, and less disease progression was observed. In addition, differences in the response rates were observed based on the HER1 and HER2 expression status of the tumors, lending a possible explanation to observed endocrine therapy resistance. The trial demonstrated that neoadjuvant letrozole is not only safe but superior to tamoxifen in the treatment of postmenopausal women with hormone receptor-positive, locally advanced breast cancer and proposed potentially useful biomarkers for measuring treatment responsiveness [63].

Table 2 lists the key features of the randomized prospective trials examining letrozole in the neoadjuvant setting.

Anastrozole (Arimidex)

A phase I study by Dixon et al. (2000) examined the efficacy of neoadjuvant anastrozole in postmenopausal women with highly ER-positive locally advanced or large breast cancers. Patients received either 1 or 10 mg of anastrozole daily over 3 months and effects on tumor volume reduction were examined by ultrasound. They observed a median reduction in tumor volume of 75.5% for both dosage groups combined, which resulted in a conversion to

Table 2 Prospective randomized trials of neoadjuvant therapy with letrozole

Study (number of patients)	Patient characteristics	Regimen	Duration of treatment (months)	Median follow-up (months)	Time to progression	ORR	OS/DFS
Dixon et al. (n=24) [103]	Post, ER(+)/rich, LABC	LET 2.5 vs 10 mg	3	3	NA	83% for 2.5 vs 66.6% for 10 mg	NA/NA
Miller et al. (n=47) [104]	Post, ER(+)	LET 2.5 or 10 mg vs ANA 1 or 10 mg vs TAM 40 mg	3	3	NA	NS	NA/NA
Eiermann et al. (n=337) [105]	Post, ER(+) ±PgR(+)	LET 2.5 mg vs TAM 20 mg	4	1.5	NA	LET 55% vs TAM 36%, $P<0.001$	NA/NA
Femara Study P025 (n=907) [106]	Post, LABC	LET 2.5 mg vs TAM 20 mg	Until PD	24	LET 9.4 months vs TAM 6.0 months, $P<0.0001$	LET 32% vs TAM 21%, $P = 0.0002$	Median OS LET 34 months vs TAM 30 months, $P = 0.53$
Letrozole P024 (n=324) [107]	Post, ER(+) ± PgR(+), ineligible for BCS	LET 2.5 mg vs TAM 20 mg	4	60	NA	LET 60% vs TAM 41%, $P = 0.004$	NA/NA

LET, letrozole; TAM, tamoxifen; ANA, anastrozole; LABC, locally advanced breast cancer; BCS, breast-conserving surgery; Post, postmenopausal; ORR, overall response rate (CR + PR); PD, progression of disease; LR, local recurrence; OS, overall survival; DFS, disease-free survival; NS, not significant; NA, not analyzed.

breast-conserving surgery in 15 out of the 17 patients initially felt to require mastectomy [64]. In a follow-up study, these tumors were stained for erbB2. There was no observed difference in clinical response in relation to erbB2 status, and changes in Ki67 and PgR did not differ between tumors that were erbB2 3+ versus those that were erbB2 negative or 1+ [65].

A later study by Milla-Santos and colleagues evaluated response rates in postmenopausal women with hormone receptor-positive, locally advanced tumors. One hundred and twelve women were treated with neoadjuvant anastrozole (1 mg daily) over a 3-month treatment period preceding their planned surgery. Following pathological analysis of surgical specimens, they reported a 12% CR rate and a 71% PR rate resulting from a 3-month course of neoadjuvant anastrozole [66].

Anastrozole Versus Tamoxifen

Anastrozole has been compared to tamoxifen in two randomized, double-blind trials evaluating postmenopausal breast cancer patients with metastatic disease and either positive or unknown hormone receptor status. The Tamoxifen or Arimidex Randomized Group Efficacy and Tolerability (TARGET) study conducted in European centers demonstrated comparable times to disease progression (8.3 versus 8.2 months, respectively) and rates of CR, PR, and disease stabilization in the tamoxifen and anastrozole study arms [67]. Conversely, the North American Study by Nabholtz et al. (2000) demonstrated that anastrozole was significantly superior to tamoxifen in terms of time to disease progression (11.1 versus 5.6 months, $P = 0.005$) and clinical benefit rates [68]. Reasons for the discrepancies in reported results may stem from the patient populations enrolled, as 45% of the patients in the European study versus 89% in the North American study were known hormone receptor positive. Later analysis of the combined data from the two studies after an 18.2-month follow-up demonstrated that anastrozole to be equivalent to tamoxifen in terms of time to progression, but retrospective subgroup analysis demonstrated anastrozole to be superior to tamoxifen in terms of time to progression in the receptor-positive subgroup (10.7 versus 6.4 months). Similarly, while anastrozole had similar objective response rates, the clinical benefit rates (CR, PR, and disease stabilization) were higher (57.1 versus 52%) [69]. It is thus suggested from retrospective analysis that anastrozole is superior to tamoxifen in terms of time to progression in patients with receptor-positive tumors.

The Immediate Preoperative Anastrozole, Combination or Tamoxifen (IMPACT) study was designed to be the neoadjuvant counterpart of the Arimidex, Tamoxifen Alone, or in Combination (ATAC) trial. This study compared anastrozole (1 mg daily) to tamoxifen (20 mg daily) versus anastrozole plus tamoxifen. This multicenter, randomized double-blind trial recruited 330 postmenopausal women with ER- and PgR-positive large, operable, or advanced breast cancers and monitored them during a 3-month neoadjuvant treatment course. The primary study end point was objective tumor response rate. Secondary end points included incidence of breast-conserving surgery, while subsequent analyses allowed measurement of key biomarkers for treatment response, notably hormone receptor expression and proliferation and apoptotic rates. Clinical response rates were similar in the anastrozole and tamoxifen treatment arms (37 versus 36%, respectively) and the combination treatment arm (39%). However, the clinical response rate was significantly increased in the anastrozole arm as compared to the tamoxifen arm in erbB2-positive patients (58 versus 22%, P = 0.09), suggesting that anastrozole is preferred over tamoxifen in erbB2-positive breast cancer patients [70]. These results mirrored those seen in similar studies analyzing letrozole versus tamoxifen in erbB2-positive tumors. In addition, more patients that received neoadjuvant anastrozole were able to undergo breast-conserving surgery as compared to those who received tamoxifen (46 versus 22%, P = 0.03) [71].

The study of Preoperative Arimidex Compared with Tamoxifen (PROACT) trial continued to analyze neoadjuvant anastrozole compared to tamoxifen. The study randomized 451 postmenopausal women with ER-positive breast cancer to receive either neoadjuvant anastrozole (n = 228) or tamoxifen (n = 223) over a 3-month period preceding surgery. Of note, 137 patients in the study received concomitant neoadjuvant chemotherapy, so subgroup analysis was performed to assess responses with endocrine therapy alone. Tumor response rates, defined in the trial as shrinkage by >30% of the largest tumor diameter, were 36.2% in the anastrozole arm versus 26.5% in the tamoxifen arm (P = 0.07) [72].

Table 3 further describes the key prospective randomized trials of neoadjuvant anastrozole.

Exemestane

A randomized phase II trial of the European Organization for the Research and Treatment of Cancer (EORTC Breast Group) (2001) compared exemestane to tamoxifen in 117 previously untreated breast cancer patients with positive or unknown hormone receptor status. The overall response rate was significantly better for exemestane than tamoxifen (44.6 versus 14.3%) [73]. An ongoing EORTC phase III trial is comparing the efficacy and time to disease progression of exemestane versus tamoxifen [74].

A phase II study by Dixon and colleagues (2001) evaluated the efficacy of neoadjuvant exemestane (25 mg daily for 3 months) in 12 postmenopausal women with ER-positive operable and locally advanced breast cancers. They observed median reductions in clinical and radiographic tumor volumes of 82.5–85.5%. Neoadjuvant exemestane resulted in conversion from planned

Table 3 Prospective randomized trials of neoadjuvant therapy with anastrozole

Study (number of patients)	Patient characteristics	Regimen	Duration of treatment (months)	Median follow-up (months)	Time to progression (months)	ORR	OS/DFS
Milla-Santos et al. (n=238) [108]	Post, ER(+), LABC	ANA 1 mg mg vs TAM 40 mg	3	13.3	ANA 18 months vs TAM 7 months, $P<0.01$	83% for ANA vs 56% for TAM, $P< 0.001$	ANA 17.4 months vs TAM 16 months, $P = 0.003$)/ NA
TARGET (n=668) [109]	Post, HR(+) or unknown, LABC or metastatic	ANA 1 mg vs TAM 20 mg	Until PD	19	NS	NS	NA/NA
Arimidex Study Group (n=353) [110]	Post, LABC	ANA 1 mg vs TAM 20 mg	Until PD	17.2	ANA 11.1 months vs TAM 5.6 months, $P = 0.005$	NA	NA/NA
IMPACT (n=330) [111]	Post, ER(+)	ANA 1 mg + TAM placebo vs TAM 20 mg + ANA placebo vs ANA 1 mg + TAM 20 mg	3	3	NA	NS	NA/NA
PROACT (n=451) [112]	Post, ER(+) ± PgR(+), LABC	ANA 1 mg + TAM placebo vs TAM 20 mg + ANA placebo	3	3	NA	NS	NA/NA

ANA, anastrozole; TAM, tamoxifen; Post, postmenopausal; LABC, locally advanced breast cancer; BCS, breast-conserving surgery; ORR, overall response rate (CR + PR); PD, progression of disease; LR, local recurrence; OS, overall survival; DFS, disease-free survival; NS, not significant; NA, not analyzed.

mastectomy to breast-conserving surgery in 10 out of 12 patients, resulting in an 83.3% rate for conservative surgery [75].

Two phase I studies have evaluated combined neoadjuvant chemoendocrine approaches using exemestane in combination with standard chemotherapy. Preclinical studies provided the first evidence that exemestane increases the pathological response rate to neoadjuvant epirubicin when administered concomitantly. The first study examined 16 patients with locally advanced breast cancers treated with exemestane (25 mg daily) and concomitant increasing doses of epirubicin (25, 30, and 35 mg/m^2 per week) for 8–12 weeks. From the 10 evaluable patients, they observed 2 clinical CR, 4 clinical PR, 3 with stable disease, and 1 with disease progression. Breast-conserving surgery was able to be performed in 66% of the patients, and they reported one case each with a pathological CR and PR [76]. A similar study treated 11 patients with locally advanced breast cancer with daily exemestane (25 mg) and concomitant increasing doses of docetaxel (20, 25, and 30 mg/m^2 per week) for 8–12 weeks. From the nine evaluable patients, Lichtenegger and colleagues noted 78% with clinical PR which translated into 78 and 22% with grade 1 and 2 pathological responses, respectively [77]. Phase II studies analyzing both agents in conjunction with neoadjuvant exemestane are currently in the works.

A multicenter Spanish phase II trial (2002) evaluated the efficacy of neoadjuvant exemestane (25 mg daily) for 6 months in 33 postmenopausal breast cancer patients. They observed a 50% radiographic partial response, and 10 patients previously evaluated for mastectomy were able to undergo breast-conserving surgery [78].

Miller et al. (2002) performed in vivo and in situ studies in 12 postmenopausal women with untreated large or locally advanced ER-rich tumors. The effect of exemestane (25 mg daily) for 3 months on aromatization peripherally and in breast cancer and surrounding normal tissue was determined. Immediately before starting therapy, patients received an 18-h infusion of radioactively labeled androgen and estrogen, followed by a wedge biopsy. This procedure was repeated after the 3-month treatment period, and the data were used to calculate peripheral and local aromatization. Neoadjuvant exemestane treatment was associated with a marked reduction in aromatization peripherally and in non-malignant breast tissue in all patients and in the breast tumor in all but one patient. Clinical and radiographic reduction in tumor volume ranged from 82.5 to 85.5%, resulting in subsequent conversion to breast-conserving surgery in 8 of 10 patients. Clinical benefits were accompanied by a marked reduction in cellular proliferation and PgR expression. These data again supported the use of exemestane as neoadjuvant therapy for breast cancer in postmenopausal women [79].

Final results from the German Neoadjuvant Aromasin Initiative (GENARI) trial (2003), a phase II study with exemestane, demonstrated a partial clinical response rate of 37% and no pathological CRs following 16 weeks of treatment [80]. A similar phase II study examined the effects of 4–5 months of neoadjuvant exemestane (25 mg daily) on postmenopausal, operable ER-positive breast cancer. Using the RECIST criteria (described below) for evaluation, they reported clinical CR and PR rates of 5.9 and 64.7%, respectively, with 23.5% demonstrating stable disease. In addition, breast-conserving surgery was possible in 45.2% [81].

A multicenter phase II trial of the Saitama Breast Cancer Clinical Study Group (SBCCSG-03) in Japan has evaluated the efficacy and tolerability of 4 months of neoadjuvant exemestane in 44 postmenopausal patients with ER-positive and/or PgR-positive, stage II to IIIB breast cancer measuring ≥3 cm. Breast-conserving surgery was performed in 27 (90%) of 30 patients that underwent surgery at 4 months, and a pathological response was observed in 13 (43%) of those patients. A clinical response was seen in 27 (66%) of 41 evaluable patients. Though their study lacks long-term follow-up, with an incidence of adverse events recorded as ≥10%, their findings suggested that neoadjuvant exemestane is not only effective but well tolerated in postmenopausal women with ER-positive breast cancer [82].

Table 4 summarizes the key features of trials evaluating exemestane in the neoadjuvant setting.

Comparison Between AIs: The ACOSOG Z1031 Trial

In 2006 the American College of Surgeons Oncology Group (ACOSOG) Z1031 trial opened for accrual (Fig. 1). The trial is currently accruing postmenopausal women with stage II/III ER-positive breast cancer who are randomized to receive neoadjuvant anastrozole (1 mg daily), exemestane (25 mg daily), or letrozole (2.5 mg daily) for 16–18 weeks preceding their planned surgery. With planned accrual to 375 patients over 3 years, the trial is designed not only to compare neoadjuvant anastrozole, exemestane, and letrozole with regard to radiographic response rates and safety, but to determine which of the three agents will be targeted in a future phase III study comparing neoadjuvant AIs with neoadjuvant chemotherapy [83]. Using an algorithm that considers both clinical and radiographic response rates, Z1031 will validate results from the IMPACT trial in addition to examining these other end points.

Pathologic response rates will be determined by analysis of both pre- and post-treatment primary tumor samples and patient blood samples in a central laboratory. Treatment effects will be analyzed in an effort to establish a molecular signature or gene expression profile that is predictive of AI treatment response and resistance. Tumor samples will be subjected to the Oncotype DX assay to determine a recurrence score and analyzed for ER, PgR, HER2, and Ki67.

Table 4 Prospective randomized trials of neoadjuvant therapy with exemestane

Study (number of patients)	Patient characteristics	Regimen	Duration of treatment (months)	Median follow-up (months)	Time to progression (months)	ORR	OS/DFS
EORTC (n=117) [113]	Post, LABC	TAM 20 mg vs EXE 25 mg	Until PD	24	NA	EXE 41% vs 17% TAM	NA/NA
Tubiana-Hulin et al. (n=42) [114]	Post, HR(+), LABC	EXE 25 mg	4–5	4	NA	73%	NA/NA
SBCCSG-03 (n=44) [115]	Post, HR(+), LABC	EXE 25 mg	4	4	N/A	66%	NA/NA

EXE, exemestane; TAM, tamoxifen; Post, postmenopausal; LABC, locally advanced breast cancer; ORR, overall response rate (CR + PR); PD, progression of disease; LR, local recurrence; OS, overall survival; DFS, disease-free survival; NS, not significant; NA, not analyzed

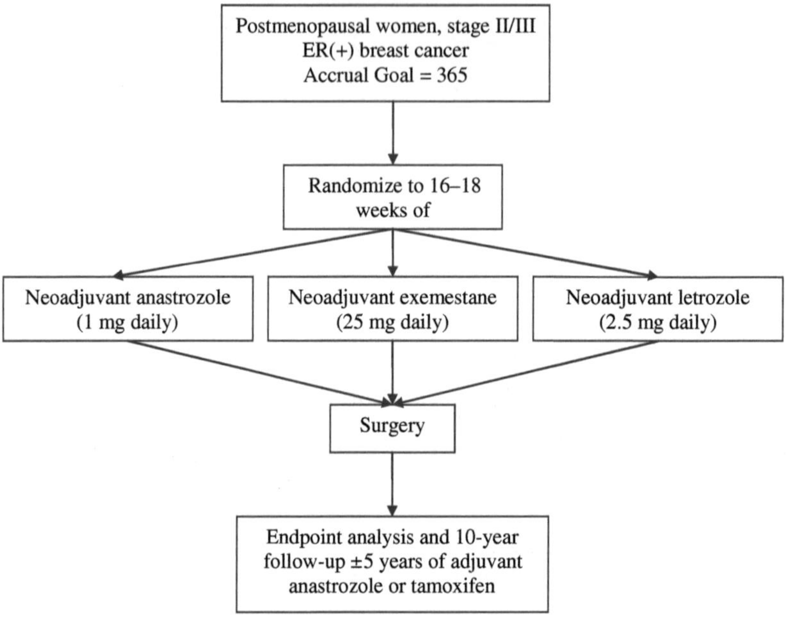

Fig. 1 ACOSOG Z1031 trial schema

Measurement of Response to Neoadjuvant Hormonal Therapy

Clinical Response

Clinical response is a subjective measurement of treatment efficacy, as demonstrated by that equivalent clinical responses observed among all three treatment arms in the IMPACT trial, a finding that was attributed to difficulties in assessing small tumors [84]. Measurement of tumor response by radiographic imaging offers another alternative to quantify and compare response to treatment, and as demonstrated in the letrozole P024 study, mammographic tumor measurements do allow for comparison of treatment effects. Both mammography and ultrasound have been shown to correlate well with actual tumor sizes, with one limitation of the latter being operator dependence. MRI has also been suggested by the National Cancer Institute but awaits validation. With regard to assessing response criteria, the NCI currently favors breast tumor evaluation with the RECIST criteria or Response Evaluation Criteria in Solid Tumors. This method evaluates the change in a measurable lesion as determined by ruler or micrometer caliper in a single dimension [85]. While attempts have been to standardize tumor measurements, bi-dimensional measurements are still obtained and reported in neoadjuvant endocrine therapy trials.

Surgical Outcome

The best argument in favor of neoadjuvant endocrine therapy is the observation that it has been shown to improve surgical outcomes in terms of tumor downsizing and subsequent conversion to breast-conserving surgery. In the letrozole P024 trial, treatment with letrozole improved rates of breast-conserving surgery over tamoxifen [86]. Though more subjective, reports on the rates of conversion to breast-conserving surgery in cases where mastectomy was deemed unavoidable are a potentially measurable outcome for comparisons of neoadjuvant endocrine therapeutic response.

Pathologic Response

Pathologic complete response, or pCR, is defined as the disappearance of all invasive disease in the breast and regional nodes. Pathological partial response, or pPR, is defined as a 51–99.9% reduction in measurable disease. A pathological CR is a validated surrogate end point in the context of neoadjuvant chemotherapy trials. A pathological CR, however, is uncommon in endocrine therapy trials to have comparative value. Other criteria have thus been adopted as alternatives to describe the treatment effects and allow comparisons among neoadjuvant endocrine therapy trials.

Examination of the Ki67 data from the letrozole P024 trial, in which approximately 50% of tumors demonstrated a post-treatment Ki67 level of ≥1% (the detection limit), has suggested a complete cell cycle arrest in response to treatment, as such a dramatic drop in Ki67 levels suggests that those tumors must have been entirely estrogen dependent. Tao and colleagues have suggested that a cell cycle CR can be interpreted as a pathological CR in the neoadjuvant endocrine setting. That is, Ki67 is a variable that can be easily measured in post-treatment specimens and identifies a specific tumor to be highly responsive to treatment. Further analysis has statistically linked ER expression to cell cycle CR [87]. At higher levels of ER positivity, cell cycle CRs were more common with letrozole (69%) than tamoxifen (40%, P = 0.0002) [88]. This suggests that cell cycle CR may be an alternative method to determine efficacy of endocrine therapy where pathological CR is not valid.

Caution must be exercised in biomarker end point analysis, however, for as also demonstrated in the P024 trial, observed early changes in tumor cell proliferation following neoadjuvant treatment with letrozole did not accurately predict subsequent clinical response. Changes in proliferation seen at later times can be the consequence of response and may be associated with early resistance. High expression of c-erbB2 did not hinder tumor responses to neoadjuvant treatment with letrozole but was associated with high tumor proliferation before and during treatment [89]. It remains to be determined whether these characteristics confer subsequent resistance to treatment and early relapse in the adjuvant setting.

Gene Expression Profiling

Patient Profiling Using Microarrays

Selection of endocrine therapy requires the identification of markers that accurately predict response and resistance. Microarray analysis of tumor RNA is an extremely powerful tool which allows global gene expression to be measured. When used in combination with neoadjuvant treatment, sequential biopsies may be analyzed and results correlated with clinical and pathological response. Several studies are examining the potential of RNA microarrays in patients receiving neoadjuvant endocrine therapy to identify the molecular signatures associated with tumor sensitivity and resistance. Miller and colleagues have analyzed clinical response in postmenopausal women with large, ER-rich breast cancers who received a 3-month course of treatment with neoadjuvant letrozole. Their objectives were to discover genes that change with estrogen deprivation—specifically, those whose change in expression differ between tumors which are either responsive or resistant to treatment. Using tumor RNA from pre- and post-treatment tissue, a total of 91 down-regulated genes have been identified that are functionally associated with cell cycle progression, particularly mitosis [90]. Their results indicate that molecular profiling of early changes with neoadjuvant treatment offers the opportunity to distinguish between clinically responsive and resistant tumors and provides important information about the heterogeneity of endocrine resistance [91].

Similar studies of expression profiling using cDNA arrays on ER-positive tumor tissue preceding and following neoadjuvant treatment with anastrozole or letrozole have also demonstrated profound changes in expression of proliferation-related genes as well as many classical estrogen-dependent genes such as TFF1, CCND1, PDZK1, and AGR2. The changes in gene expression have been integrated into a Global Index of Dependence on Estrogen (GIDE), which enumerates the genes changing by at least twofold with therapy. The GIDE varied markedly between tumors and related significantly to pretreatment levels of HER2 and changes in immunohistochemically detected Ki67 [92]. This study also demonstrated the existence of transcriptional signatures associated with neoadjuvant AI use. Larger data sets using this approach should enable identification of estrogen-dependent molecular changes, which are the key determinants of benefit or resistance to endocrine therapy.

The Oncotype DX Assay

Patients diagnosed with axillary node-negative ER-positive breast cancer have an excellent prognosis, yet at least 15% of them fail after 5 years of tamoxifen treatment. A patient-specific prognostic assay to identify those patients that would benefit the most from chemotherapy in addition to tamoxifen, or those best treated by tamoxifen alone, would avoid overtreatment and undue morbidity. Neoadjuvant trials have established biomarkers for responsiveness and resistance to adjuvant treatment, which has led to molecular assays to predict prognosis in breast cancer. This is exemplified in the emergence of the Oncotype DX assay. The assay is a reverse transcription-PCR genomic test that predicts the likelihood of breast cancer recurrence in early-stage, node-negative, ER-positive breast cancer and thus those patients most likely to appreciate benefit from adjuvant endocrine or chemotherapy. The assay uses a stepwise approach of going through independent model-building and validation sets to generate a 21-gene Recurrence Score (RS), which is based on monitoring of mRNA expression levels of 16 cancer-related genes in relation to five reference genes. The RS is used to stratify patients into low- (RS<11), intermediate- (11–25), and high-risk (>25) categories. The RS provides a more accurate, reproducible measure of breast cancer aggressiveness, therapeutic responsiveness, and prognosis than standard measures. It does not require fresh tissue, and its application to pooled RNA samples from fixed paraffin-embedded tissues has demonstrated precision and reproducibility [93]. Clinically validated among the patient subsets in the NSABP B-14 and B-20 trials, the assay now serves as a clinical adjunct in determining those patients most likely to benefit from adjuvant tamoxifen (low RS) or chemotherapy (high RS) [94]. The RS identified approximately 50% of the patients who had excellent prognosis after tamoxifen alone and suggested that high-risk patients identified by RS would preferentially benefit from chemotherapy. A prospective study—the Trial Assigning Individualized Options for Treatment (Rx) (TAILORx)—is currently accruing in North America and will examine whether chemotherapy is required for the intermediate-risk group defined by the RS [95].

Current Recommendations

Neoadjuvant endocrine therapy trials for breast cancer are now accepted investigational approaches for oncology group and pharmaceutical company-based research programs. A 2007 update from the American Society of Clinical Oncology recommends CA 15-3, CA 27.29, carcinoembryonic antigen, ER, PR, human epidermal growth factor receptor 2, urokinase plasminogen activator, and plasminogen activator inhibitor 1 for clinical use as tumor markers in breast cancer, with insufficient evidence to support the use of DNA/ploidy by flow cytometry, p53, cathepsin D, cyclin E, proteomics, certain multiparameter assays, detection of bone marrow micrometastases, and circulating tumor cells [96]. Data from ongoing trials are needed to further assess the efficacy of such markers, how exactly they should be applied to patient management, and the role they should play in determining candidates for neoadjuvant endocrine treatment.

Future Directions

Despite data collected from previous and ongoing studies, neoadjuvant endocrine therapy is not being administered routinely to patients outside the setting of clinical trials. Neoadjuvant endocrine treatment with AIs has evolved from being an experimental effort to palliate women with locally advanced breast cancer unsuitable for surgery or chemotherapy to representing a viable and possibly preferred alternative for postmenopausal women with hormone receptor-positive large tumors or locally advanced breast cancer.

The absence of a large validation study comparing patients receiving neoadjuvant endocrine therapy to those receiving neoadjuvant chemotherapy or immediate surgery continues to be a major hurdle in the routine adoption of first-line endocrine therapy. Ellis and colleagues have proposed a trial similar to NSABP B18 to investigate neoadjuvant AIs versus immediate surgery or neoadjuvant AIs versus neoadjuvant chemotherapy [97]. This type of trial could help to demonstrate that neoadjuvant endocrine therapy improves OS beyond that observed with traditional postoperative chemotherapy. In the interim, studies of neoadjuvant endocrine therapy will continue to serve as platforms for biomarker discovery as well as a forum in which to test new potential therapeutic agents, with promise of contributing to our understanding of the molecular basis for observed therapeutic responses to endocrine agents.

References

1. Rossouw E, Anderson GL, Prentice RL, et al., for Writing Group for the Women's Health Initiative. Risks and benefits of estrogen plus progestin in healthy postmenopausal women: principal results from the Women's Health Initiative. JAMA 2002;288:321–333.
2. Chlebowski RT, Hendrix SL, Langer RD, et al. Influence of estrogen plus progestin on breast cancer and mammography in healthy postmenopausal women: the Women's Health Initiative randomized trial. JAMA 2003;289:3243–3253.
3. Million Women Study Collaborators. Breast cancer and hormone-replacement therapy in the Million Women Study. Lancet 2002;362;419–427.
4. Abrial C, Mouret-Reynier MA, Cure H, et al. Neoadjuvant endocrine therapy in breast cancer. The Breast 2006;15:9–19.
5. Goldhirsch A, Wood WC, Gelber RD, et al, 10th St. Gallen conference. progress and promise: highlights of the international expert consensus on the primary therapy of early breast cancer 2007. Ann Oncol. 2007;18(7):1133–1144.
6. Mauriac L, Debled M, Durand M, et al. Neoadjuvant tamoxifen for hormone-sensitive non-metastatic breast carcinomas in early postmenopausal women. Ann Oncol 2002;13:293–298.
7. Dixon JM, Jackson J, Renshaw L, et al. Neoadjuvant tamoxifen and aromatase inhibitors: comparisons and clinical outcomes. J Steroid Biochem Mol Biol 2003;86:295–299.
8. Dixon JM, Anderson TJ, Miller WR. Neoadjuvant endocrine therapy of breast cancer: a surgical perspective. Eur J Cancer 2002;38(17):2214–2221.
9. Jordan VC. Tamoxifen: a most unlikely pioneering medicine. Nat Rev Drug Discov 2003;2:205–213

10. Jones LW, Haykowsky M, Pituskin EN, et al. Cardiovascular reserve and risk profile of postmenopausal women after chemoendocrine therapy for hormone receptor-positive operable breast cancer. The Oncologist 2007;12:11.
11. Buzdar A. The ATAC (Arimidex, Tamoxifen, Alone or in Combination) trial in postmenopausal women with early breast cancer—updated efficacy results based on a median follow-up of 47 months. San Antonio Breast Cancer Symposium 2002; abstr. 13.
12. Braithwaite RS, Chlebowski RT, Lau J, et al. Meta-analysis of vascular and neoplastic events associated with tamoxifen. J Gen Intern Med. 2003;18(11):937–947.
13. Coller JK, Krebsfaenger N, Klein K, et al. Large interindividual variability in the in vitro formation of tamoxifen metabolites related to the development of genotoxicity. Br J Clin Pharmacol 2004;57:105–111.
14. Early Breast Cancer Trialists' Collaborative Group. Effects of chemotherapy and hormonal therapy for early breast cancer on recurrence and 15-year survival: an overview of the randomized trials. Lancet 2005;365:1687–1717.
15. Johnson MD, Zuo H, Lee KH, et al. Pharmacologic characterization of 4-hydroxy-N-desmethyl tamoxifen, a nover active metabolite of tamoxifen. Breast Cancer Res Treat 2004;85:151–159.
16. Miller WR. Aromatase activity in breast tissue. J Steroid Biochem Mol 1991;39:783–90.
17. Dixon JM, Jackson J, Renshaw L, et al. Neoadjuvant tamoxifen and aromatase inhibitors: comparisons and clinical outcomes. J Steroid Biochem Mol Biol 2003;86:295–299.
18. Thurlimann B, Beretta K, Bacchi M, et al. First-line fadrozole HCI (CGS16949A) versus tamoxifen in postmenopausal women with advanced breast cancer. Prospective randomized trial of the Swiss Group for Clinical Cancer Research SAKK 20/88. Ann Oncol 1996;7:471–9.
19. Tominaga T, Adachi I, Sasaki Y, et al. Double-blind randomized trial comparing the nonsteroidal aromotase inhibitors letrozole and fadrozole in postmenopausal women with advanced breast cancer. Ann Oncol 2003;14:62–1470.
20. Silva E, Gatalica Z, Snyder C, et al. Hereditary breast cancer: Part II. Management of hereditary breast cancer: implications of molecular genetics and pathology. Breast J 2007. [Epub ahead of print]
21. Fitzgibbons P. Prognostic factors in breast cancer: College of American Pathologists Consensus Statement 1999. Arch Pathol Lab Med 2000;124:966.
22. Bast R, et al. 2000 update of recommendations for the use of tumor markers in breast and colorectal cancer: clinical practice guidelines of the American Society of Clinical Oncology. J Clin Oncol 2000;19:1865.
23. Gokhale S, Rosen D, Sneige N, et al, Assessment of two automated imaging systems in evaluating estrogen receptor status in breast carcinoma. Appl Immunohistochem Mol Morphol 2007;15(4):451–455.
24. Green S, Walter P, Greene G, et al. Cloning of the human estrogen receptor cDNA. J Steroid Biochem 1986;24:77–83.
25. Fuqua SA, Schiff R, Parra I, et al. Estrogen receptor beta protein in human breast cancer: correlation with clinical tumor parameters. Cancer Res 2003;63:2434–2439.
26. Dixon JM, Jackson J, Renshaw L, et al. Neoadjuvant tamoxifen and aromatase inhibitors: comparisons and clinical outcomes. J Steroid Biochem Mol Biol 2003;86:295–299.
27. Jordan VC, O'Malley BW. Selective estrogen-receptor modulators and antihormonal resistance in breast cancer. J Clin Oncol 2007;25(36):5815–5824.
28. Omoto Y, Kobayashi S, Inoue S, et al. Evaluation of estrogen receptor beta wild-type and variant protein expression, and relationship with clinicopathological factors in breast cancers. Eur J Cancer 2002;38:380-6.2000;92:179–181.
29. Mann S, Laucirica R, Carlson N, et al. Estrogen receptor beta expression in invasive breast cancer. Human Pathol 2001;32:113–118.

30. Vinayagam R, Sibson DR, Holcombe C, et al. Association of estrogen receptor beta 2 (ERβ2/ERβcx) with outcome of adjuvant endocrine treatment for primary breast cancer – a retrospective study. BMC Cancer 2007;18(7):131.
31. Esslimani-Sahla M, Simony-Lafontaine J, Kramar A, et al. Estrogen receptor ß (ERß) level but not its ERßcx variant helps to predict tamoxifen resistance in breast cancer. Clin Cancer Res 2004;10:5769–5776.
32. Jensen EV, Cheng G, Palmieri C, et al. Estrogen receptors and proliferation markers in primary and recurrent breast cancer. Proc Natl Acad Sci USA 2001;98: 15197–15202.
33. Miller WR, Anderson TJ, Dixon JM, et al. Estrogen receptor beta and neoadjuvant therapy with tamoxifen: prediction of response and effects of treatment. Br J Cancer 2006;94(9):1333–8.
34. Knight W, Osborne C, McGuire W. Hormone receptors in primary and advanced breast cancer. Clin Endocrinol Metab 1980;9:361.
35. Bezwoda W, Esser J, Dansey R, et al. The value of estrogen and progesterone receptor determinations in advanced breast cancer. Cancer 1991;68:867.
36. Pertschuk L, Feldman J, Eisenberg K, et al. Immunocytochemical detection of progesterone receptor in breast cancer with monoclonal antibody. Cancer 1988;62:342.
37. Leo JC, Lin VC. The activities of progesterone receptor isoform A and B are differentially modulated by their ligands in a gene-selective manner. Int J Cancer 2008;122(1):230–243.
38. Ellis MJ, Coop A, Singh B, et al. Letrozole inhibits tumor proliferation more effectively than tamoxifen independent of HER1/2 expression status. Cancer Res 2003;63:6523–6531.
39. Tao Y, Klause A, Vickers A, et al. Clinical and biomarker endpoint analysis in neoadjuvant endocrine therapy trials. J Ster Biochem Mol Biol 2005;95:91–95.
40. Dowsett M, Smith IE, Ebbs SR, et al., IMPACT Trialists Group. Prognostic value of Ki67 expression after short-term presurgical endocrine therapy for primary breast cancer. J Natl Cancer Inst 2007;99(2):167–170.
41. Akashi-Tanaka S, Omatsu M, Shimizu C, et al. Favorable outcome in patients with breast cancer in the presence of pathological response after neoadjuvant endocrine therapy. Breast 2007;16(5):482–488.
42. Pierce JH, Arnstein P, DiMarco E, et al. Oncogenic potential of erbB-2 in human mammary epithelial cells. Oncogene 1991;6:1189–1194.
43. Slamon DJ, Godolphin W, Jones LA, et al. Studies of the HER-2/neu proto-oncogene in human breast and ovarian cancer. Science 1989;244:707–712.
44. Ellis MJ, Coop A, Singh B, et al. Letrozole is more effective neoadjuvant endocrine therapy than tamoxifen for ERB1- and/or ERB2-positive, estrogen receptor-positive primary breast cancer: evidence from a phase III randomized trial. J Clin Oncol 2001;19(18):3808–3816.
45. Preece PE, Wood RA, Mackie CR, et al. Tamoxifen as initial sole treatment of localized breast cancer in elderly women: a pilot study. BMJ 1982;284:869–870.
46. Bates T, Riley DL, Houghton J, et al. Breast cancer in elderly women: a cancer research campaign trial comparing treatment with tamoxifen and optimal surgery with tamoxifen alone. Br J Surg 1991;78:591–594.
47. Van Dalsen AD, De Vries J. Treatment of breast cancer in elderly patients. J Surg Oncol 1995;60:80–82.
48. Tan SM, Cheung KL, Willsher PC, et al. Locally advanced primary breast cancer: medium-term results of a randomized trial of multimodal therapy versus initial hormone therapy. Eur J Cancer 2001;37:2331–2338.
49. Gazet JC, Ford HT, Coombes RC, et al. Prospective randomized trial of tamoxifen vs. surgery in elderly patients with breast cancer. Eur J Surg Oncol 1994;20:207–214.
50. Mustacchi G, Ceccherini R, Milani S, et al. Tamoxifen alone versus adjuvant tamoxifen for operable breast cancer of the elderly: long-term results of the phase III randomized controlled multicenter GRETA trial. Ann Oncol 2003;14(3):414–420.

51. Fentiman IS, Christiaens MR, Paridaens R, et al. Treatment of operable breast cancer in the elderly: a randomised clinical trial EORTC 10851 comparing tamoxifen alone with modified radical mastectomy. Eur J Cancer. 2003;39(3):309–316.
52. Dixon JM, Love CDB, Bellamy COC, et al. Letrozole as primary medical therapy for locally advanced and large operable breast cancer. Breast Cancer Res Treat 2001;66:191–199.
53. Paepke S, Tulusan A, Kiesel L, et al. A multi-center study of pre-operative treatment with letrozole for optimal duration of treatment in postmenopausal women with ER and/or PgR positive breast cancer. Proc ASCO 2003 (abstr. 321).
54. Renshaw L, Murray J, Young O, et al. Is there an optimal duration of neoadjuvant letrozole therapy? San Antonio 2004 (abstr. 405).
55. Miller WR, White S, Dixon JM, et al. Proliferation, steroid receptors and clinical/pathological response in breast cancer treated with letrozole. Br J Cancer. 2006;Apr 10;94(7):1051–1056.
56. Eiermann W, Paepke S, Appfelstaedt L, et al. Preoperative treatment of postmenopausal breast cancer patients with letrozole: a randomized double-blind multicenter study. Ann Oncol 2001;12(11):1505–1506.
57. Ellis MJ, Coop A, Singh B, et al. Letrozole is more effective neoadjuvant endocrine therapy than tamoxifen for ERB1- and/or ERB2-positive, estrogen receptor-positive primary breast cancer: evidence from a phase III randomized trial. J Clin Oncol 2001;19(18):3808–3816.
58. Mouridsen H, Gershanovich M, Sun Y, et al. Superior efficacy of letrozole versus tamoxifen as first-line therapy for postmenopausal women with advanced breast cancer; results of a phase III study of the International Letrozole Breast Cancer Group. J Clin Oncol 2001;19:2596–2606.
59. Mouridsen H, Gershanovich M, Sun Y, et al. Phase III study of letrozole versus tamoxifen as first-line therapy of advanced breast cancer in postmenopausal women: analysis of survival and update of efficacy from the International Letrozole Breast Cancer Group. J Clin Oncol 2003;21:2101–2109.
60. Miller WR, Dixon JM, Cameron DA, et al. Biological and clinical effects of aromatase inhibitors in neoadjuvant therapy. J Steroid Biochem Mol Biol 2001;79:103–107.
61. Miller WR, Dixon JM, Macfarlane L, et al. Pathological features of breast cancer response following neoadjuvant treatment with either letrozole or tamoxifen. Eur J Cancer 2003;39(4):462–468.
62. Ellis MJ, Coop A, Singh B, et al. Letrozole is more effective neoadjuvant endocrine therapy than tamoxifen for ERB1- and/or ERB2-positive, estrogen receptor-positive primary breast cancer: evidence from a phase III randomized trial. J Clin Oncol 2001;19(18):3808–3816.
63. Ellis MJ, Ma C. Letrozole in the neoadjuvant setting: the P024 trial. Breast Cancer Res Treat 2007;105:33–43.
64. Dixon JM, Renshaw L, Bellamy C, et al. The effects of neoadjuvant anastrozole (Arimidex) on tumor volume in postmenopausal women with breast cancer: a randomized, double-blinded, single-center study. Clin Cancer Res 2000;6:2229–2235.
65. Dixon JM, jackson J, Hills M, et al. Anatrozole demonstrates clinical and biological effectiveness in erbB2 ER positive breast cancers. San Antonio 2002 (abstr. 263).
66. Milla-Santos A, Milla I, Rallo L, et al. Anastrozole (A) as neoadjuvant (NEO) therapy for hormone-dependent locally advanced breast cancer (LABC) in postmenopausal (PM) patients (pts). Proc ASCO 2002;21 (abstr. 156).
67. Bonneterre J, Thurlimann B, Robertson JF, et al. Anastrozole versus tamoxifen as first-line therapy for advanced breast cancer in 668 postmenopausal women: results of the Tamoxifen or Arimidex Randomized Group Efficacy and Tolerability study. J Clin Oncol 2000;18:3748–3757.
68. Nabholtz JM, Buzdar A, Pollak M, et al. Anatrozole is superior to tamoxifen as first-line therapy for advanced breast cancer in postmenopausal women: results of a North

American multicenter randomized trial. Arimidex Study Group. J Clin Oncol 2000;18:3758–3767.
69. Bonneterre J, Buzdar A, Nabholtz JM, et al. Anastrozole is superior to tamoxifen as first-line therapy in hormone receptor positive advanced breast carcinoma. Cancer 2001;92:2247–2258.
70. Dixon JM, Jackson J, Renshaw L, et al. Neoadjuvant tamixifen and aromatase inhibitors: comparisons and clinical outcomes. J Steroid Biochem Mol Biol 2003;86:295–299.
71. Smith I, Dowsett M. Comparison of anastrozole vs tamoxifen alone and in combination as neoadjuvant treatment of estrogen receptor-positive (ER+) operable breast cancer in postmenopausal women: the IMPACT trial. San Antonio 2003 (abstr. 1).
72. Cataliotti L, Buzdar A, Noguchi S, et al. Efficacy of preoperative arimidex (anastrozole) compared with tamoxifen (PROACT) as neoadjuvant therapy in postmenopausal women with hormone receptor-positive breast cancer. Eur J Cancer 2004;2:46.
73. Dirix L, Piccart M, Lohrisch C, et al. Efficacy of and tolerance to exemestane versus tamoxifen in 1st line hormone therapy of postmenopausal metastatic breast cancer patients: a European Organization for the Research and Treatment of Cancer (EORTC Breast Group) Phase II trial with Pharmacia and Upjohn. Proc Am Soc Clin Oncol 200120:29a.
74. Paridaens R, Dirix L, Lohrisch C, et al. Mature results of a randomized phase II multicenter study of exemestane versus tamoxifen as first-line hormone therapy for postmenopausal women with metastatic breast cancer. Ann Oncol 2003;14(9):1391–1398.
75. Dixon JM, Anderson T, Miller WR. Phase IIb study of neoadjuvant exemestane (EXE) in locally advanced breast cancer. Proc ASCO 2001 (abstr. 1908)
76. Wolf C, Hackl W, Kuemper S, et al. Exemestane combined with epirubicin, Q1wX, as preoperative chemoendocrine treatment for patients with primary breast cancer: a phase I study. Proc ASCO 2001 (abstr. 1819).
77. Lichtenegger W, Hackl W, Huettner C, et al. Exemestane combined with weekly docetaxel as preoperative treatment for breast cancer. Proc ASCO 2001 (anstr. 1832).
78. Gil M, Barnadas A, Cirera L, et al. Exemestane as neoadjuvant treatment in patients >65 years with T>3 cm; preliminary results of a multicenter Spanish phase II trial. San Antonio 2002 (abstr. 272).
79. Miller WR, Dixon JM. Endocrine and clinical endpoints of exemestane as neoadjuvant therapy. Cancer Control 2002;9(2 Suppl):9–15.
80. Krainick U, Astner A, Jonat W, et al. Phase II study to define safety and efficacy of exemestane as preoperative therapy for postmenopausal patients with primary breast cancer—final results of the German Neoadjuvant Aromasin Initiative (GENARI). San Antonio 2003 (abstr. 239).
81. Tubiana-Hulin M, Spyratos F, Becette V, et al. Phase II study of neoadjuvant exemestane in postmenopausal patients with operable breast cancer. San Antonio 2003 (abstr. 443).
82. Takei H, Suemasu K, Inoue K, et al. Multicenter phase II trial of neoadjuvant exemestane for postmenopausal patients with hormone receptor-positive, operable breast cancer: Saitama Breast Cancer Clinical Study Group (SBCCSG-03). Breast Cancer Res Treat. 2008;107(1):87–94.
83. Ma CX, Ellis MJ. Neoadjuvant endocrine therapy for locally advanced breast cancer. Semin Oncol 2006;33:650–656. Review.
84. Smith I, Dowsett M. Comparison of anastrozole vs tamoxifen alone and in combination as neoadjuvant treatment of estrogen receptor-positive (ER+) operable breast cancer in postmenopausal women: the IMPACT trial. San Antonio 2003 (abstr. 1).
85. Gehan EA, Tefft MC. Will there be resistance to the RECIST (response evaluation criteria in solid tumors)? J Natl Cancer Inst 2000;92:179–181.
86. Wong ZW, Ellis MJ. Neoadjuvant endocrine therapy for breast cancer: an overlooked option? Oncology 2004;18;411–420.

87. Tao Y, Klause A, Vickers A, et al. Clinical and biomarker endpoint analysis in neoadjuvant endocrine therapy trials. J Steroid Biochem Mol Biol 2005;95:91–95.
88. Ellis MJ, Coop A, Singh B, et al. Letrozole is more effective neoadjuvant endocrine therapy than tamoxifen for ERB1- and/or ERB2-positive, estrogen receptor-positive primary breast cancer: evidence from a phase III randomized trial. J Clin Oncol 2001;19(18):3808–3816.
89. Miller WR, Anderson TJ, White S, et al. Growth factor signaling in clinical breast cancer and its impact on response to conventional therapies: the Edinburgh experience. Endocr Relat Cancer 2005;12 Suppl 1: S119–S123.
90. Miller WR, Larionov A, Renshaw L, et al. Aromatase inhibitors – gene discovery. J Steroid Biochem Mol Biol. 2007;106(1-5):130–142.
91. Miller WR, Larionov A, Anderson TJ, et al. Predicting response and resistance to endocrine therapy: profiling patients on aromatase inhibitors. Cancer 2008;112(3 Suppl):689–694.
92. Mackay A, Urruticoechea A, Dixon JM, et al. Molecular response to aromatase inhibitor treatment in primary breast cancer. Breast Cancer Res 2007;9(3):R37.
93. Cronin M, Sangli C, Liu ML, et al. Analytical validation of the Oncotype DX genomic diagnostic test for recurrence prognosis and therapeutic response prediction in node-negative, estrogen receptor-positive breast cancer. Clin Chem 2007;53(6):1084–1091.
94. Paik S, Shak S, Tang G, et al. A multigene assay to predict recurrence of tamoxifen-treated, node-negative breast cancer. N Engl J Med 2004;351(27):2817–2826.
95. Paik S. Development and clinical utility of a 21-gene recurrence score prognostic assay in patients with early breast cancer treated with tamoxifen. Oncologist 2007;12(6):631–635.
96. Harris L, Fritsche H, Mennel R, et al. American Society of Clinical Oncology 2007 update of recommendations for the use of tumor markers in breast cancer. J Clin Oncol 2007;25(33): 5287–5312.
97. Ellis MJ. Neoadjuvant endocrine therapy as a drug development strategy. Clin Cancer Res 2004;10:391s–395s.
98. Bates T, Riley DL, Houghton J, et al. Breast cancer in elderly women: a cancer research campaign trial comparing treatment with tamoxifen and optimal surgery with tamoxifen alone. Br J Surg 1991;78:591–4.
99. Gazet JC, Ford HT, Coombes RC, et al. Prospective randomized trial of tamoxifen vs. surgery in elderly patients with breast cancer. Eur J Surg Oncol 1994;20:207–214.
100. Tan SM, Cheung KL, Willsher PC, et al. Locally advanced primary breast cancer: medium-term results of a randomized trial of multimodal therapy versus initial hormone therapy. Eur J Cancer 2001;37:2331–2338.
101. Mustacchi G, Ceccherini R, Milani S, et al. Tamoxifen alone versus adjuvant tamoxifen for operable breast cancer of the elderly: long-term results of the phase III randomized controlled multicenter GRETA trial. Ann Oncol 2003; 414–420.
102. Fentiman IS, Christiaens MR, Paridaens R, et al. Treatment of operable breast cancer in the elderly: a randomised clinical trial EORTC 10851 comparing tamoxifen alone with modified radical mastectomy. Eur J Cancer. 2003;39(3):309–316.
103. Dixon JM, Love CDB, Bellamy COC, et al. Letrozole as primary medical therapy for locally advanced and large operable breast cancer. Breast Cancer Res Treat 2001;66:191–199.
104. Miller WR, Dixon JM, Cameron DA, et al. Biological and clinical effects of aromatase inhibitors in neoadjuvant therapy. J Steroid Biochem Mol Biol 2001;79:103–107.
105. Eiermann W, Paepke S, Appfelstaedt L, et al. Preoperative treatment of postmenopausal breast cancer patients with letrozole: a randomized double-blind multicenter study. Ann Oncol 2001;12(11):1505–1506.
106. Mouridsen H, Gershanovich M, Sun Y, et al. Phase III study of letrozole versus tamoxifen as first-line therapy of advanced breast cancer in postmenopausal women:

analysis of survival and update of efficacy from the International Letrozole Breast Cancer Group. J Clin Oncol 2003;21:2101–2109.
107. Ellis MJ, Coop A, Singh B, et al. Letrozole is more effective neoadjuvant endocrine therapy than tamoxifen for ERB1- and/or ERB2-positive, estrogen receptor-positive primary breast cancer: evidence from a phase III randomized trial. J Clin Oncol 2001;19(18):3808–3816.
108. Milla-Santos A, Milla L, Portella J, et al. Anastrozole versus tamoxifen as first-line therapy in postmenopausal patients with hormone-dependent advanced breast cancer: a prospective, randomized, phase III study. Am J Clin Oncol 2003;26(3):317–322.
109. Bonneterre J, Thurlimann B, Robertson JF, et al. Anastrozole versus tamoxifen as first-line therapy for advanced breast cancer in 668 postmenopausal women: results of the Tamoxifen or Arimidex Randomized Group Efficacy and Tolerability study. J Clin Oncol 2000;18:3748–3757.
110. Nabholtz JM, Buzdar A, Pollak M, et al. Anatrozole is superior to tamoxifen as first-line therapy for advanced breast cancer in postmenopausal women: results of a North American multicenter randomized trial. Arimidex Study Group. J Clin Oncol 2000;18:3758–3767.
111. Dowsett M, Smith IE, Ebbs SR, et al. Proliferation and apoptosis as markers of benefit in neoadjuvant endocrine therapy of breast cancer. Clin Cancer Res 2006;12(3 Pt 2):1024s–1030s.
112. Cataliotti L, Buzdar A, Noguchi S, et al. Efficacy of preoperative arimidex (anastrozole) compared with tamoxifen (PROACT) as neoadjuvant therapy in postmenopausal women with hormone receptor-positive breast cancer. Eur J Cancer 2004;2:46.
113. Paridaens R, Dirix L, Lohrisch C, et al. Mature results of a randomized phase II multicenter study of exemestane versus tamoxifen as first-line hormone therapy for postmenopausal women with metastatic breast cancer. Ann Oncol. 2003;14(9):1391–1398.
114. Tubiana-Hulin M, Becette V, Bieche I, et al. Exemestane as neoadjuvant hormonotherapy for locally advanced breast cancer: results of a phase II trial. Anticancer Res 2007;27(4C):2689–2696.
115. Takei H, Suemasu K, Inoue K, et al. Multicenter phase II trial of neoadjuvant exemestane for postmenopausal patients with hormone receptor-positive, operable breast cancer: Saitama Breast Cancer Clinical Study Group (SBCCSG-03). Breast Cancer Res Treat. 2008;107(1):87–94.

Hormone Resistance

Stephen R.D. Johnston

Introduction

About 75% of breast cancers are estrogen and/or progesterone receptor (ER, PgR) positive, and estrogen is the main stimulant in the development and growth of these tumours. Thus deprivation of estrogenic signalling has been the basis of hormonal therapy for patients with ER/PgR-positive disease. Currently available endocrine strategies include targeting the ER itself with the selective estrogen receptor modulator tamoxifen or the ER downregulator fulvestrant, as well as suppressing the amount of available ligand (estrogen) for the receptor with gonadal suppression in pre-menopausal women (ovariectomy or luteinising hormone-releasing hormone agonists), or aromatase inhibitors in post-menopausal women. Large-scale randomised trials have shown that 5 years of tamoxifen given immediately after surgery for early-stage ER+ breast cancer reduces mortality by 28% [1]. Indeed among post-menopausal women with early-stage ER+ breast cancer, endocrine therapy has actually been shown to have a greater impact on reducing annual breast cancer death rate than adjuvant chemotherapy (31% vs 20%) [2].

Given their proven efficacy and generally favourable side effect profile, endocrine therapies are widely used in the treatment of both early-stage and recurrent/metastatic breast cancer. Unfortunately, despite documented levels of ER in recurrent disease, up to 50% of patients with metastatic disease do not respond to first-line endocrine treatment (de novo resistance), while the remainder will eventually relapse despite an initial response (*acquired* resistance) [3]. In the last two decades there have been major efforts to understand the various biological mechanisms responsible for the development of endocrine resistance, with the ultimate aim of identifying new therapeutic strategies to enhance the efficacy of current treatment strategies for hormone receptor-positive breast cancer.

S.R.D. Johnston (✉)
Department of Medicine, Royal Marsden NHS Foundation Trust, Chelsea, London SW4 6JJ, UK
e-mail: stephen.johnston@rmh.nhs.uk

S.A.W. Fuqua (ed.), *Hormone Receptors in Breast Cancer*,
Cancer Treatment and Research 312, DOI 10.1007/978-0-387-09463-2_9,

Table 1 Postulated mechanisms of endocrine resistance and potential therapeutic implications for the clinic

Biological mechanism	Therapeutic options
Genomic ER related	
Loss of ER expression and/or function by growth factor suppression	Sequential growth factor ER-targeted therapy
ER silencing due to promoter hypermethylation	Demethylating agents or HDAC inhibitors
Enhanced genomic functions of ER via HER2 and AIB1 or p38MAPK	Dual ER and HER2 targeting
ER hypersensitivity to low residual estrogen levels	Continued ED + ER downregulator or growth factor inhibitor
ER mutations/variants	Rare
Pharmacological/pharmacogenomic	
Altered tamoxifen metabolism and cellular clearance, possibly related to CYP2D6 genotypes	Higher tamoxifen doses in selected patients?
Aromatase expression and function	Relevance unknown
Growth factor signalling	
Switch to ER-independent proliferation (i.e. loss CDK10 and ER-independent ERK activation)	Non-ER-targeted therapy
Growth factor-mediated activation of classical ER via AF-1 – requires ER ligand	Combined growth factor ER-targeted therapy
Enhanced non-genomic ER interaction at membrane with growth factor pathways (EGFR, IGFR, HER2)	Combined growth factor ER-targeted therapy

Various theories, each supported by pre-clinical and in some instances clinical data, have been suggested to explain endocrine resistance. These include mechanisms that have a sustained dependence on ER-mediated signalling, while others implicate growth factor-mediated mitogenic signalling which may or may not cross-talk with existing ER-signalling pathways (Table 1). Just as breast cancer is proving to be a heterogenous disease with different molecular phenotypes [4], the strong likelihood is that even in ER+ disease there will be no single unifying mechanism for endocrine resistance. Therefore, identifying which resistance mechanism is operational in an individual patient could become clinically relevant in tailoring the most appropriate subsequent therapy, e.g. non-ER-targeted treatment, further endocrine manipulation, or a combination of both. Central to all research in endocrine resistance, however, is having a clear molecular understanding of ER signalling, and in particular how current therapies modulate the ER pathway.

Modulation of ER Signalling

In the classical model of estrogenic signalling, estrogen (E2) diffuses into the cell and binds nuclear ER, which in turn activates receptor dimerisation and association with various co-activator (NCOA) and co-repressor (NCOR) proteins

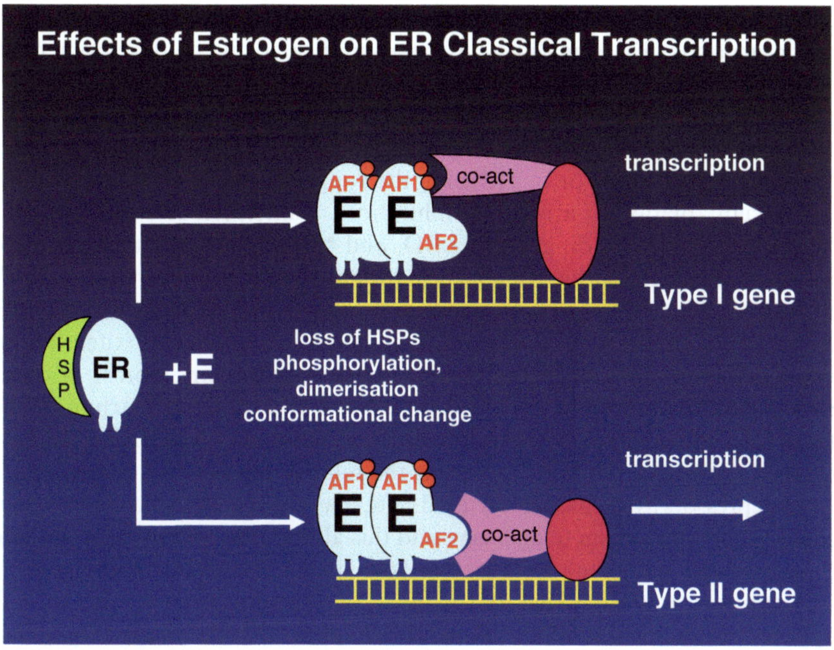

Fig. 1 Effects of estrogen on ER classical transcription

to a greater or lesser extent [5]. The activated ER binds as a dimer to estrogen response elements (ERE) in the promoters of target genes and activates gene transcription through two separate transactivation domains within ER, termed AF-1 in the amino-terminal region and AF-2 in the carboxy-terminal region [6, 7] (Fig. 1). Activation by AF-2 requires ligand (i.e. E2) binding to the ligand-binding domain (LBD), while AF-1 can be phosphorylated by growth factor receptors or other downstream effectors and may act both independently of hormone and synergistically with AF-2 to increase the efficiency of ER-transcriptional activity [8]. Studies have indicated that ERE-bound ER is subsequently ubiquitinated and targeted for proteosomal degradation, such that each ER molecule appears to be destined for only one cycle of signalling [9]. In addition to its role as a classical transcription factor, ER can also enhance transcription without direct DNA binding by participating in protein–protein interactions with other transcription factors (non-classical genomic activity) [10]. For example, ER can essentially act as a co-activator and increase the activity of the jun/fos activator protein 1 (AP-1) transcription complex [11]. In addition non-genomic functions for ER have been described whereby estrogen-bound ER interacts directly with, and phosphorylates, membrane-associated growth factor receptors [12, 13] as well as downstream effectors such as the p85 subunit of phosphoinositide-3-kinase (PI3K) [14] resulting in further pro-survival and anti-apoptotic signalling. As discussed below, a shift in the relative contribution of classical vs non-classical genomic, or non-genomic, ER signalling has been implicated in the development of endocrine resistance.

Current endocrine therapies that modulate ER signalling do so either by competitive antagonism with endogenous ligand (E2) for binding to ER (i.e. tamoxifen, fulvestrant) or by reducing the supply of available ligand for ER (i.e. ovarian ablation or aromatase inhibition). Tamoxifen acts as a competitive inhibitor upon binding to the LBD, and by preferentially recruiting co-repressors (NCORs) induces a conformational change that inactivates AF-2, but has no effect on AF-1 transcriptional activity [15] (Fig. 2) Because ER activity in the breast is predominantly mediated via AF-2, tamoxifen has an overall antagonist effect in the breast, but may act as an agonist in other tissues primarily driven by AF-1, such as bone and the endometrium of the uterus [16]. Alterations in the relative contributions of AF-1/AF-2 to ER-mediated gene transcription, as well as the relative amounts of co-activators and co-repressors available in individual cells, may shift the balance of tamoxifen activity from antagonism to agonism, and this also has been implicated in some mechanisms of tamoxifen resistance (see below).

By contrast, it is envisaged that removal of all endogenous ligands for ER might prevent activation of all ER-mediated transcriptional events, regardless of whether AF-1 or AF-2 regulated (Fig. 3). Clearly the success of such a

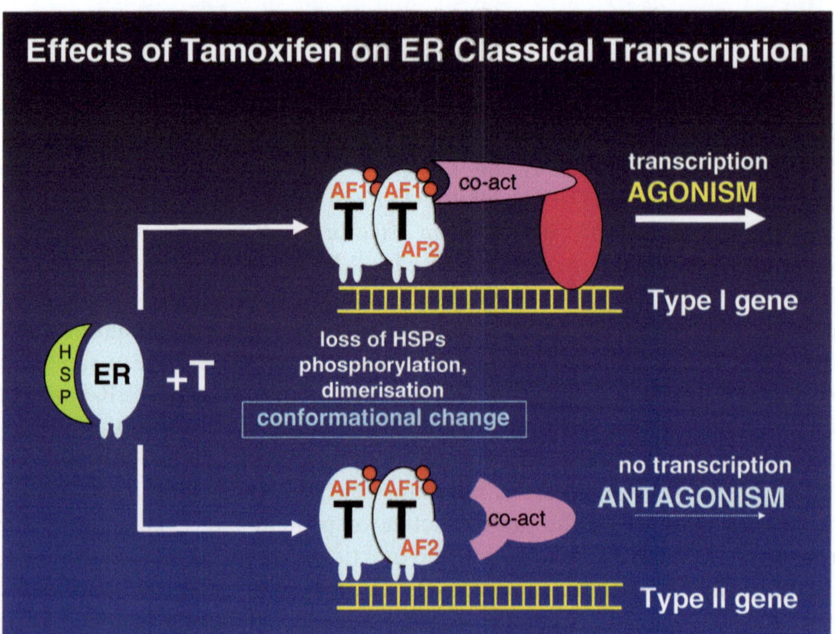

Fig. 2 Effects of tamoxifen on ER classical transcription

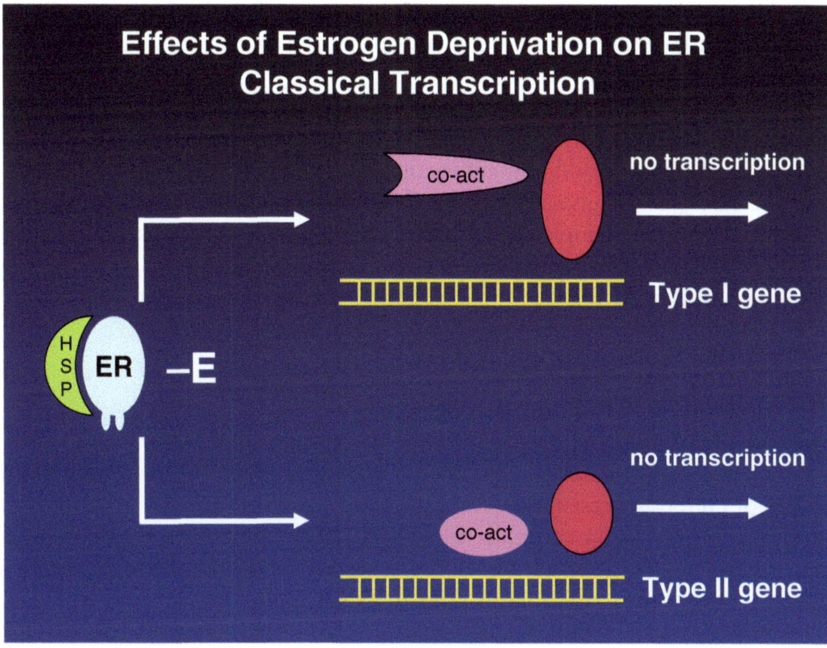

Fig. 3 Effects of estrogen deprivation on ER classical transcription

strategy depends on achieving near complete estrogen deprivation, especially as residual amounts of endogenous estradiol might be sufficient to still activate the receptor [17]. Model systems have helped understand the differences in mode of action between estrogen deprivation and antiestrogens such as tamoxifen. In the MCF-7 xenograft model in which human hormone-sensitive ER+ breast cancer cells are established as tumours in athymic oophorectomised mice, the tumours require exogenous estradiol support for their growth [18]. We have previously shown that removal of all estradiol support, which in this model provides complete estrogen deprivation similar to that achieved with third generation aromatase inhibitors, was superior to tamoxifen with greater tumour regressions and prolonged time to re-growth. Moreover, molecular analysis of the treated tumours revealed that estrogen-regulated genes were more effectively switched off by estrogen deprivation than by tamoxifen [19], with a greater induction of apoptosis and more substantial inhibition of cell proliferation. Analogous results have been reported by others demonstrating that aromatase inhibitors (AIs) were more effective than tamoxifen in MCF-7 xenografts in which the cells had been transfected with the human aromatase gene [20]. These laboratory data mirror evidence from the clinic that in post-menopausal women with ER+ breast cancer AIs are clinically superior to tamoxifen when given adjuvantly upfront [21]. This supports the notion that estrogen deprivation may overcome some of the mechanisms of tamoxifen-specific resistance, which in turn may relate to specific pharmacological or pharmacodynamic features of acquired resistance to antiestrogen drugs.

Thus an understanding of ER signalling, and how this is modulated both by its natural ligands and by various endocrine therapies, provides the basis for investigating the changes that might account for hormonal resistance. In essence, these are likely to involve either loss or alteration of ER function, pharmacological/pharmacodynamic changes to individual drug therapies, or enhanced growth factor/mitogenic signalling with or without interaction with the ER-signalling pathway. Evidence for each of these mechanisms is presented below.

ER Function in Hormone Resistance

Most in vitro and clinical observations suggest that even following the development of endocrine resistance, ER signalling continues to play an important role in the proliferation of breast cancer [22]. The clinic biopsies of tumours from breast cancer patients who have relapsed on an antiestrogen show a functional ER that is still able to bind to DNA [23], while women who have become refractory to tamoxifen or non-steroidal aromatase inhibitors actually respond to further endocrine manipulation with the ER-alpha downregulator fulvestrant [24], indicating that ER-mediated signalling remains functional. As discussed later in this chapter, there is an increasing body of evidence that cross-talk with growth factor and downstream mitogenic pathways can augment the genomic and non-genomic functions of ER.

Loss of ER

While ER expression is an obligate requirement for sensitivity to endocrine therapy, loss of ER either due to the clonal selection of ER-negative cells or due to transcriptional suppression of ER gene expression could account for acquired endocrine resistance associated with progressive disease. We and others have shown in sequential paired biopsies from patients treated with tamoxifen that ER loss over time might account for hormonal resistance in a minority of patients [22, 25, 26] (Fig. 4). PgR loss during endocrine therapy occurs more frequently, and when this occurs the tumour often takes on a more aggressive course [27]. Laboratory studies have suggested that transcriptional repression of the PgR gene by signalling through the insulin-like growth factor (IGFR) and epidermal growth factor receptor families (EGFR/HER2) may be the cause of PgR downregulation in some tumours [28].

ER silencing as a result of promoter hypermethylation has been documented in a proportion of breast cancers [29]. Importantly, this process has been shown to be reversible. Demethylating agents or histone deacetylase (HDAC)

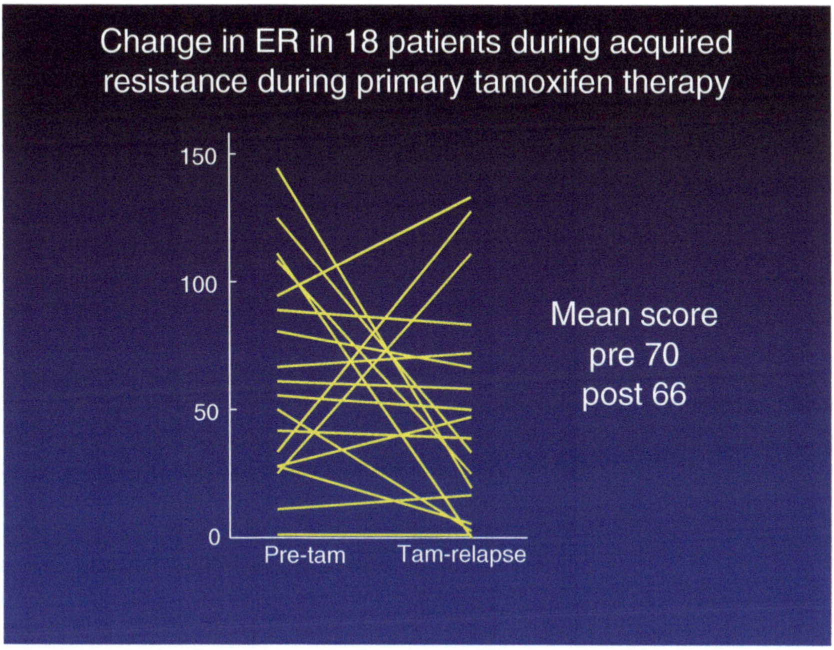

Fig. 4 Change in ER expression by immunohistochemistry (histoscore) in 18 patients during development of acquired resistance to tamoxifen therapy (from [22])

inhibitors can reactivate expression of a functional ER in cell lines with ER silencing due to promoter methylation [30, 31]. These observations are quite provocative and have obvious clinical implications for a proportion of patients with ER– tumours who might potentially benefit from endocrine therapy if ER expression could be reactivated using a demethylating agent. A trial of tamoxifen in combination with a HDAC inhibitor in patients who have relapsed after endocrine therapy is ongoing to investigate whether the HDAC inhibitor may restore endocrine sensitivity by enhancing/restoring ER expression.

There is some evidence that enhanced peptide growth factor signalling due to overexpression of HER2 can directly suppress ER expression, which in turn may eventually lead to complete loss of ER [32]. ER+ cell lines stably transfected with full-length HER2 demonstrate downregulation in ER, while quantitative measurements of ER levels in tumour samples show consistently lower levels of the receptor among patients with HER2-amplified breast cancer [33]. Furthermore, interruption of hyperactive mitogen-activated protein kinase (MAPK) signalling or epidermal growth factor receptor (EGFR) has been shown to re-induce ER expression both in cell lines and in xenograft models [34, 35]. In fact, in a small study of 10 ER–/HER2+ patients treated with trastuzumab, three patients acquired ER expression in sequential biopsies during treatment [36]. Furthermore, studies with the dual EGFR/HER2 tyrosine kinase inhibitor lapatinib have shown that long-term treatment was associated with an adaptive increase in ER signalling [37]. As discussed later in this chapter, the dynamic interaction between ER and growth factor signalling certainly supports using ER and growth factor-targeted therapies in combination, or in fact in sequence, as one may sensitise to the other and thus enhance/retain endocrine responsiveness longer than would otherwise occur.

The degree to which complete loss of ER secondary to peptide growth factor signalling may contribute to acquired endocrine resistance needs further confirmation from serial clinical samples from women who have relapsed on endocrine therapy. Likewise it is unclear whether this is always a reversible phenomenon or whether tumours bypass endocrine pathways and permanently switch to ER-independent signalling. A recent report using an in vitro RNA interference (RNAi) screening approach in tamoxifen-treated ER+ MCF-7 breast cancer cells has identified key modifiers of tamoxifen sensitivity that induce signalling which bypasses ER [38]. In particular, loss of cyclin-dependent kinase 10 (CDK10) via gene silencing may induce resistance to ER signalling and overcome the G1-cell cycle arrest caused by tamoxifen. The mechanism for this appears to involve release of the ETS2 transcription factor (normally suppressed by CDK10), which in turn activates c-RAF-1 and ERK 1/2 signalling independent of any upstream growth factors. This results in enhanced cell proliferation that does not involve any activation of ER-alpha or any ER-regulated genes. As such, this represents a novel ER-independent means by which cells may escape regulation from tamoxifen – the authors confirmed the possible significance of their finding in two clinical data sets whereby low CDK10 expression in primary breast cancers was associated with a statistically shorter time to distant relapse/overall survival. Further prospective studies are required to see if loss of CDK10 is a reliable biomarker of endocrine resistance in ER+ breast cancer.

Potentiation of Genomic ER Activity

ER transcription is tightly regulated by the balance of NCOAs/NCORs within individual cells. Mitogenic signalling can alter the expression of some of these co-regulators thereby enhancing both classical and non-classical genomic ER transcription. The co-activator NCOA3, also known as AIB1 (amplified in breast cancer-1) is overexpressed in 50% of breast carcinomas and amplified in 5% of tumours [39]. Among untreated ER+ patients, AIB1 expression is associated with an improved survival. In contrast, in HER2-amplified breast cancer AIB1 has been associated with a poorer outcome with tamoxifen – this might be explained by the fact that HER2 activates AIB1 and enhances the agonist effects of tamoxifen [40, 41]. Similarly, decreased levels of NCORs have been shown to enhance tamoxifen agonism by shifting the balance towards ER-transcriptional activity [42]. These data suggest that mitogenic signalling via other pathways (i.e. HER2) can alter the ratio of NCOAs/NCORs and result in an altered response of

ER to endogenous E2 or to exogenous tamoxifen, in particular enhancing an agonist response. Whether profiling tumours by measuring the levels of various transcription co-regulators may offer useful predictive information regarding endocrine responsiveness has not been clearly established.

The hormonally regulated cell cycle regulator cyclin D1 is overexpressed/amplified in 50/25% of ER+ human breast cancers. As a transducer of both ER and growth factor-mediated cell cycle progression, cyclin D1 emerged as another potentiator of ER genomic activity that might account for endocrine resistance in some tumours. In addition, experimental data have suggested that cyclin D1 could interact directly with ER via recruitment of members of the SRC (steroid receptor co-activators) family of NCOAs in the absence of endogenous ligand [43]. However, clinical data regarding any causal relationship between cyclin D1 and endocrine responsiveness are conflicting [44, 45].

In addition to directly binding with DNA and increasing classical genomic transcription of ER-dependent genes, ligand-bound ER may also complex with other transcriptional factors, such as fos/jun via AP-1 non-classical genomic activity. Stress and/or cytokine signalling pathways can contribute to AP-1 signalling, and thus have been associated with resistance to tamoxifen. Laboratory and clinical studies suggest that elevated levels of phosphorylated jun N-terminal kinase (JNK) are associated with tamoxifen resistance, and preliminary data have also implicated activated p38 MAPK [46]. The p38 MAPK is activated by a variety of environmental stresses including ionizing radiation, heat, oxidative stress, inflammatory cytokines (TNF family), growth factor receptors such as HER2, and tissue ischemia (hypoxia). In endometrial cancer cells estrogen and tamoxifen both stimulate p38 MAPK activity. In turn, p38 MAPK signalling has been reported to phosphorylate ER (Thr^{311}), inhibit ER nuclear export, enhance ER's interaction with co-activators, and increase the estrogen agonist activity of tamoxifen-bound ER. Although the mechanisms by which signalling through these pathways might contribute to tamoxifen resistance in clinical breast cancer are not well defined, preliminary evidence in human tumours and MCF-7 xenografts has suggested an association of p38 MAPK with hormonal resistance [46]. In tissue microarrays (TMAs) from 39 patients with paired biopsies before and after acquired resistance to tamoxifen, all ER+ tumours that overexpressed HER2 originally or at resistance expressed high levels of phosphorylated p38 MAPK. In three patients, ER+ tumours that were initially HER2– had converted to HER2+ at the time of relapse on tamoxifen, including conversion to FISH+ in two cases (Fig. 5). In the pre-treatment and tamoxifen-resistant specimens there were strong correlations between phosphorylated p38 MAPK and phosphorylated ERK1/2 MAPK. In the tamoxifen-resistant xenograft tumours high ER expression was preserved, and, like the clinical samples, there was a striking increase in phosphorylated p38 MAPK. These data support the concept that adaptive changes in ER genomic signalling occur during development of hormonal resistance to tamoxifen and implicate various cross-talk between mitogenic signalling and ER pathways in the underlying process.

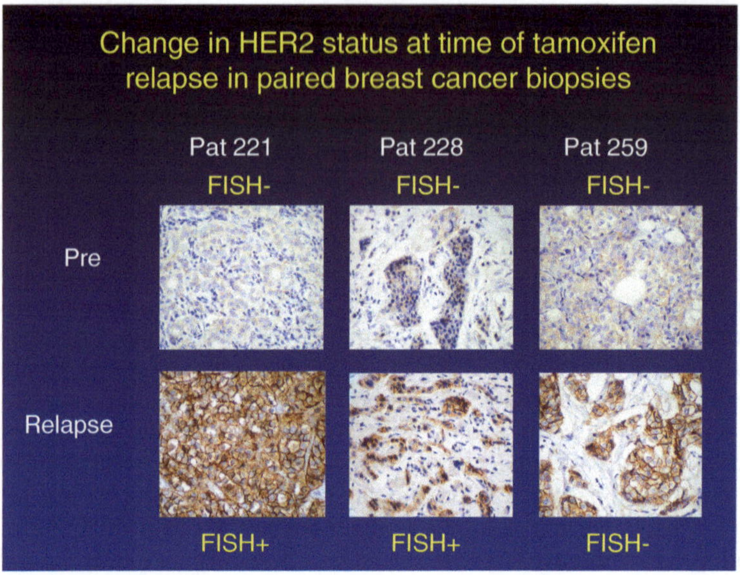

Fig. 5 Change in HER2 status at time of tamoxifen relapse in paired breast cancer biopsies during acquisition of resistance to tamoxifen (from [46])

Hypersensitive ER Signalling Following Prolonged Estrogen Deprivation

Although loss of ER may occur in some tumours during prolonged endocrine therapy, it is clear that in many instances signalling through ER is retained. In particular, the biological mechanisms contributing to resistance following long-term estrogen deprivation (LTED) using aromatase inhibitors or gonadal suppression have been associated with retention and enhanced ER signalling. Adaptation to LTED may lead to upregulation in ER, and in vitro models have shown that part of the adaptive process involves an increase in ER expression and E2 hypersensitivity to very low levels of residual estrogen [47]. Data from several groups support this hypersensitivity concept as a means of escape from estrogen deprivation. While wild-type MCF-7 cells respond maximally to doses of estradiol of c. 10^{-11} to 10^{-10} M, cells exposed to LTED adapt and instead respond maximally at c. 10^{-13} M [17, 48, 47]. In part, this is caused by an adaptive increase in ER expression and function, but there is additional evidence for increased ‘cross-talk’ between various growth factor receptor-signalling pathways and ER at the time of relapse, with ER becoming activated and super-sensitised by a number of different intracellular kinases, including mitogen-activated protein kinases (MAPKs) and the insulin-like growth factor (IGF)/AKT pathway [49]. Increased expression of HER2/HER3, MAPK, and IGFR signalling in cells that become resistance to LTED may activate residual and enhanced levels of ER in a manner similar to that observed in acquired tamoxifen-resistant cells. Evidence to support this is provided by increased levels of ER phosphorylated at Ser 118, together with increase in pp90RSK which is one of the kinases thought to be involved in ER activation. Proof of principle has then been provided by evidence that ER-mediated gene transcription (which is enhanced 10-fold in these cells that become sensitive to LTED) can be abrogated by a number of different approaches to interrupt upstream signalling, including gefitinib, the MEK inhibitor UO126, and the ER downregulator fulvestrant which degrades receptor [47]. Thus, it would appear that the ER remains an integral part of signalling, even following failure of aromatase inhibitors.

ER Mutations/Variants

Until recently little evidence has been found for significant mutations in the ER gene in human breast cancer patients [50–52]. A mutation has been described in the ER in tamoxifen-resistant xenografts of the human MCF-7 breast cancer cell line. The mutation (tyr351asp) leads to the tumours being growth-stimulated by tamoxifen [53] but has not been found in human breast carcinomas. An estrogen hypersensitive ER mutant (lys303arg) has been reported in a large proportion of atypical breast hyperplasias and breast carcinomas, which may result in an agonist response to tamoxifen or sensitisation to the low levels of residual estrogen with aromatase inhibitors [54]. If confirmed by others this may play a role in acquired resistance to tamoxifen or estrogen deprivation.

Pharmacological Mechanisms of Hormonal Resistance

Tamoxifen

Measurements of intratumoural levels of tamoxifen have shown that women with acquired resistance to tamoxifen have lower levels than sensitive controls [55]. Whether low intracellular levels of tamoxifen are attributable to decreased influx of the drug or increased efflux via a membrane pump such as p-glycoprotein has not been established. However, this mechanism is likely a minor contributor to tamoxifen resistance as clinical samples have consistently demonstrated that tamoxifen saturates ER with greater than 99.9% occupancy [56].

The cytochrome P450 2D6 enzyme is required to convert tamoxifen to its more potent metabolite, endoxifen. It has been suggested that reduced activity of this enzyme may lead to lower circulating levels of endoxifen, and thus reduce the therapeutic efficacy of tamoxifen. Approximately 7–10% of the population may be classified as poor metabolisers of tamoxifen due to CYP2D6 variants (i.e. the biallelic polymorphism CYP2D6*4), which in turn may be associated with fewer hot flushes and a decreased level of circulating endoxifen. In a retrospective analysis of an adjuvant tamoxifen trial, the CYP2D6*4 genotype was associated with an increased risk of relapse among tamoxifen-treated women [57]. Similarly, CYP2D6 inhibitors, such as the selective serotonin reuptake inhibitor antidepressants, frequently used to treat post-menopausal hot flushes, also decrease endoxifen levels leading some to suggest that these agents should be avoided in tamoxifen-treated women [57, 58]. Whether women with homozygous CYP2D6 variants would benefit from higher doses of tamoxifen or an alternate endocrine therapy has not been investigated. Likewise, routine testing for CYP2D6 genotypes is not recommended at this time in the clinical setting, but as further studies report this host factor could become a recognised mechanism for tamoxifen-specific resistance that would be screened for prospectively.

Aromatase

In post-menopausal women, the only source of estradiol is from the aromatisation of adrenal androgens. While peripheral conversion in adipose tissue contributes to measurable levels of circulating estradiol, local production via tumoural aromatase activity results in 10- to 20-fold higher estradiol concentrations in the tumour than in plasma [59]. Variations in tumour aromatase levels could therefore contribute to responsiveness to AIs. A small study suggested that the level of intratumoural aromatase activity could predict the response to the first-generation aromatase inhibitor, aminoglutethemide [60]. However, more recent studies have shown no correlation between mRNA aromatase levels and response to AIs [61].

A number of single nucleotide polymorphisms (SNPs) have been identified in the aromatase gene (CYP19) and the CYP3A enzymes that metabolise aromatase inhibitors, although most do not translate into a clinically significant variation in circulating estradiol levels [62]. One SNP has been shown in vitro to reduce affinity of the aromatase enzyme for exemestane [63]; however, there is no clinical evidence to date that genetic variations in CYP19 lead to resistance to aromatase inhibition in vivo.

Growth Factor Signalling and Hormonal Resistance

Membrane peptide growth factor receptors such as the epidermal growth factor receptor (EGFR), the human epidermal receptors-2 (HER2), or the insulin growth factor 1 receptor (IGF1R) have been implicated in endocrine resistance. Overexpression of HER2 due to gene amplification occurs in approximately 15–20% of all human breast cancers [64] and has been associated with poor prognosis and de novo resistance to tamoxifen in the neoadjuvant setting [65]. Similarly, EGFR is overexpressed in a number of breast cancers and has also been associated with poor response to tamoxifen [65]. Importantly, cell models of acquired resistance to both tamoxifen and estrogen deprivation (ED) have shown that the development of resistance over time is associated with an adaptative upregulation in growth factor-signalling pathways, whereby cells enhance their dependence on EGFR- or HER2-signalling pathways [47].

Activation of these membrane receptors stimulates two major intracellular kinase signalling cascades – the ras/mitogenic-activated protein kinase (MAPK) pathway and the phosphatidylinositol 3-kinase (PI3K)/Akt pathway (Fig. 6). These pathways activate downstream effectors leading to a cascade of signals involved in malignant growth and survival, and can be involved in endocrine resistance by a number of mechanisms including downregulation and loss of ER expression (described above), a total switch to ER-independent growth using these pathways, or bi-directional cross-talk between ER and mitogenic signalling. This latter 'cross-talk' mechanism in particular involves synergistic interaction between ER and mitogenic signalling resulting in enhanced genomic and non-genomic functions of ER.

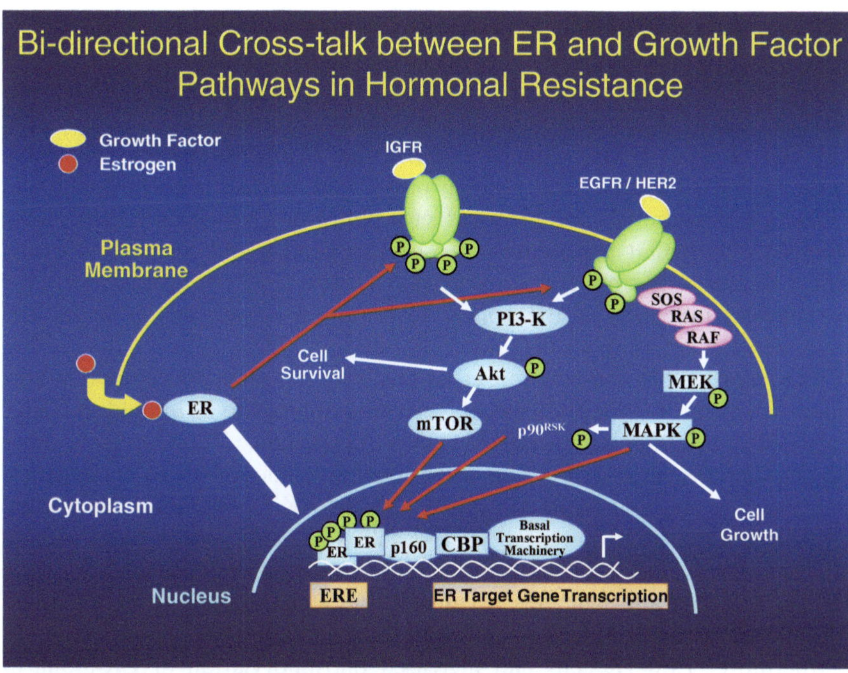

Fig. 6 Bi-directional cross-talk that may become operational between ER and growth factor pathways in hormonal resistance

Cross-Talk via Classical ER Transcription Mechanisms

Growth factor-mediated activation of MAPK or Akt can potentiate E2-mediated ER classical transcriptional activity by directly phosphorylating AF-1 [66]. Importantly, both MAPK and Akt have been shown to phosphorylate ER within AF-1, at serine 118 and serine 167, respectively, in the absence of E2, thereby contributing to ligand-independent ER transactivation [67, 68] (Fig. 6). Other downstream effectors of peptide growth factor receptors have also been shown to activate ER such as protein kinase A and the cyclin E-cdk-2 complex [6].

An increase in AF-1 transcription may predict for differential sensitivity to endocrine agents. Tamoxifen may quite efficiently block AF-2-mediated transcription; however, in tumours that exhibit high levels of AF-1 activity driven by mitogenic signalling, tamoxifen may act as an agonist [16]. This is supported by the high rate of primary tamoxifen resistance observed in neoadjuvant trials of HER2-amplified breast cancer [65]. There are some data to suggest that E2 deprivation using an aromatase inhibitor or ER downregulation using fulvestrant may therefore be a more effective anti-cancer strategy in EGFR/HER2+ breast cancer [65, 69, 70].

Enhanced Non-genomic Role for ER in Cross-Talk

Conversely, in addition to its effects on transcription, estrogen-bound ER has also been shown to result in non-genomic effects via rapid activation of EGFR [12], IGF1R [13], HER2 [71], or the cleavage of membrane-bound growth factor receptor ligands, such as EGF or TGF-alpha [72]. This bi-directional interaction between ER and growth factor pathways creates a self-reinforcing synergistic loop that potentiates pro-survival signals and may allow breast cancer to escape normal endocrine responsiveness (Fig. 6). Furthermore, the extranuclear functions of ER appear to require a ligand, and both E2 and tamoxifen can act as agonists [12].

Importantly, this non-genomic cross-talk does not seem operational in hormone-sensitive ER+ MCF-7 cells, its relevance appears to be limited to HER2 amplified or cell lines with acquired endocrine resistance [73]. Our group have recently demonstrated that in tamoxifen-resistant clones of MCF-7 cells (Tam-1R) there are elevated levels of phosphorylated AKT and ERK1/2-activated p90RSK compared to parental MCF-7 cells (Wt) [74]. While there was no change in the overall level of ER-alpha between the two cell lines, ER location was shifted to extranuclear sites in Tam-1R cells with co-localisation of ER and HER2 demonstrated by immunoprecipitation and confocal analysis (Fig. 7). Furthermore, Tam-1R cells had increased phosphorylation of ER-alpha at ser167 which was not inhibited by siRNA blockade of AKT or ERK1/2. In contrast, HER2 tyrosine kinase inhibition resulted in re-localisation of ER to

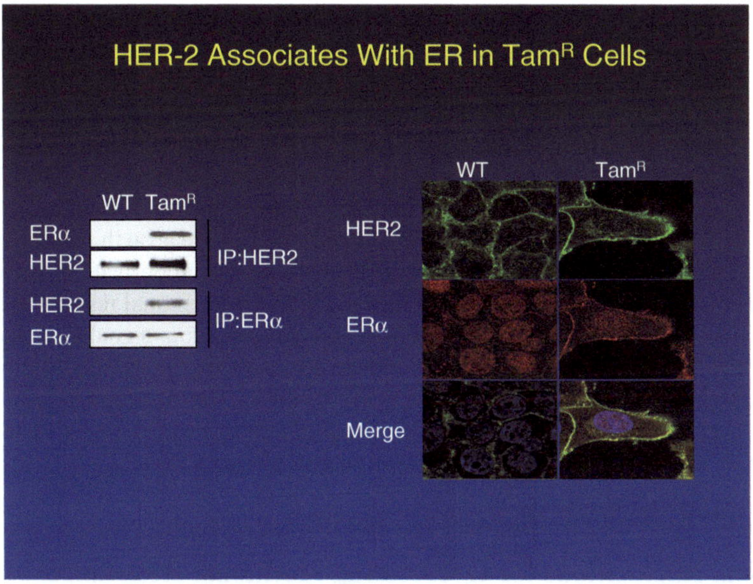

Fig. 7 HER2 associates with ER in tamoxifen-resistant cells as determined by immunoprecipitation and confocal analysis of parental vs tamoxifen-resistant MCF-7 cells (from [74], with permission from Dr Lesley-Ann Martin)

the nucleus and restoration of endocrine responsiveness. Unfortunately, while supported by extensive in vitro models, the clinical relevance of the non-genomic actions of ER and its interaction with membrane peptide growth factor receptors remain somewhat controversial, and membrane and/or cytoplasmic ER has yet to be conclusively demonstrated in clinical samples.

Cross-Talk as Mechanism of Resistance to Estrogen Deprivation

Recent laboratory research with ER+ breast cancer cells into the mechanisms of resistance to long-term estrogen deprivation (LTED) has demonstrated that various growth factor pathways and oncogenes involved in the signal transduction cascade become activated and utilised by breast cancer cells to bypass normal endocrine responsiveness [75, 76]. Pre-clinical data indicate that exposure to LTED (analogous to that caused by AIs) and subsequent development of acquired resistance may be accompanied by adaptive increases in ER gene expression and intercellular signalling, resulting in hypersensitivity to low estradiol levels [47, 77–79]. There is evidence for increased 'cross-talk' between various growth factor receptor-signalling pathways and ER at the time of relapse on LTED, with ER becoming activated and super-sensitised by a number of different intracellular kinases, including mitogen-activated protein kinases (MAPKs), epidermal growth factor receptor (EGFR) and HER2/HER3 signalling, and the insulin-like growth factor (IGF)/AKT pathway [49, 79]. In cells resistant to long-term estrogen deprivation (LTED-R), ER-mediated gene transcription is enhanced 10-fold in these cells, but can be abrogated by a number of different approaches to interrupt upstream signalling including the EGFR tyrosine kinase inhibitor gefitinib, MEK inhibitors, and the ER downregulator fulvestrant which degrades ER protein [47].

Thus, it would appear that both ER and various peptide growth factors are an integral part of signalling even following failure of estrogen deprivation therapies, and that a possible successful approach to overcoming hormonal resistance could involve the use of the ER downregulator fulvestrant or various signal transduction inhibitors (STIs) to remove ER and/or activation of 'cross-talk' ER signalling, respectively. Furthermore as discussed below, evidence is now emerging that such drugs may be more effective when given in combination with existing endocrine therapies in an attempt to delay or prevent resistance occurring.

Clinical Implications for Overcoming Hormonal Resistance

The clinical implications of a retained, albeit an altered or hyperactive, ER-signalling pathway with or without 'cross-talk' activation of peptide growth factor pathways are that further endocrine therapies can be used after development of hormonal resistance, either alone or in combination with novel signalling agents. Pre-menopausal patients who respond and relapse after estrogen withdrawal by ovarian suppression can respond, at the time of subsequent relapse, to further suppression of estrogen levels by the addition of an aromatase inhibitor [80]. This suggests that the initial resistance was to acquisition of enhanced sensitivity to residual post-menopausal levels of estrogen, which can be overcome by further reducing circulating levels in these patients. This has been further supported by a recent clinical trial showing that women who have relapsed on an AI respond to more potent endocrine manipulation using the irreversible aromatase inhibitor exemestane or ER downregulation with fulvestrant [24].

Fulvestrant Targeting Activated ER in Hormonal Resistance

Fulvestrant is a novel type of estrogen receptor (ER) antagonist that unlike tamoxifen has no known agonist effects [81]. Fulvestrant binds to the ER but due to its steroidal structure and long side chain induces a different conformational shape with the receptor to that achieved by the non-steroidal antiestrogen tamoxifen. Because of this, fulvestrant prevents ER dimerisation and leads to the rapid degradation of the fulvestrant–ER complex, producing the loss of cellular ER. Thus fulvestrant, unlike tamoxifen, inhibits ER binding with DNA and produces abrogation of estrogen-sensitive gene transcription [82]. It has been shown that due to its unique mechanism of action, fulvestrant delays the emergence of acquired resistance compared with tamoxifen in an MCF-7 hormone-sensitive xenograft model [83]. The lack of agonist effects means that fulvestrant did not support the growth of tumours that became resistant to, and subsequently stimulated by, tamoxifen.

Clinical data from three phase II studies in a total of 293 post-menopausal women with advanced breast cancer suggest some modest efficacy for fulvestrant in a second/third-line setting [84, 85, 86]. In these three studies clinical benefit rates (i.e. that include objective tumour responses and stable disease for at least 6 mo) of 30, 44, and 35%, respectively, have been reported. Many of these patients had progressed on prior treatment with several endocrine agents, and these results imply that disease progression after non-steroidal aromatase inhibitors may not preclude subsequent treatment with fulvestrant. This was confirmed in the large randomised phase III 'Evaluation of Faslodex vs Exemestane Clinical Trial' (EFECT) study that demonstrated similar efficacy for fulvestrant vs exemestane in patients who have progressed on treatment with non-steroidal AIs [24].

Recent pre-clinical data have suggested that the efficacy of fulvestrant, especially in the setting of endocrine resistance where activated ER signalling may be dominant, may critically depend on the background estrogen environment in which the cells exist. Recent experiments with tamoxifen-stimulated breast cancer xenografts demonstrated paradoxical effects on tumour growth dependent on whether fulvestrant was administered in the presence or absence of estrogen [87]. While wild-type MCF-7 xenografts were growth stimulated by estrogen and inhibited both by tamoxifen and fulvestrant, in contrast long-term tamoxifen-treated (MCF-7TAMLT) tumours which became resistant and growth stimulated by tamoxifen were inhibited by estradiol. The addition of fulvestrant to estradiol-treated tumours reversed these effects and actually stimulated growth of MCF-7TAMLT tumours. However, when fulvestrant was given to these tumours on its own in a low-estradiol environment, tumours did not grow. Similar results have been reported in LTED-R cells in vitro where maximal growth inhibition of cells was observed with a dose of 10^{-8} M fulvestrant, yet the titration back of increasing amounts of estradiol resulted in re-growth of cells which fulvestrant was no-longer able to effectively antagonise [88].

On the basis of these findings, phase III clinical trials of fulvestrant are currently in progress that will investigate additional roles for fulvestrant in breast cancer therapy either following prior non-steroidal AI treatment or in combination with AIs (to maintain low estradiol levels) as first-line therapy. The comparator for several of these studies is the steroidal aromatase inactivator exemestane which in phase II studies has shown some efficacy following progression on non-steroidal AIs [89]. An ongoing phase III trial (SoFEA) will compare progression-free survival in patients who have progressed on a non-steroidal AI and who are subsequently treated with either fulvestrant plus continued anastrozole or with fulvestrant alone. Secondary aims include a comparison of fulvestrant vs exemestane and an examination of biological markers of response. In addition, two trials (FACT and SWOG 226) will compare the efficacy of a combination of fulvestrant plus anastrozole with anastrozole alone in the first-line setting. As AIs move forward into the adjuvant setting the results of these trials will help define optimal sequencing of endocrine therapies, and in particular whether fulvestrant used alone or in combination with aromatase inhibitors is the most effective strategy [90].

Endocrine Therapy in Combination with Anti-growth Factor Receptor Therapies

Growth factor signalling has been extensively implicated in endocrine resistance, and in some cases the interaction between ER and mitogenic pathways can be described as a dynamic inverse relationship, where inhibition of one results in compensatory increase in the other. As discussed above this is supported by pre-clinical and clinical data showing that growth factor inhibition may increase ER expression or function and re-sensitise breast cancer cells to endocrine therapy and would support combination or, in fact, sequential treatment. Alternatively, growth factor signalling can interact synergistically with ER and augment both genomic and non-genomic functions of the receptor. This would provide a strong rationale for simultaneous blockade of both ER and mitogenic pathways using various signal transduction inhibitors (STIs).

For hormone-resistant breast cancer, in particular ER+ cells that overexpress HER2, the strategy of combined STIs and endocrine therapy may be more effective than using STIs alone in this setting. Most of the experimental data in support of this concept has come from HER2+ tamoxifen-resistant models rather than LTED-resistant scenarios, but similar principles may apply. It has been shown that signal transduction blockade using a HER2 tyrosine kinase inhibitor (AG1478) or a MAPK inhibitor (UO126) may abrogate antiestrogen resistance, while combined treatment with tamoxifen and STI was significantly more effective than either therapy alone, not only at inhibiting estrogen-mediated gene transcription and tumour colony survival in vitro, but also at delaying tumour xenograft growth in vivo [91]. Others have shown that hormone-resistant MCF-7 cells with upregulated HER2 signalling are sensitive to the TKI gefitinib, and that combined therapy of gefitinib and tamoxifen provided maximal growth inhibition and significantly delayed the time to progression of the disease [92]. Using an in vivo model of MCF-7/HER2 overexpressing xenografts, similar effects were seen with gefitinib combined with estrogen deprivation, which provided greater inhibition of growth and substantially delayed acquired resistance compared with estrogen deprivation alone [35].

Based on the evidence outlined above, a number of trials were initiated with either the HER2 monoclonal antibody trastuzumab or the EGFR/HER2 tyrosine kinase inhibitors (TKIs) gefitinib, erlotinib, or lapatinib in combination with endocrine therapy (Table 2) [93]. While some of these trials are in patients

Table 2 Reported results from clinical trials of combinations of endocrine therapies with targeted biological agents in ER+ post-menopausal breast cancer

Clinical setting	Trial phase and number patients	Intervention	Clinical endpoints	Biological correlates	Author and reference
Combination with gefitinib (GEF) or erlotinib (ERL)					
MBC Hormone-refractory	**II** $N=15$	ANA + GEF	PR = 0 SD = 0	None available (NA)	Mita et al. [94]
MBC Hormone-sensitive	**II** $N=150$	LET + ERL	CBR = 11/20 so far	Will record EGFR/HER2 and ER phosphorylation	Mayer et al. [95]
MBC Hormone-sensitive	**II RCT** $N=206$ Stratum 1	TAM vs TAM + GEF	PFS 10.9 mo (TAM + GEF) vs 8.8 mo (TAM), $p=0.31$ CBR 50.5% (TAM + GEF) vs 45.5% (TAM), $p=0.74$	To be conducted	Osborne et al. [99]
Neoadjuvant EBC	**II RCT** $N=206$	ANA vs ANA + GEF × 16 weeks	ORR = 61% (ANA) vs 48% (ANA + GEF), $p=0.067$	Reduction in Ki67=83.6% (ANA) vs 77.4% (ANA + GEF), $p=0.164$	Smith et al. [96]
Pre-operative EBC EGFR+ only	**II RT** $N=56$	GEF vs GEF + ANA × 4–6 weeks	ORR=50% (GEF) vs 54% (ANA + GEF)	Reduction in Ki67 = 92.4% (GEF) vs 98% (ANA + GEF), $p=0.005$	Polychronis et al. [97]
Combination with trastuzumab (TRAS)					
HER2+ MBC (note: all pts were TRAS and AI naïve)	**II** $N=33$	TRAS + LET	PR = 26% SD = 26%	NA	Marcom et al. [100]
HER2+ MBC (all pts were IHC 3+ or FISH+)	**III RCT** $N=207$	ANA vs ANA + TRAS	PFS = 2.4 mo (ANA) vs 4.8 mo (ANA + TRAS), $p=0.0016$ ORR = 6.8% (ANA) vs 20.3% (ANA + TRAS), $p=0.018$	NA	Mackey et al. [101]

Table 2 (continued)

Clinical setting	Trial phase and number patients	Intervention	Clinical endpoints	Biological correlates	Author and reference
Combination with lapatinib (LAP)					
MBC (all cancers)	**I** $N=17$	LAP + LET	4 SD including 1 breast cancer	NA	Chu et al. [103]
Combination with farnesyltransferase inhibitors: tipifarnib (TIP)					
MBC Hormone resistant	**I** $N=12$	TAM + TIP	PR = 2/12 SD>6 mo = 1/12	NA	Lebowitz et al. [110]
MBC Tamoxifen resistant	**I** $N=20$	TAM + TIP	PR = 1/20 SD>6 mo = 4/20	NA	Dalenc et al. [109]
MBC Tamoxifen resistant	**II RCT** $N=120$	LET vs LET + TIP	PR = 38% (LET) vs 30% (LET + TIP) CBR = 62% (LET) vs 49% (LET + LAP)	NA	Johnston et al. [111]
Combination with mTOR inhibitors: everolimus (EVE) or temsirolimus (TEM)					
MBC	**II** $N=92$	LET vs LET + TEM 10 mg daily vs LET + TEM 30 mg intermittent	ORR = 45% (LET) vs 33% (LET + TEM10) vs 40% (LET + TEM30) PFS = 11.6 mo (LET) vs 11.5 mo (LET + TEM10) vs 13.2 mo (LET + TEM30)	NA	Baselga et al. [118]

Table 2 (continued)

Clinical setting	Trial phase and number patients	Intervention	Clinical endpoints	Biological correlates	Author and reference
Pre-operative EBC	**II RCT** $N=270$	LET vs LET + EVE 10 mg/d × 4 mo	Clin ORR 68% (LET + EVE) vs 59% (LET) Clin USS 58% (LET + EVE) vs 47% (LET)	If High S6Kinase ORR 82% (LET = EVE) vs 68% (LET)	Baselga et al. [120] Gardner et al. [121]
MBC	**III RCT** $N=992$	LET vs LET + TEM 30 mg intermittent	ORR = 24% (LET) vs 24% (LET + TEM) SD = 19% (LET) vs 16% (LET + TEM) PFS = 9.2 mo (LET) vs 9.2 mo (LET + TEM)	NA	Chow et al. [119]

MBC: metastatic breast cancer; EBC: early (primary) breast cancer;
RCT: randomized controlled trial; RT: randomized trial;
PR: partial response; SD: stable disease >6 mo;
ORR: objective response rate (PR + CR); CBR: clinical benefit rate (ORR + stable disease >6 mo);
USS: ultrasound; PFS: progression-free survival; OS: overall survival;
TAM: tamoxifen; EVE: everolimus; TEM: temsirolimus; TIP: tipifarnib; TRAS: trastuzumab;
ANA: anastrozole; LET: letrozole; GEF: gefitinib; ERL: erlotinib.

with established hormonal resistance where activated growth factor pathways may be operative, many of the trials are in the first-line ER+ hormone-sensitive setting in combination with an aromatase inhibitor, where clinical and experimental data have shown that TKIs alone may have limited activity. Therefore, the primary endpoint for these trials is to investigate whether time to disease progression (TTP) can be significantly prolonged by the addition of an STI to endocrine therapy, thus delaying the emergence of resistance as demonstrated in various pre-clinical models described above.

Gefitinib and erlotinib are both small-molecule tyrosine kinase inhibitors of the ATP-binding site of the EGFR and have been shown to delay the development of tamoxifen resistance in vitro [92]. Two studies have explored the potential benefit for combining either gefitinib or erlotinib with an aromatase inhibitor (Table 2) [94, 95]. Neither study showed significant clinical efficacy. More definitive answers to the question of combined EGFR inhibition with endocrine therapy might be obtained by studying homogenous tumour populations in the early (primary) breast cancer setting. However, a randomised neoadjuvant trial of anastrozole alone or in combination with gefitinib given for 3 months prior to surgery in 206 post-menopausal patients with ER+ primary breast cancer was also negative (Table 2) [96]. This study also failed to select patients for EGFR overexpression, although molecular studies of tumour specimens obtained pre- and post-treatment will be crucial to explain response/resistance to both therapies. In contrast, a pre-operative trial of gefitinib vs gefitinib combined with anastrozole for 4–6 weeks prior to surgery was conducted in women with known ER+ and EGFR+ primary breast cancer [97]. This study showed that both treatments effectively reduced the size of breast tumours and levels of ER phosphorylation, and that combined treatment induced the greatest reduction in tumour proliferation. These studies of EGFR therapies illustrate the importance of selecting tumours with the known target for combined STI–endocrine therapy, although the reported rates for EGFR expression in primary breast cancer do vary quite dramatically among studies (range 15–90%) [98].

The results of a randomised, double-blind placebo-controlled phase II trial of tamoxifen with/without gefitinib in 290 patients with ER+ metastatic breast cancer were recently presented [99]. This study set out to prove the pre-clinical concept that combination therapy could delay the onset of acquired resistance to endocrine therapy, as demonstrated both in vitro [72] and in xenograft models in vivo [35, 92]. Patient's disease was either endocrine naïve or had developed greater than a year after completion of adjuvant tamoxifen (Stratum 1, $n = 206$), or had developed during or after AI therapy (Stratum 2 $n = 84$). In the endocrine naïve patients (Stratum 1) there was a numerical increase in progression-free survival from 10.9 to 8.8 months (hazard ratio 0.84, 95% CI 0.59–1.18, $p = 0.31$) which met the pre-defined criterion of a 5% improvement in PFS. Clinical benefit rate was also numerically superior (50.5 vs 45.5%). Patients that had been pre-exposed to AIs did not gain any benefit from the combination, suggesting that difference in patient populations is crucial in selecting an appropriate population to test in these studies. Further randomised trials in metastatic disease of gefitinib and anastrozole vs anastrozole alone are in progress to see if a delay in acquired resistance to estrogen deprivation can be delivered by combined therapy, again as previously demonstrated in xenograft models [35].

HER2 signalling may repress expression of ER directly via hyperactivated MAPK [34], and clinical evidence exists that trastuzumab may restore both ER expression and endocrine responsiveness in advanced breast cancer [36]. A phase II clinical trial of letrozole and the monoclonal antibody trastuzumab in patients with ER+/HER2+ metastatic breast cancer revealed that the combination was well tolerated and had a clinical benefit rate (PR + SD) of 50% [100] (Table 2). A randomised phase II trial in 207 patients with known ER+/HER2+ metastatic breast cancer recently reported a doubling of progression-free survival with the addition of trastuzumab over anastrozole alone (4.8 mo vs 2.4 mo, $p = 0.0016$) [101]. Ongoing studies remain looking at trastuzumab in combination with aromatase inhibitors, although a three-arm randomised trial of trastuzumab, an aromatase inhibitor, or the combination is required to confirm whether the combination actually offers an additive benefit.

Lapatinib is a potent oral tyrosine kinase inhibitor of both EGFR and HER2. As a dual inhibitor it may have the potential for greater anti-tumour effect than strategies targeting a single receptor, and in vitro data have demonstrated that estrogen deprivation significantly enhances the antiproliferative effects of lapatinib in HER2-amplified breast cancer cell lines [37, 102]. A phase I study has shown that the combination of lapatinib with letrozole was well tolerated with toxicities consisting mainly of grade 1–2 diarrhoea, nausea, rash, and fatigue [103], while a small phase II trial of lapatinib and tamoxifen was designed on the basis of pre-clinical evidence that lapatinib can significantly enhance sensitivity to tamoxifen in cell lines with acquired tamoxifen resistance [102, 104]. A phase III trial has completed recruitment of 1200 patients with metastatic ER+ breast cancer who were randomised to receive either letrozole alone or letrozole combined with lapatinib. Importantly, patients were selected regardless of their known EGFR/HER2 status in the primary tumour, but were stratified according to the time interval since adjuvant tamoxifen (> or <6 months). This large study may offer an important insight into the subgroups of patients most likely to benefit from a lapatinib–endocrine combination, such as known HER2+/ER+ breast cancer with potential de novo endocrine resistance (at least 200 such patients should be included in the study) or tumours that might develop acquired resistance to letrozole during treatment due to adaptive HER2 upregulation. To identify the latter, all patients had serum taken at baseline entry for assessment of circulating extracellular domain (ECD) HER2 which has been reported to be a predictor of poorer outcome with endocrine therapy, with sero-conversion occurring during endocrine therapy in up to 25% of patients with ER+ metastatic disease treated with either letrozole or tamoxifen [105, 106]. Thus, correlative biomarker studies will be crucial to the interpretation of which ER+ tumours derive benefit from combined STI–endocrine therapy.

Endocrine Therapy Combined with Farnesyltransferase Inhibitors

Interfering with the downstream effectors of growth factor receptors has emerged as another effective anti-tumour strategy. Ras proteins are membrane-bound GTP-binding proteins that are frequently aberrantly expressed in breast cancer [107], and act as mitogenic switches between growth factors receptors and downstream intracellular signalling via Raf/MAPK. This reaction is catalysed by the farnesyltransferase enzyme. FTIs such as tipifarnib and lonafarnib were developed in an effort to interrupt this pathway by inhibiting farnesylation, the first step in Ras activation. Based on encouraging results in cell line and tumour xenograft models [108] trials have been conducted in combination with tamoxifen or aromatase inhibitors (Table 2). Again, small phase I/II studies that included patients with endocrine resistance suggested evidence of efficacy [109, 110]. Unfortunately a larger randomised phase II study of letrozole alone or in combination with tipifarnib failed to show added benefit for the combination [111]. Mistakes in this trial included underpowering with inappropriate clinical endpoints of response rate rather than disease stabilisation. However, the true target for FTIs remains poorly understood, with up to 30 proteins that require farnesylation having a role in cellular growth and survival [112].

Endocrine Therapy Combined with mTOR Antagonists

The PI3K/Akt/mTOR pathway is activated by a number of growth factors, including insulin, insulin-like growth factor I (IGF-1), basic fibroblast growth factor (bFGF), EGF, and vascular epidermal growth factor (VEGF). Inhibiting this key effector of multiple pro-survival signals has therefore emerged as a viable therapeutic strategy in cancer. Mutations in the catalytic domain of PI3K have been identified in 20–25% of breast cancers [113, 114]. A further 15–35% of breast cancer patients demonstrate reduced expression of PTEN (phosphatase and tensin homolog deleted on chromosome Ten), a known inhibitor of the PI3K/AKT pathway which may be associated with poor prognosis in patients with ER+ breast cancer treated with tamoxifen [115, 116]. As such these cancers may be resistant to strategies targeting upstream growth factor receptors, but particularly sensitive to PI3K or mTOR inhibition. Furthermore, preclinical studies have demonstrated that the combination of letrozole with an mTOR inhibitor results in synergistic growth inhibition and apoptosis in ER+ breast cancer cell models [117].

While PI3K inhibitors are still in the early stages of development, mTOR inhibitors have been tested in breast cancer in combination with endocrine therapies (Table 2). A randomised phase II study of letrozole alone or in combination with another inhibitor, temsirolimus, has also been reported [118]. Preliminary results suggested a modest benefit to the combination in terms of median progression-free survival (13.2 mo vs 11.6 mo). Unfortunately, the resulting large phase III randomised trial of letrozole alone or in combination with temsirolimus in 992 post-menopausal women was terminated early after an interim analysis demonstrated a lack of benefit for the combination [119]. As with gefitinib, the inability to identify patients in whom the tumours demonstrate dependence on PI3K-mTOR activation severely limited the likelihood of success for this large phase III trial. Likewise, concern has been expressed that mTOR inhibition may induce a feedback loop via S6kinase and IGFR which enhances further Akt activation, thus overcoming the effects of mTOR inhibition.

Further studies in the neoadjuvant setting have evaluated the benefit of adding the mTOR inhibitor everolimus (RAD-001) to letrozole [120]. In a randomised phase II study in 270 post-menopausal women with ER+ primary operable breast cancer (>2 cm in size), the combination of letrozole 2.5 mg/day and everolimus 10 mg/day for 4 months pre-surgery resulted in a significantly greater tumour shrinkage as judged by ultrasound (58 vs 47%, $p = 0.03$) and a greater reduction in cell proliferation as measured by changes in Ki-67 after 15 days therapy. In associated biomarker studies to determine those tumours most likely to respond to combined mTOR antagonists and AI, elevated levels of one of the downstream biomarkers of mTOR activation (pS6240 kinase) was associated with a greater chance of response to the combination (odds ratio 2.1) [121]. These types of clinical studies in primary breast cancer are more likely to yield informative biomarker data than correlative studies in advanced disease, and as such may help select appropriate patients for combination strategies which attempt to overcome endocrine resistance pathways.

Conclusion

A number of theories have been proposed as contributing to endocrine resistance, and it is unlikely that there is any single dominant mechanism in the clinic. As discussed in this chapter pre-clinical evidence exists to support a number of valid hypotheses, including loss/repression of ER and various pharmacological/pharmacogenetic host factors that may account for resistance to tamoxifen. However, there is an increasing body of evidence to suggest that ER signalling survives, and that growth factor receptor and downstream kinases often operate in conjunction with ER to account for both de novo and acquired endocrine resistance. The nature of the interaction between ER and mitogenic signalling likely varies over time and from one patient to another. In some activated growth factor-mediated signalling suppresses ER expression and function, raising the possibility that growth factor-targeted therapy may directly restore endocrine responsiveness. In other cases, ER and growth factor signalling may interact synergistically providing the basis for combination strategies. Unlike tamoxifen resistance, relatively less is known about the mechanisms underpinning resistance to long-term estrogen deprivation, although as more post-menopausal women are receiving first-line adjuvant treatment with AIs, this question will become increasingly relevant. Both growth factor signalling and E2 hypersensitivity have been shown to contribute and would suggest that continued ED with an AI might be a superior approach to growth factor targeting alone.

Despite the strong pre-clinical data and rationale, translation of these hormone resistance hypotheses into clinical studies of combined STI and endocrine therapies has yielded disappointing results to date, which may be in part attributable to a poor selection of patients. It is unlikely that patients will respond to combination with specific inhibitors unless the intended target is a significant driver of endocrine-resistant growth. Conversely, while significant overexpression of HER2 is a known requirement for benefit from trastuzumab, further studies are needed to determine whether more moderate receptor expression or activation may be relevant in the setting of endocrine resistance. A number of trials are currently exploring the benefit of various targeted agents in combination or in sequence with endocrine therapy and include biological analyses that may shed further light on the clinically relevant mechanisms of endocrine resistance. Integrating these biological studies into ongoing clinical trails, together with appropriate and intelligent combinations of various signalling agents together, may ultimately be the smart way to combat the various hormonal resistance pathways that cancer cells utilise to survive.

References

1. Early Breast Cancer Trialists' Collaborative Group. Tamoxifen for early breast cancer: an overview of the randomised trials. Lancet. 1998;351:1451–67.
2. Early Breast Cancer Trialists' Collaborative Group. Effects of chemotherapy and hormonal therapy for early breast cancer on recurrence and 15-year survival: an overview of the randomised trials. Lancet. 2005;365:1687–717.
3. Ring A, Dowsett M. Mechanisms of tamoxifen resistance. Endocrinol Relat Cancer. 2004;11:643–58.
4. Sorlie T, Perou CM, Tibshirani R, et al. Gene expression patterns of breast carcinomas distinguish tumor subclasses with clinical implications. Proc Natl Acad Sci U S A. 2001;98:10869–74.
5. Shibata H, Spencer TE, Onate SA, et al. Role of co-activators and co-repressors in the mechanism of steroid/thyroid receptor action. Recent Prog Horm Res. 1997;52:141–64.
6. Ali S, Coombes RC. Endocrine-responsive breast cancer and strategies for combating resistance. Nat Rev Cancer. 2002;2:101–12.
7. Kumar V, Green S, Stack G, Berry M, Jin JR, Chambon P. Functional domains of the human estrogen receptor. Cell. 1987;51:941–51.
8. Glaros S, Atanaskova N, Zhao C, Skafar DF, Reddy KB. Activation function-1 domain of estrogen receptor regulates the agonistic and antagonistic actions of tamoxifen. Mol Endocrinol. 2006;20:996–1008.
9. Reid G, Hubner MR, Metivier R, et al. Cyclic, proteasome-mediated turnover of unliganded and liganded ERalpha on responsive promoters is an integral feature of estrogen signaling. Mol Cell. 2003;11:695–707.

10. Osborne CK, Schiff R. Estrogen-receptor biology: continuing progress and therapeutic implications. J Clin Oncol. 2005;23:1616–22.
11. Kushner PJ, Agard DA, Greene GL, et al. Estrogen receptor pathways to AP-1. J Steroid Biochem Mol Biol. 2000;74:311–7.
12. Fan P, Wang J, Santen RJ, Yue W. Long-term treatment with tamoxifen facilitates translocation of estrogen receptor alpha out of the nucleus and enhances its interaction with EGFR in MCF-7 breast cancer cells. Cancer Res. 2007;67:1352–60.
13. Kahlert S, Nuedling S, van Eickels M, Vetter H, Meyer R, Grohe C. Estrogen receptor alpha rapidly activates the IGF-1 receptor pathway. J Biol Chem. 2000;275:18447–53.
14. Simoncini T, Hafezi-Moghadam A, Brazil DP, Ley K, Chin WW, Liao JK. Interaction of oestrogen receptor with the regulatory subunit of phosphatidylinositol-3-OH kinase. Nature. 2000;407:538–41.
15. Metzger D, Losson R, Bornert JM, Lemoine Y, Chambon P. Promoter specificity of the two transcriptional activation functions of the human oestrogen receptor in yeast. Nucleic Acids Res. 1992;20:2813–7.
16. Tzukerman MT, Esty A, Santiso-Mere D, et al. Human estrogen receptor transactivational capacity is determined by both cellular and promoter context and mediated by two functionally distinct intramolecular regions. Mol Endocrinol. 1994;8:21–30.
17. Masamura S, Santner SJ, Heitjan DF, Santen RJ. Estrogen deprivation causes estradiol hypersensitivity in human breast cancer cells. J Clin Endocrinol Metab. 1995;80:2918–25.
18. Osborne CK, Hobbs K, Clark GM. Effect of estrogens and antiestrogens on growth of human breast cancer cells in athymic nude mice. Cancer Res. 1985;45:584–90.
19. Johnston SR, Boeddinghaus IM, Riddler S, et al. Idoxifene antagonizes estradiol-dependent MCF-7 breast cancer xenograft growth through sustained induction of apoptosis. Cancer Res. 1999;59:3646–51.
20. Brodie A, Jelovac D, Long BJ. Predictions from a preclinical model: studies of aromatase inhibitors and antiestrogens. Clin Cancer Res. 2003;9:455S–9S.
21. Baum M, Budzar AU, Cuzick J, et al. Anastrozole alone or in combination with tamoxifen versus tamoxifen alone for adjuvant treatment of postmenopausal women with early breast cancer: first results of the ATAC randomised trial. Lancet. 2002;359:2131–9.
22. Johnston SR, Saccani-Jotti G, Smith IE, et al. Changes in estrogen receptor, progesterone receptor, and pS2 expression in tamoxifen-resistant human breast cancer. Cancer Res. 1995;55:3331–8.
23. Johnston SR, Lu B, Dowsett M, et al. Comparison of estrogen receptor DNA binding in untreated and acquired antiestrogen-resistant human breast tumors. Cancer Res. 1997;57:3723–7.
24. Gradishar WJ, Chia S, Piccart M, on behalf of the EFECT writing committee. Fulvestrant versus exemestane following prior non-steroidal aromatase inhibitor therapy: first results from EFECT, a randomized, phase III trial in postmenopausal women with advanced breast cancer. Breast Cancer Res Treat. 2006; 100 Suppl 1: Abstract 12.
25. Encarnacion CA, Ciocca DR, McGuire WL, Clark GM, Fuqua SA, Osborne CK. Measurement of steroid hormone receptors in breast cancer patients on tamoxifen. Breast Cancer Res Treat. 1993;26:237–46.
26. Kuukasjarvi T, Kononen J, Helin H, Holli K, Isola J. Loss of estrogen receptor in recurrent breast cancer is associated with poor response to endocrine therapy. J Clin Oncol. 1996;14:2584–9.
27. Gross GE, Clark GM, Chamness GC, McGuire WL. Multiple progesterone receptor assays in human breast cancer. Cancer Res. 1984;44:836–40.
28. Petz LN, Ziegler YS, Schultz JR, Nardulli AM. Fos and Jun inhibit estrogen-induced transcription of the human progesterone receptor gene through an activator protein-1 site. Mol Endocrinol. 2004;18:521–32.
29. Giacinti L, Claudio PP, Lopez M, Giordano A. Epigenetic information and estrogen receptor alpha expression in breast cancer. Oncologist. 2006;11:1–8.

30. Yang X, Phillips DL, Ferguson AT, Nelson WG, Herman JG, Davidson NE. Synergistic activation of functional estrogen receptor (ER)-alpha by DNA methyltransferase and histone deacetylase inhibition in human ER-alpha-negative breast cancer cells. Cancer Res. 2001;61:7025–9.
31. Ferguson AT, Lapidus RG, Baylin SB, Davidson NE. Demethylation of the estrogen receptor gene in estrogen receptor-negative breast cancer cells can reactivate estrogen receptor gene expression. Cancer Res. 1995;55:2279–83.
32. Creighton CJ, Hilger AM, Murthy S, Rae JM, Chinnaiyan AM, El-Ashry D. Activation of mitogen-activated protein kinase in estrogen receptor alpha-positive breast cancer cells in vitro induces an in vivo molecular phenotype of estrogen receptor alpha-negative human breast tumors. Cancer Res. 2006;66:3903–11.
33. Konecny G, Pauletti G, Pegram M, et al. Quantitative association between HER-2/neu and steroid hormone receptors in hormone receptor-positive primary breast cancer. J Natl Cancer Inst. 2003;95:142–53.
34. Oh AS, Lorant LA, Holloway JN, Miller DL, Kern FG, El-Ashry D. Hyperactivation of MAPK induces loss of ERalpha expression in breast cancer cells. Mol Endocrinol. 2001;15:1344–59.
35. Massarweh S, Osborne CK, Jiang S, et al. Mechanisms of tumor regression and resistance to estrogen deprivation and fulvestrant in a model of estrogen receptor-positive, HER-2/neu-positive breast cancer. Cancer Res. 2006;66:8266–73.
36. Munzone E, Curigliano G, Rocca A, et al. Reverting estrogen-receptor-negative phenotype in HER-2-overexpressing advanced breast cancer patients exposed to trastuzumab plus chemotherapy. Breast Cancer Res. 2006;8(1):R4 Epub 2005 Dec 7.
37. Xia W, Bacus S, Hegde P, et al. A model of acquired autoresistance to a potent ErbB2 tyrosine kinase inhibitor and a therapeutic strategy to prevent its onset in breast cancer. Proc Natl Acad Sci U S A. 2006;103:7795–800.
38. Iorns E, Turner NC, Elliott R, et al. Identification of CDK10 as an Important Determinant of Resistance to Endocrine Therapy for Breast Cancer. Cancer Cell. 2008;13:91–104.
39. Bautista S, Valles H, Walker RL, et al. In breast cancer, amplification of the steroid receptor coactivator gene AIB1 is correlated with estrogen and progesterone receptor positivity. Clin Cancer Res. 1998;4:2925–9.
40. Osborne CK, Bardou V, Hopp TA, et al. Role of the estrogen receptor coactivator AIB1 (SRC-3) and HER-2/neu in tamoxifen resistance in breast cancer. J Natl Cancer Inst. 2003;95:353–61.
41. Kirkegaard T, McGlynn LM, Campbell FM, et al. Amplified in breast cancer 1 in human epidermal growth factor receptor – positive tumors of tamoxifen-treated breast cancer patients. Clin Cancer Res. 2007;13:1405–11.
42. Lavinsky RM, Jepsen K, Heinzel T, et al. Diverse signaling pathways modulate nuclear receptor recruitment of N-CoR and SMRT complexes. Proc Natl Acad Sci U S A. 1998;95:2920–5.
43. Zwijsen RM, Buckle RS, Hijmans EM, Loomans CJ, Bernards R. Ligand-independent recruitment of steroid receptor coactivators to estrogen receptor by cyclin D1. Genes Dev. 1998;12:3488–98.
44. Kenny FS, Hui R, Musgrove EA, et al. Overexpression of cyclin D1 messenger RNA predicts for poor prognosis in estrogen receptor-positive breast cancer. Clin Cancer Res. 1999;5:2069–76.
45. Han S, Park K, Bae BN, et al. Cyclin D1 expression and patient outcome after tamoxifen therapy in estrogen receptor positive metastatic breast cancer. Oncol Rep. 2003;10:141–4.
46. Gutierrez MC, Detre S, Johnston SR, et al. Molecular changes in tamoxifen-resistant breast cancer: relationship between estrogen receptor, HER-2, and p38 mitogen-activated protein kinase. J Clin Oncol. 2005;23:2469–76.
47. Martin LA, Farmer I, Johnston SR, Ali S, Marshall C, Dowsett M. Enhanced estrogen receptor (ER) alpha, ERBB2, and MAPK signal transduction pathways operate during

the adaptation of MCF-7 cells to long term estrogen deprivation. J Biol Chem. 2003;278:30458–68.
48. Santen R, Jeng MH, Wang JP, et al. Adaptive hypersensitivity to estradiol: potential mechanism for secondary hormonal responses in breast cancer patients. J Steroid Biochem Mol Biol. 2001;79:115–25.
49. Jeng MH, Yue W, Eischeid A, Wang JP, Santen RJ. Role of MAP kinase in the enhanced cell proliferation of long term estrogen deprived human breast cancer cells. Breast Cancer Res Treat. 2000;62:167–75.
50. Karnik PS, Kulkarni S, Liu XP, Budd GT, Bukowski RM. Estrogen receptor mutations in tamoxifen-resistant breast cancer. Cancer Res. 1994;54:349–53.
51. Anderson TI, Wooster R, Laake K, et al. Screening for ESR mutations in breast and ovarian cancer patients. Hum Mutat. 1997;9:531–6.
52. Dowsett M, Daffada A, Chan CM, Johnston SR. Oestrogen receptor mutants and variants in breast cancer. Eur J Cancer. 1997;33:1177–83.
53. Wolf DM, Jordan VC. The estrogen receptor from a tamoxifen stimulated MCF-7 tumor variant contains a point mutation in the ligand binding domain. Breast Cancer Res Treat. 1994;31:129–38.
54. Fuqua SA, Wiltschke C, Zhang QX, et al. A hypersensitive estrogen receptor-alpha mutation in premalignant breast lesions. Cancer Res. 2000;60:4026–9.
55. Johnston SR, Haynes BP, Smith IE, et al. Acquired tamoxifen resistance in human breast cancer and reduced intra-tumoral drug concentration. Lancet. 1993;342:1521–2.
56. Dowsett M, Haynes BP. Hormonal effects of aromatase inhibitors: focus on premenopausal effects and interaction with tamoxifen. J Steroid Biochem Mol Biol. 2003;86:255–63.
57. Goetz MP, Rae JM, Suman VJ, et al. Pharmacogenetics of tamoxifen biotransformation is associated with clinical outcomes of efficacy and hot flashes. J Clin Oncol. 2005;23:9312–8.
58. Goetz MP, Knox SK, Suman VJ, et al. The impact of cytochrome P450 2D6 metabolism in women receiving adjuvant tamoxifen. Breast Cancer Res Treat. 2007;101:113–21.
59. Chetrite GS, Cortes-Prieto J, Philippe JC, Wright F, Pasqualini JR. Comparison of estrogen concentrations, estrone sulfatase and aromatase activities in normal, and in cancerous, human breast tissues. J Steroid Biochem Mol Biol. 2000;72:23–7.
60. Miller WR, Anderson TJ, Jack WJ. Relationship between tumour aromatase activity, tumour characteristics and response to therapy. J Steroid Biochem Mol Biol. 1990;37:1055–9.
61. Lin Z RS, Cotterill H, Rademaker A, Khan S, Haynes B, Dowsett M, Bulun SE, Innes J, Hern RA, Smith I. Messenger RNA levels of estrogen-related genes in malignant breast tumor tissue predict responsiveness to aromatase inhibitors. Breast Cancer Res Treat. 2006; 100 (1): Abstract 14.
62. Dunning AM, Dowsett M, Healey CS, et al. Polymorphisms associated with circulating sex hormone levels in postmenopausal women. J Natl Cancer Inst. 2004;96:936–45.
63. Ma CX, Adjei AA, Salavaggione OE, et al. Human aromatase: gene resequencing and functional genomics. Cancer Res. 2005;65:11071–82.
64. Slamon DJ, Clark GM, Wong SG, Levin WJ, Ullrich A, McGuire WL. Human breast cancer: correlation of relapse and survival with amplification of the HER-2/neu oncogene. Science. 1987;235:177–82.
65. Ellis MJ, Coop A, Singh B, et al. Letrozole is more effective neoadjuvant endocrine therapy than tamoxifen for ErbB-1- and/or ErbB-2-positive, estrogen receptor-positive primary breast cancer: evidence from a phase III randomized trial. J Clin Oncol. 2001;19:3808–16.
66. Chen D, Washbrook E, Sarwar N, et al. Phosphorylation of human estrogen receptor alpha at serine 118 by two distinct signal transduction pathways revealed by phosphorylation-specific antisera. Oncogene. 2002;21:4921–31.

67. Kato S, Endoh H, Masuhiro Y, et al. Activation of the estrogen receptor through phosphorylation by mitogen-activated protein kinase. Science. 1995;270:1491–4.
68. Campbell RA, Bhat-Nakshatri P, Patel NM, Constantinidou D, Ali S, Nakshatri H. Phosphatidylinositol 3-kinase/AKT-mediated activation of estrogen receptor alpha: a new model for anti-estrogen resistance. J Biol Chem. 2001;276:9817–24.
69. Dowsett M, Ebbs SR, Dixon JM, et al. Biomarker changes during neoadjuvant anastrozole, tamoxifen, or the combination: influence of hormonal status and HER-2 in breast cancer – a study from the IMPACT trialists. J Clin Oncol. 2005;23:2477–92.
70. Smith IE, Dowsett M, Ebbs SR, et al. Neoadjuvant treatment of postmenopausal breast cancer with anastrozole, tamoxifen, or both in combination: the Immediate Preoperative Anastrozole, Tamoxifen, or Combined with Tamoxifen (IMPACT) multicenter double-blind randomized trial. J Clin Oncol. 2005;23:5108–16.
71. Chung YL, Sheu ML, Yang SC, Lin CH, Yen SH. Resistance to tamoxifen-induced apoptosis is associated with direct interaction between Her2/neu and cell membrane estrogen receptor in breast cancer. Int J Cancer. 2002;97:306–12.
72. Knowlden JM, Hutcheson IR, Jones HE, et al. Elevated levels of epidermal growth factor receptor/c-erbB2 heterodimers mediate an autocrine growth regulatory pathway in tamoxifen-resistant MCF-7 cells. Endocrinology. 2003;144:1032–44.
73. Osborne CK, Shou J, Massarweh S, Schiff R. Crosstalk between estrogen receptor and growth factor receptor pathways as a cause for endocrine therapy resistance in breast cancer. Clin Cancer Res. 2005;11:865s–70s.
74. Pancholi S, Lykkesfeldt A, Banerjee S, Farmer I, Leary A, Johnston S, Dowsett M, Martin LA. ERBB2 influences the subcellular localization of the estrogen receptor in tamoxifen resistant MCFF7 cells leading to the activation of AKT and $p90^{RSK}$. Endocrinol Relat Cancer. 2008; (in press).
75. Johnston SR, Dowsett M. Aromatase inhibitors for breast cancer: lessons from the laboratory. Nat Rev Cancer. 2003;3:821–31.
76. Nicholson RI, McClelland RA, Robertson JF, Gee JM. Involvement of steroid hormone and growth factor cross-talk in endocrine response in breast cancer. Endocrinol Relat Cancer. 1999;6:373–87.
77. Chan CM, Martin LA, Johnston SR, Ali S, Dowsett M. Molecular changes associated with the acquisition of oestrogen hypersensitivity in MCF-7 breast cancer cells on long-term oestrogen deprivation. J Steroid Biochem Mol Biol. 2002;81:333–41.
78. Jeng MH, Shupnik MA, Bender TP, et al. Estrogen receptor expression and function in long-term estrogen-deprived human breast cancer cells. Endocrinology. 1998;139:4164–74.
79. Shim WS, Conaway M, Masamura S, et al. Estradiol hypersensitivity and mitogen-activated protein kinase expression in long-term estrogen deprived human breast cancer cells in vivo. Endocrinology. 2000;141:396–405.
80. Dowsett M, Stein RC, Coombes RC. Aromatization inhibition alone or in combination with GnRH agonists for the treatment of premenopausal breast cancer patients. J Steroid Biochem Mol Biol. 1992;43:155–9.
81. Wakeling AE, Dukes M, Bowler J. A potent specific pure antiestrogen with clinical potential. Cancer Res. 1991;51:3867–73.
82. Dauvois S Fau, White R, White R Fau, Parker MG, Parker MG. The antiestrogen ICI 182780 disrupts estrogen receptor nucleocytoplasmic shuttling.
83. Osborne CK, Coronado-Heinsohn EB, Hilsenbeck SG, et al. Comparison of the effects of a pure steroidal antiestrogen with those of tamoxifen in a model of human breast cancer. J Natl Cancer Inst. 1995;87:746–50.
84. Perey LP, Paridaens R, Hawle H, et al. Clinical benefit of fulvestrant in postmenopausal women with advanced breast cancer and primary or acquired resistance to aromatase inhibitors: final results of phase II Swiss Group for Clinical Cancer Research Trial (SAKK 21/00). Ann Oncol. 2007;18(1):64–9.

85. Steger GG, Bartsch R, Wenzel C, et al. Fulvestrant in pre-treated patients with advanced breast cancer: a single centre experience. Eur J Cancer. 2005;41(17):2655–61.
86. Ingle JR, Suman VJ, Rowland KM, et al. Fulvestrant in women with advanced breast cancer after progression on prior aromatase inhibitor therapy: North Central Cancer Treatment Group Trial N0032. J Clin Oncol. 2006;24(7):1052–6.
87. Osipo C, Gajdos C, Liu H, Chen B, Jordan VC. Paradoxical action of fulvestrant in estradiol-induced regression of tamoxifen-stimulated breast cancer. J Natl Cancer Inst. 2003;95:1597–608.
88. Martin LA, Pancholi S, Chan CM, et al. The anti-oestrogen ICI 182,780, but not tamoxifen, inhibits the growth of MCF-7 breast cancer cells refractory to long-term oestrogen deprivation through down-regulation of oestrogen receptor and IGF signalling. Endocrinol Relat Cancer. 2005;12:1017–36.
89. Lonning PE, Bajetta E, Murray R, et al. Activity of exemestane in metastatic breast cancer after failure of non-steroidal aromatase inhibitors: a phase II trial. J Clin Oncol. 2000;18:2234–44.
90. Johnston SRD. Fulvestrant and the sequential endocrine cascade for advanced breast cancer. Br J Cancer. 2004;90 Suppl 1:S15–8.
91. Kurokawa H, Lenferink AE, Simpson JF, et al. Inhibition of HER2/neu (erbB-2) and mitogen-activated protein kinases enhances tamoxifen action against HER2-overexpressing, tamoxifen-resistant breast cancer cells. Cancer Res. 2000;60:5887–94.
92. Shou J, Massarweh S, Osborne CK, et al. Mechanisms of tamoxifen resistance: increased estrogen receptor-HER2/neu cross-talk in ER/HER2-positive breast cancer. J Natl Cancer Inst. 2004;96:926–35.
93. Johnston SR, Leary A, Martin LA, Smith IE, Dowsett M. Enhancing endocrine response with novel targeted therapies : why have the clinical trials to date failed to deliver on the preclinical promise? Cancer. 2008;112:710–7.
94. Mita M, Bono J, Mita A. A phase II and biologic correlative study investigating anastrozole (A) in combination with gefitinib (G) in postmenopausal patients with estrogen receptor positive (ER) metastatic breast carcinoma (MBC) who have previously failed hormonal therapy. Breast Cancer Res Treat. 2005;94 Suppl 1: Abstract 1117.
95. Mayer I, Ganja N, Shyr Y, Muldowney N, Arteaga C. A phase II trial of letrozole plus erlotinib in post-menopausal women with hormone-sensitive metastatic breast cancer: preliminary results of toxicities and correlative studies. Breast Cancer Res Treat. 2006;100 Suppl 1: Abstract 4052.
96. Smith IE, Walsh G, Skene A, et al. A phase II placebo-controlled trial of neo-adjuvant anastrozole alone or with gefitinib in early breast cancer. J Clin Oncol. 2007;25:3816–22.
97. Polychronis A, Sinnet HD, Hadjiminas D, et al. Pre-operative gefitinib versus gefitinib and anastrozole in postmenopausal patients with oestrogen-receptor positive and epidermal growth factor receptor positive primary breast cancer: a double blind placebo-controlled phase II randomised trial. Lancet Oncol. 2005;6:383–91.
98. Atkins D, Reiffen KA, Tegtmeier CL, Winther H, Bonato MS, Storkel S. Immunohistochemical detection of EGFR in paraffin-embedded tumor tissues: variation in staining intensity due to choice of fixative and storage time of tissue sections. J Histochem Cytochem. 2004;52:893–901.
99. Osborne K, Neven P, Dirix L, Mackey J, Robert J, Underhill C, Gutierrez C, Magill P, Hargreaves L. Randomized phase II study of gefitinib (IRESSA) or placebo in combination with tamoxifen in patients with hormone receptor positive metastatic breast cancer. Breast Cancer Res Treat. 2007;106 Suppl 1: Abstract 2067.
100. Marcom PK, Isaacs C, Harris L, et al. The combination of letrozole and trastuzumab as first or second-line biological therapy produces durable responses in a subset of HER2 positive and ER positive advanced breast cancers. Breast Cancer Res Treat. 2007;102:43–9.

101. Mackey JR, Kaufman B, Clemens M, et al. Trastuzumab prolongs progression-free survival in hormone-dependent and HER2-positive metastatic breast cancer. Breast Cancer Res Treat. 2006;100 Suppl 1: Abstract 3.
102. Leary AF, Martin LA, Lykkesfeldt AE, Dowsett M, Johnston SRD. Enhancing endocrine responsiveness using the dual EGFR/HER2 tyrosine kinase inhibitor lapatinib in cell models of endocrine resistance. Breast Cancer Res Treat. 2006;100 Suppl 1: Abstract 303.
103. Chu Q, Cianfrocca ME, Murray N, Oslund M, Nelson LM, Rowinsky E, Schwartz G, Goldstein LJ, Loftiss JI, Paul E, Koch KM, Pandite L. A phase I and pharmacokinetic study of Lapatinib in combination with letrozole in patients with advanced cancer. Clin Cancer Res. 2008 Jul 15;14(14):4484–90.
104. Chu I, Blackwell K, Chen S, Slingerland J. The dual ErbB1/ErbB2 inhibitor, lapatinib (GW572016), cooperates with tamoxifen to inhibit both cell proliferation- and estrogen-dependent gene expression in antiestrogen-resistant breast cancer. Cancer Res. 2005;65:18–25.
105. Fehm T, Becker S, Duerr-Stoerzer S, et al. Determination of HER2 status using both serum HER2 levels and circulating tumour cells in patients with recurrent breast cancer whose primary tumour status was HER2 negative or of unknown HER2 status. Breast Cancer Res. 2007;9(5):R74.
106. Lipton A, Ali SM, Leitzel K, et al. Serum HER-2/neu and response to the aromatase inhibitor letrozole versus tamoxifen. J Clin Oncol. 2003;21:1967–72.
107. Clark GJ, Der CJ. Aberrant function of the Ras signal transduction pathway in human breast cancer. Breast Cancer Res Treat. 1995;35:133–44.
108. Martin LA, Head JE, Pancholi S, et al. The farnesyltransferase inhibitor R115777 (tipifarnib) in combination with tamoxifen acts synergistically to inhibit MCF-7 breast cancer cell proliferation and cell cycle progression in vitro and in vivo. Mol Cancer Ther. 2007;6:2458–67.
109. Dalenc F, Lacroix-Tikri M, Mourey L. Tipifarnib with tamoxifen as a rescue for tamoxifen acquired clinical resistance for metastatic ER and/or PgR positive breast cancer after relapse under tamoxifen. Preliminary results. Breast Cancer Res Treat. 2005;94:S241.
110. Lebowitz PF, Eng-Wong J, Widemann BC, et al. A phase I trial and pharmacokinetic study of tipifarnib, a farnesyltransferase inhibitor, and tamoxifen in metastatic breast cancer. Clin Cancer Res. 2005;11:1247–52.
111. Johnston SR, Semiglazov VF, Manikhas GM, et al. A phase II, randomized, blinded study of the farnesyltransferase inhibitor tipifarnib combined with letrozole in the treatment of advanced breast cancer after antiestrogen therapy. Breast Cancer Res Treat. 2007; Epub Sept 13.
112. Appels NM, Beijnen JH, Schellens JH. Development of farnesyl transferase inhibitors: a review. Oncologist. 2005;10:565–78.
113. Wu G, Xing M, Mambo E, et al. Somatic mutation and gain of copy number of PIK3CA in human breast cancer. Breast Cancer Res. 2005;7:R609–16.
114. Bachman KE, Argani P, Samuels Y, et al. The PIK3CA gene is mutated with high frequency in human breast cancers. Cancer Biol Ther. 2004;3:772–5.
115. Saal LH, Holm K, Maurer M, et al. PIK3CA mutations correlate with hormone receptors, node metastasis, and ERBB2, and are mutually exclusive with PTEN loss in human breast carcinoma. Cancer Res. 2005;65:2554–9.
116. Shoman N, Klassen S, McFadden A, Bickis MG, Torlakovic E, Chibbar R. Reduced PTEN expression predicts relapse in patients with breast carcinoma treated by tamoxifen. Mod Pathol. 2005;18:250–9.
117. Boulay A, Rudloff J, Ye J, et al. Dual inhibition of mTOR and estrogen receptor signaling in vitro induces cell death in models of breast cancer. Clin Cancer Res. 2005;11:5319–28.

118. Baselga J, Roche H, Fumoleau P, et al. Treatment of postmenopausal women with locally advanced or metastatic breast cancer with letrozole alone or in combination with temsirolimus: a randomized, 3-arm, phase 2 study. Breast Cancer Res Treat. 2005;94 Suppl 1: Abstract 1068.
119. Chow LS, Sun Y, Jassem J, Baselga J, Hayes DF, Wolff AC, et al. Phase 3 study of temsirolimus with letrozole or letrozole alone in postmenopausal women with locally advanced or metastatic breast cancer. Breast Cancer Res Treat. 2006;100 Suppl 1: Abstract 6091.
120. Baselga J, Semiglazov V, van Dam P, Manikhas A, Bellet M, Mayordomo J, Campone M, Kubista E, Greil R, Bianchi G, Steinseifer J, Molloy B, Tokaji E, Dixon JM, Jonat W, Rugo HS. Phase II double-blind randomized trial of daily oral RAD001 (everolimus) plus letrozole (LET) or placebo (P) plus LET as neoadjuvant therapy for ER+ breast cancer. Beast Cancer Res Treat. 2007;106 Suppl 1: Abstract 2066.
121. Gardner H, Bandaru R, Barret C, et al. Biomarker analysis of a phase II double-blind randomised trial of daily oral RAD001 (Everolimus) plus letrozole or placebo plus letrozole as neoadjuvant therapy for patients with estrogen receptor positive breast cancer. Breast Cancer Res Treat. 2007;106 Suppl 1: Abstract 4006.

Strategies of Hormonal Prevention

Yuxin Li and Powel H. Brown

Introduction

Breast cancer is the most common cancer in women excluding skin cancer. Estimated by the National Cancer Institute, one in eight women in the United States will develop breast cancer during their lifetime. The high risk of this disease had prompted extensive studies in breast cancer prevention and treatment. With aggressive screening to detect early breast cancer and significant advances in treatment, breast cancer mortality rate has declined dramatically. However, it remains the second leading cause of cancer death in women, exceeded only by lung cancer [1]. In contrast to the progressions in detection and treatment, the incidence of breast cancer in the United States has been increased by almost 40% in an 18-year period (1980–1999), and showed a declining trend in recent years. The decreased incidence of breast cancer was observed mainly in women aged 50 years or older and was more evident in estrogen receptor (ER)-positive cancers than in ER-negative cancers. Ravdin et al. have proposed that the decline of breast cancer incidence might be related to the drop of hormone replacement therapy among postmenopausal women in the United States [2]. The influence of hormonal medication on breast cancer incidence is a strong evidence of using endocrine interventions to prevent the development of breast cancer.

Mammary carcinogenesis was noted to be a hormonally dependent process more than a century ago. The association of estrogen with breast cancer has been recognized since Beatson first demonstrated that bilateral oophorectomy could benefit premenopausal women with inoperable breast cancer in 1896 [3]. Subsequent investigations implicated that estrogen is a key factor for the initiation and promotion of breast cancer, suggesting the potential

P.H. Brown (✉)
Lester and Sue Smith Breast Center, Baylor College of Medicine, Houston, TX, USA
e-mail: pbrown@bcm.tmc.edu

S.A.W. Fuqua (ed.), *Hormone Receptors in Breast Cancer*,
Cancer Treatment and Research 312, DOI 10.1007/978-0-387-09463-2_10,

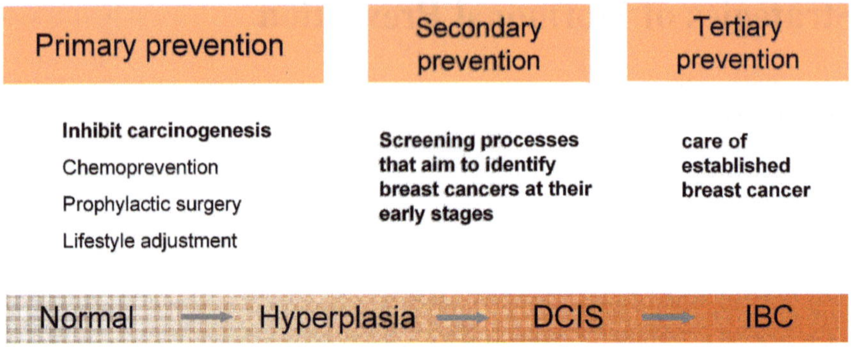

Fig. 1 Breast cancer prevention approaches

therapeutic and preventive effects of antiestrogenic agents. Therefore, strategies to reduce the estrogen exposure to breast tissue, or to antagonize the estrogen activity, represent the mainstream in the current breast cancer prevention studies.

Currently available approaches to prevent breast cancer can be categorized into enhanced surveillance, lifestyle adjustment, prophylactic surgery, and chemoprevention. Enhanced surveillance includes regular self-examination, clinical breast examination, and annual mammography. This is secondary prevention approach that aims to detect breast cancer at the earlier stages (Fig. 1). However, it has no role to inhibit mammary carcinogenesis. Prevention of mammary carcinogenesis will rely on the primary prevention approaches that include lifestyle adjustment, prophylactic surgery, and chemoprevention. All of these strategies have involved hormonal changes or modulation of hormonal signaling pathways as the underlying mechanisms.

Lifestyle Adjustments

Lifestyle adjustments are considered as safe and natural processes to reduce the risk of breast cancer. The idea of lifestyle adjustment originated from promising data of observational studies. A comparison of breast cancer incidence across geographic regions demonstrated a tremendous variation in incidence in which more than 5-fold difference was observed between low-risk and high-risk areas [4]. Moreover, migration studies showed that breast cancer rates increased in persons who moved from low-risk area to high-risk area [5], suggesting that environmental exposures and lifestyle changes contribute substantially to the risk of breast cancer. Abundant epidemiological data suggest that early pregnancy, physical activity, or dietary factor may prevent the development of breast cancer.

Early Pregnancy

Extensive epidemiological and clinical data indicate that women who have early full-term pregnancy (especially before the age of 20 or 24 years) have a significant reduction in their lifetime risk of developing breast cancer, and additional pregnancies increase the protection [6]. This phenomenon is consistently observed in both human and rodents [7, 8], suggesting that hormonal changes during the pregnancy is attributed to the protection of breast tissue from carcinogenesis. At present, the mechanism by which parity protects against breast cancer is not fully understood. It is suggested that this protective effect could result from terminal differentiation of a subpopulation of mammary epithelial cells at increased risk of carcinogenesis. The induction of pregnancy-driven differentiation could be induced by either the hormonal milieu of pregnancy [9] or the environmental milieu and alterations in the immunological profile of the host [10, 11]. The Russo group have described the normal mammary tissue as consisting of the undifferentiated lobules type 1 (Lob 1), the more-developed lobules type 2 and 3, and lobules type 4 which occur during pregnancy and lactation. After menopause, the breast regresses to Lob 1 in both nulliparous and parous women. It was postulated that the Lob 1 in breast of nulliparous women, which had not gone through the full process of differentiation, contains a high concentration of reproducing progenitor cells (also called "stem cells 1"). These stem cells 1 are susceptible to neoplastic transformation when exposed to carcinogenetic events. In contrast, Lob 1 in postmenopausal parous breast contains a different group of reproducing progenitor cells called "stem cells 2," which are refractory to neoplastic transformation. The early pregnancy-induced mammary differentiation changes the genomic signature in Lob 1 and shifts the stem cell 1 to stem cell 2; these changes with genomic expression may be the mechanism by which early pregnancy prevents breast cancer [12]. In addition, Trichopoulos et al. have postulated that the number of mammary stem cells was reduced through the process of terminal differentiation after the first full-term pregnancy, which has also contributed to the breast cancer risk reduction [13]. Clearly, clarifying the underlying mechanism of early pregnancy protection could help us develop new hormonal strategies to reduce the risk of breast cancer.

Physical Activity and Breast Cancer

During the past 20 years, numerous observational studies have demonstrated that women who exercise regularly have a reduced risk of developing breast cancer than sedentary women. However, there are a number of studies that reported no relation between physical activity and risk of breast cancer. The inconsistent findings may be attributable to the large heterogeneity in study design, exposure measurements, sample populations, and other aspects.

Recently, Monninkhof et al. have performed the meta-analysis of 19 cohort studies and 29 case–control studies concerning physical activity and breast cancer risk published between 1994 and 2006 [14]. The number of cases ranged from 46 to 3,424 in cohort studies and from 81 to 6,888 in case–control studies. These observational studies have been scored by quality assessment according to three important sources of error (selection, misclassification, and confounding bias). Thus, studies were classified into higher or lower quality groups based on the median study quality score. In cohort studies, the three studies assessing total activity show inconsistent results. About 8 of the 17 cohort studies on leisure time activities showed a decreased breast cancer risk (RR<0.8) and the other 9 reported no association. In general, the lower quality studies show greater risk reductions than the higher quality studies. Risk reduction in higher quality studies ranged from 21 to 39%. In case–control studies, four of the six studies assessing total activity demonstrated a decrease in breast cancer risk (RR<0.8) ranging from 21 to 52%. A total of 14 out of 28 case–control studies on leisure time activity observed a reduced risk ranging from 23 to 65%. Overall, physical activity is associated with a modest (15–20%) risk reduction on breast cancer. When menopausal status was considered, majority studies assessing risk among postmenopausal women showed reduced risk ranging from 20 to 80%. In contrast, in premenopausal women, the evidence is much weaker and judged as indecisive. Evidence for a dose–response relationship was observed in approximately half of the higher quality studies that reported a reduced risk. The results of the trend analysis of 17 case–control studies suggest a 6% reduction in risk per hour physical activity per week assuming that activity would be sustained over a longer period of time.

Lahmann et al. have analyzed 9 studies which include 218,169 premenopausal and postmenopausal women aged 20–80 years from European Prospective Investigation into Cancer and Nutrition (EPIC) cohort studies [15]. During 6.4 years of follow-up, 3,423 incident invasive breast cancers were identified. Overall, increasing total physical activity was associated with a reduction in breast cancer risk among postmenopausal women. Interestingly, only household activity was associated with a significantly reduced risk in both postmenopausal (HR: 0.81, 95% CI = 0.70–0.93, p = 0.001) and premenopausal (HR: 0.71, 95% CI = 0.55–0.90, p = 0.003) women. Occupational activity and recreational activity were not significantly related to breast cancer risk in either premenopausal or postmenopausal women.

Multiple physiological responses to physical activity have been postulated to be attributed to the reduced risk of breast cancer [16]. These include decreased body fat and sex hormone, decreased insulin and IGFs, enhanced immune function, decreased adipocytokines, decreased mammographic density, and improved antioxidant defense systems. Among them, changes in sex hormones are perhaps the most consistently cited mechanism for the association between physical activity and breast cancer. McTiernan et al. have conducted a 12-month randomized controlled exercise trial in postmenopausal women [17]. Moderate-intensity exercise was associated with significant decrease of serum estrogen level (3.8–8.2% after 3 months of exercise), which was proportional to the degree of body fat loss. Decreased body fat will result in less substrate for estrogen and testosterone production and lead to less tissue capable of aromatization of the adrenal androgens to estrogens.

Diet and Breast Cancer

Dietary factors are thought to be important factors for the geographic change in incidence rates of breast cancer [18]. An interesting group of dietary factors is the natural phenolic compound group, which potentially can act as steroid action modulator. Phytoestrogens, which include flavonoids, tannins, stilbenoids, and lignans, are a broad group of plant-derived phenolic compounds that can bind to ER and mimic the effects of estrogen, although with low potency. Multiple epidemiologic data suggest a decreased risk of breast cancer in women from countries with high phytoestrogen consumption [19]. This has been followed by in vitro and in vivo animal studies suggesting a potential role for phytoestrogen in reducing the risk of breast cancer [20]. However, recent reviews have failed to provide strong evidence showing phytoestrogens can prevent breast cancer [21]. Several randomized clinical trials are being conducted to evaluate the preventive effect of phytoestrogens on breast cancer. In addition to phytoestrogens, a randomized controlled trial run by the Women's Health Initiative demonstrated that low-fat diet was associated with a 9% reduction (HR: 0.91, 95% CI = 0.83–1.01) in breast cancer risk over a 8.1-year average follow-up; however, this reduction did not reach statistical significance ($p = 0.09$) [22, 23].

The majority of epidemiologic studies on diet and breast cancer are case–control studies which are retrospective and constitute with recall bias, selection bias, and other bias. Recently, more data from prospective cohort studies have become available. Given the wealth of studies, Michels et al. have reviewed prospective cohort studies on diet and breast cancer incidence [24]. The review covers the wide range of nutritional factors including fat intake, fruit and vegetable consumption, antioxidant vitamins (vitamins A, C, E, and beta-carotene), serum antioxidants, carbohydrate intake and glycemic load, dairy and vitamin D consumption, heterocyclic amines, soy products, green tea, and others. To date, there is no association that is consistent, strong, and statistically significant between diet and breast cancer incidence, except for regular alcohol consumption and weight gain. A recent pooled analyses of six prospective cohort studies showed that consumption of each additional 10 g of alcohol per day was associated with a 9% (95% CI = 4–13%) increase in the risk of breast cancer [25]. Similarly, analysis of pooled data from seven prospective cohort studies demonstrated an association between high body mass index (BMI) and breast cancer [26]. This study showed increased breast cancer risk in postmenopausal women with high BMI, with a relative risk (RR) of 1.26 (95% CI = 1.09–1.46) for postmenopausal women with a BMI above 28 kg/m compared to postmenopausal women with a BMI of less than 21 kg/m [26].

Prophylactic Surgeries

Prophylactic surgeries consist of bilateral mastectomy and bilateral oophorectomy. These are highly invasive approaches that are only applied to women with extremely high risk of breast cancer, such as hereditary breast cancer. Unlike familial breast cancer, which has one or more first- and/or second-degree relatives affected by breast cancer, but lacks the Mendelian inheritance pattern, hereditary breast cancer is developed from women who carry a mutated phenotype of a specific gene segregating with a Mendelian inheritance pattern [27, 28]. These cancers account for 5–10% of all breast cancers. Majority (75%) of hereditary breast cancer patients carry the mutation of BRCA1 (breast cancer gene no. 1) or BRCA2 genes [29]. It is estimated that BRCA mutations occurred in 10% of breast cancers diagnosed in women younger than 40 years. Mutation of either gene has a markedly increased risk of developing breast and/or ovarian cancer during their lifetime, particularly at younger ages. BRCA1/BRCA2 mutations confer the lifetime risk of breast cancer from 54 [30] to 85% [31] and the lifetime risk of ovarian cancer from 20 to 54% [30, 32].

Owing to their extremely high risk of developing breast cancer, some BRCA mutation carriers may consider accepting bilateral mastectomy, which is the most effective method to prevent breast cancer. Recently, both Rebbeck and Hartmann showed that women with BRCA mutations could benefit from bilateral prophylactic mastectomy [33, 34]. However, mastectomy is not 100% effective. Previous reports indicated that mastectomy reduced the risk of breast cancer by 90–100% [35–37]. Breast cancers developed after prophylactic mastectomy were from the nipple-areolar complex, elsewhere in the breast, or metastatic locations. In a large case study done at Mayo clinic [38], 7 out of 639 women who accepted subcutaneous mastectomy developed breast cancer. Only one patient had cancer in the nipple, and the other six had cancer in the breast (one patient), chest wall (three patients), breast above areola (one patient), and the bone marrow (one patient). Cancer that developed after mastectomy is probably the result of inadequate removal of all the mammary tissues. Any amount of residual mammary gland will have significant risk to develop cancer. Metastatic disease is probably a result of the spread of cancer before the surgery.

Considering the high risk of developing both breast cancer and ovarian cancer in BRCA mutation carriers, and the poor prognosis of ovarian cancer, application of the bilateral oophorectomy in these patients is a reasonable modality. More women with BRCA mutations will prefer oophorectomy than mastectomy due to the more acceptable cosmetic outcome and the preventive effect for both ovarian and breast cancers. The idea of oophorectomy to prevent breast cancer originated from accumulating observations showing the close relationship of ovary function and breast cancer, which was noted more than a century ago. It was Albert Schinzinger, a German surgeon, who first proposed surgical oophorectomy (surgical removal of ovaries) as treatment for advanced breast cancer and prophylaxis against local recurrence after he observed that the prognosis for breast cancer appeared better in older women than in younger women [39]. In 1895, George Thomas Beatson first conducted bilateral oophorectomy in a premenopausal woman with metastatic breast cancer. Follow-up observation showed that this patient experienced a complete clinical remission and survived 4 years after surgery [3]. Influenced by this result, English surgeon Stanley Boyd first applied oophorectomy as adjuvant treatment for breast cancer. As he described, “my working hypothesis is that internal secretion of the ovaries in some cases favors the growth of the cancer.” In 1900, he reported that one-third of breast cancer patients benefited from ovarian ablation. Although these clinical data were not very encouraging, they did imply a strong relationship between estrogen and the development of breast cancer. In 1992, the Early Breast Cancer Trialists’ Collaborative Group reported a meta-analysis of clinical trials of adjuvant oophorectomy by radiation or surgery, which indicated that ovary ablation in breast cancer patients showed long-term benefits including increased disease-free and overall survival. Results of several following adjuvant trials have given direct evidence of clinical benefits of oophorectomy in breast cancer patients, particularly in patients whose cancers express hormone receptors [40–42].

The effectiveness of prophylactic oophorectomy in BRCA mutation carriers was demonstrated in recent studies. Rebbeck et al. have reported that bilateral oophorectomy in BRCA1 or BRCA2 carriers reduced the risk of breast cancer by 50% [43, 44]. In a multicenter retrospective study of 551 women with BRCA1 or BRCA2 mutations, 259 women had accepted prophylactic oophorectomy and 292 had not. After a mean follow-up of 8.8 years, 6 women (2.3%) among those who accepted the surgery received a diagnosis of stage I ovarian cancer, while 58 women (19.9%) in the control group were diagnosed with ovarian cancer. In a subgroup of 241 women with no history of breast cancer or prophylactic mastectomy, the incidence of breast cancer was reduced from 42.3% (60 out of 142 women who did not accept prophylactic surgery) to 21.2% (21 out of 99 women who had accepted bilateral oophorectomy). Similarly, Kauff et al. conducted a study in 170 BRCA mutation carriers identified between 1995 and 2001 [45]. During a mean follow-up of 24.2 months, 3 of the 98 (3.1%) women who chose salpingo-oophorectomy developed breast cancer, compared to 8 of the 72 (11.1%) women who did not choose the surgery. These studies indicated that bilateral oophorectomy reduced the risk of breast cancer by ~50% in BRCA mutation carriers. In addition, most hereditary ovarian cancers occur at the age around 50 years in BRCA1 carriers [46]. Therefore, prophylactic oophorectomy is recommended for older women who complete childbearing. This is supported by Deborah Schrag et al. who have shown that oophorectomy may be delayed by 10 years in 30-year-old BRCA carriers with little loss of life expectancy [47]. Although prophylactic surgeries are highly effective to prevent breast cancer, the invasive nature has limited their extensive clinical usage as a prevention approach.

Chemoprevention

Given the modest effect of lifestyle adjustments and high invasive nature of prophylactic surgeries, recent breast cancer prevention studies have focused heavily on chemoprevention. Chemoprevention was first defined by Michael Sporn as "prevention of cancer by the use of pharmacological agents (natural or synthetic) to inhibit or reverse the process of carcinogenesis" [48]. By nature, any biologically active agent is likely to have some adverse effects especially with long-term use. Chemopreventive agents are given to healthy women who have much lower tolerance to toxicity than cancer patients. Therefore, the decision to consider chemoprevention of breast cancer will require careful balancing of its benefits and harms for each woman. Clearly, individual risk of breast cancer will be the primary factor for the physician to select the right women who will be benefited from chemoprevention.

Breast Cancer Risk Assessment Tools

The assessment of women's risk for breast cancer challenges all physicians. To quantify the individual risk of breast cancer, a number of statistical models have been developed. The most commonly used risk assessment models are Gail model and Claus model.

Gail model was developed by Mitchell Gail in 1989, who used data from 284,780 predominately white women in the Breast Cancer Detection and Demonstration Project (BCDDP) [49]. The model estimated the overall risk of breast cancer based on six risk factors: age (valid for women aged 35 years and above), age at first menstrual period, age of first live birth, number of first-degree relatives with breast cancer, number of previous breast biopsies, and breast pathology exhibiting atypical hyperplasia. The validity of Gail model was first verified by the Texas Breast Screening Project [50], in which Gail model performed well. In another validation study of the Gail model using data from the Nurses Health Study (NHS), the model did well in predicting breast cancer risk, but had only 58% discriminatory power [51]. This means that a woman chosen randomly from the cohort of breast cancer patients has only a 58% chance to have a higher Gail index than a woman who remained disease free. The 58% of power is only slightly better than guess, which gives 50%. Therefore, Gail model is good to predict the number of breast cancers in a large group of women, but cannot predict which specific women will get breast cancer with significant accuracy. In spite of that, Gail model is still the clinical standard for breast cancer risk assessment in the prevention setting. It was the main eligibility criteria for enrolling women in the NSABP P1 trial, which demonstrated the chemopreventive effect of tamoxifen. The Breast Cancer Risk Assessment Tool, which is based on the Gail index, is available online through the website of National Cancer Institute (http://www.nci.nih.gov/bcrisktool). It is widely used for counseling and determining eligibility for breast cancer prevention trials. However, the NCI Breast Cancer Risk Assessment Tool is not designed for African American women. To more accurately predict risk in African American women, data from the Women's Contraceptive and Reproductive Experiences (CARE) study and the Surveillance Epidemiology and End Results (SEER) program were used to develop a modified model called CARE model [52]. The CARE model was validated with data from the Women's Health Initiative. It gives more accurate risk projection of breast cancer for African American women than the currently available NCI Breast Cancer Risk Assessment Tool.

A major limitation of Gail model is the negligence of family histories, which are significant in predicting breast cancer risk. In contrast, the other commonly used model, Claus model, is based entirely on family history [53]. Claus model was derived from the Cancer and Steroid Hormone (CASH) case–control study which includes 4,730 breast cancer patients and 4,688 matched controls. This model is based on the premise that breast cancer is transmitted as an autosomal dominant trait from either maternal or paternal inheritance. Both first-degree and second-degree relatives as well as the ages of breast cancer onset were taken into account. Risk can be estimated as lifetime likelihood of developing breast cancer or the probability of developing breast cancer during a 10-year interval.

Besides Gail and Claus models, there are several models that can predict the probability of BRCA mutations, which imply an extremely high risk of developing breast cancer and ovarian cancer. They are most useful for women who have both breast and ovarian cancers in their family members. These models include the Couch [54], Frank [55], and BRCAPRO models [56]. The Couch model was one of the earliest models that attempted to assess the risk of BRCA1 mutation. The Frank model calculated the risk of mutations of both BRCA1 and BRCA2 genes. Both models only assess the risk of BRCA mutations, but not the risk of developing breast cancer. The BRCAPRO model will calculate the probabilities of either carrying a BRCA mutation or of developing breast and ovarian cancers at a given age.

Recently, Tyrer and Cuzick have developed a Tyrer–Cuzick model which calculates the mutation probability of BRCA genes and a low-penetrance gene and then refines the maximum likelihood calculation by incorporating personal risk factors such as age at menopause and menarche, weight, height, age, use of hormonal replacement therapy, and previous benign breast biopsies [57]. It is being used as a risk assessment tool in the current International Breast Cancer Intervention Study (IBIS)-2 prevention trial. Although the Tyrer–Cuzick model has combined both Gail and Claus models, it is still far less satisfactory to many physicians. More recently, a group of investigators interested in breast cancer prevention met in St. Gallen, Switzerland, to form an ongoing group called the

Breast Cancer Prevention Collaborative Group (BCPCG) [58]. The BCPCG critically analyzed and selected additional risk factors that could be further examined by multivariate analysis in future studies. These risk factors include mammographic density, plasma hormone levels, bone density and fracture history, history of weight gain, age of menopause, body mass index (BMI), and waist–hip ratio. The BCPCG believed that incorporation of additional risk factors could improve existing models and will ultimately lead to a more favorable risk/benefit ratio in future breast cancer prevention studies.

Quantitative risk assessment models are extensively used in the clinics to assess the risk of women to develop breast cancer. But these models are not standard for the clinicians to decide whether to initiate chemoprevention. Histological identification of atypia, a premalignant mammary lesion, confers a 2- to 10-fold increased risk of developing breast cancer in a number of clinical studies [59–63]. Moreover, women with atypical ductal hyperplasia had a better response to tamoxifen in the NSABP P1 trial [64], in which a 86% risk reduction was observed, suggesting that atypia can predict either increased risk of breast cancer or the increased benefits from tamoxifen treatment. Methods used clinically to identify atypia changes include surgical biopsy, nipple aspirate fluid (NAF), random fine-needle aspiration (rFNA), and ductal lavage (DL). Surgical biopsy is more accurate to find atypia lesions, but is more invasive and often used in women with mammographic abnormality. Atypia found in NAF represents an ~2-fold increase in the risk of breast cancer [60]. However, NAF cannot be obtained from every woman and only very limited amount of cells can be collected for cytological examination. Ductal lavage, a safe and minimally invasive technique, yields more mammary epithelial cells than NAF, but fewer cells than rFNA [65]. Compared to NAF, ductal lavage demonstrated a 3-fold sensitivity in the detection of atypia [65]. Fabian et al. [63] have found that atypia found on rFNA carries a 5-fold increased risk of breast cancer. Both rFNA and ductal lavage were cost-effective in high-risk women for breast cancer preventive interventions [66]. These histological examinations provide invaluable tools for the clinicians in screening high-risk women who could benefit from chemoprevention.

Chemoprevention Using Hormonal Intervention

The fundamental concern to develop chemopreventive agents is to understand the carcinogenesis process to identify the most relevant target. Estrogen is known to play a critical role in the development and growth of breast cancer. The accumulating understanding of estrogen signaling and the identification of estrogen receptors ultimately led to the design of drugs targeting ERs [67]. Selective estrogen receptor modulators (SERMs) represent the major group of compounds that block ER signaling. Unlike estrogens, which are uniformly agonists toward ERs, the SERMs exert selective agonist or antagonist effects on

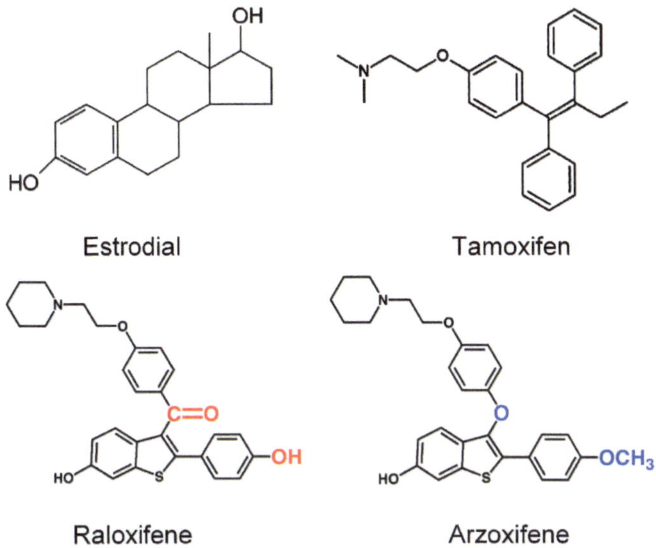

Fig. 2 Chemical structures of estrogen and SERMs

ERs depending on the target tissues [68]. Compared to the structure of natural estrogen 17β-estradiol, SERMs lack the steroid structure of estrogen, but possess a tertiary structure that allows them to bind to ER (Fig. 2). The selective activity of SERMs is due to a distinct conformational change of the SERM–ER complex and/or differential recruitment of transcriptional co-regulators, which result in activation, repression, or silencing of transcription of ER-target genes in specific tissues [69]. Currently, there are several SERMs that have been approved for clinical use or are under development (Fig. 2). Among them, tamoxifen is the prototypical SERM for breast cancer treatment and prevention.

Tamoxifen: National Surgical Adjuvant Breast and Bowel Project P-1 Trial

Tamoxifen is the first antiestrogenic agent that was approved for the treatment of breast cancer [70]. It has estrogen antagonist effect to breast, but remains as an estrogen agonist at bone and uterus (Fig. 3). In several adjuvant studies, tamoxifen was found to reduce the incidence of contralateral breast cancer by nearly 50% as a secondary endpoint [71–73]. These observations implicated that giving tamoxifen to healthy high-risk women would produce equivalent results, and ultimately led to a series of cancer prevention trials including four major trials outlined in Fig. 4.

The largest tamoxifen prevention trial is the National Surgical Adjuvant Breast and Bowel Project (NSABP) P-1 trial. From 1992 to 1997, 13,388 women with high risk of breast cancer were recruited and randomly assigned to receive

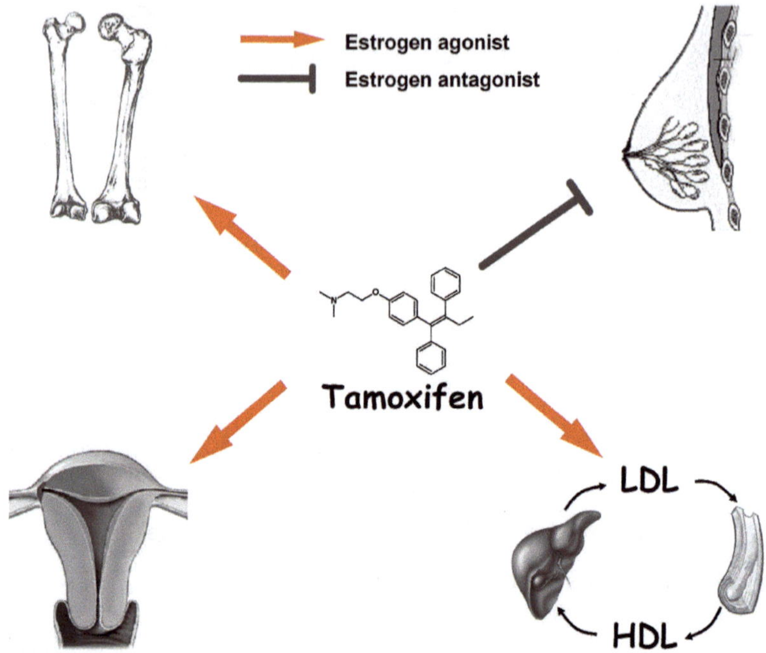

Fig. 3 Tissue-specific activity of tamoxifen

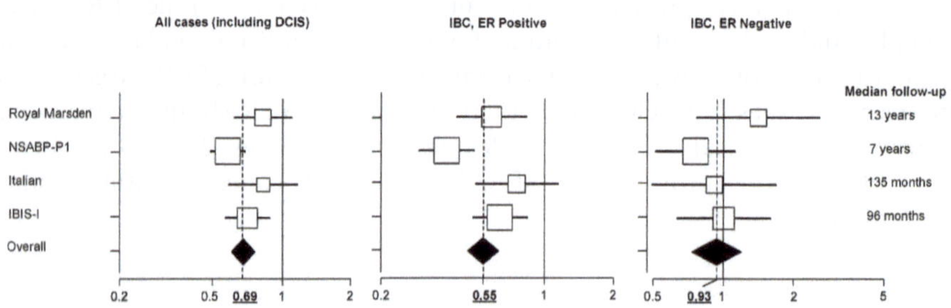

Fig. 4 Meta-analysis of four tamoxifen prevention trials. All data were obtained from published reports. The graphs were plotted using the Comprehensive Meta Analysis (Version 2) software

either placebo or tamoxifen (20 mg/day) for 5 years. The initial report showed that tamoxifen reduced the risk of invasive breast cancer by 49% after an average of 47.7 months of follow-up [64]. Recent updated data result in a 43% risk reduction of invasive breast cancer after an average of 74 months of follow-up [74]. The cumulative rate of invasive breast cancer was reduced from 42.5 per 1,000 women in the placebo group to 24.8 per 1,000 women in the tamoxifen group (risk ratio: 0.57, 95% CI = 0.46–0.70). Tamoxifen substantially reduced the risk of invasive breast cancer every year after 7 years of follow-up, suggesting that the preventive effect persists even many years after completing tamoxifen intake. Risk was reduced in all subgroups with different ages, history of preinvasive breast cancer, and levels of predicted risk of breast cancer. The risk was reduced by 36% in women aged 49 years or younger, 43% in those aged 50–59 years, and 51% in those aged 60 years or older. This suggested that tamoxifen is effective in both premenopausal and postmenopausal women. When estrogen receptor status was considered, tamoxifen only reduced the risk of ER-positive breast cancer (Fig. 4). ER-positive breast cancer was reduced by 62% (4.58 per 1,000 vs 1.74 per 1,000). However, there was no statistical difference in the rates of ER-negative breast cancer between these two groups (1.06 per 1,000 vs 1.39 per 1,000).

Another benefit from tamoxifen treatment is the beneficial effect on bones. In the P1 trial, women who received tamoxifen had reduced bone fractures from hip, spine, and radius. There was a 32% reduction in hip fractures, 31% reduction in Colles' fractures (distal radius fracture), and 25% reduction in spine fracture. Since tamoxifen has estrogen agonist effect on the uterus, long-term use of this agent confers increased risk of developing endometrial cancer. Based on the observation through 7 years of follow-up, tamoxifen increased risk of invasive endometrial cancer by 3.28-fold, from 4.68 per 1,000 women in the placebo group to 15.64 per 1,000 women in the tamoxifen group [74]. This increased risk is only observed in women aged 50 years or older and not in younger women aged below 50 years. Most endometrial cancers were at International Federation of Gynecology and Obstetrics (FIGO) stage I. Another major side effect of tamoxifen is thromboembolic events including stroke, pulmonary embolism, and deep-vein thrombosis. Although tamoxifen increased the incidence of stroke (RR: 1.42, 95% CI = 0.97–2.08) and deep-vein thrombosis (RR: 1.44, 95% CI = 0.91–2.30), the increases were not statistically significant. The incidence of pulmonary embolism was statistically increased by tamoxifen (RR: 2.16, 95% CI = 1.08–4.51).

While endometrial cancer and thromboembolic events are the two most severe adverse effects of tamoxifen, they are not the major complaints from the women who received tamoxifen due to their very low incidence rate. The only difference noted between women who took tamoxifen and placebo is related to hot flush and vaginal discharge. Hot flushes occurred in 45.7% of women who received tamoxifen and 28.7% of women in the placebo group. Vaginal discharge was reported in 29.0% of women in the tamoxifen group, as compared with 13.0% in the placebo group. About 8% more women in the tamoxifen group than the placebo group reported that their hot flushes were extremely bothersome, and 2% complained about the vaginal discharge in the same manner. Because of the promising data from NSABP P1 trial, the US Food and Drug Administration (FDA) has approved the clinical usage of tamoxifen to prevent breast cancer in high-risk women.

Other Tamoxifen Prevention Trials

Before the P1 trial was started, a pilot prevention trial was initiated at the Royal Marsden Hospital, London, UK, in 1986 [75]. This trial recruited 2,494 healthy women at an increased risk of breast cancer based on family history. The first efficacy analysis published in 1998 reported no reduction in breast cancer incidence when the tamoxifen arm was compared with the placebo arm (tamoxifen, 34; placebo, 36; RR = 1.06). However, in 2007, a 20-year follow-up (median follow-up = 13 years) report showed that the risk of ER-positive breast cancer was not statistically significantly lower in the tamoxifen arm than in the placebo arm during the 8-year treatment period (tamoxifen, 30; placebo, 39; HR = 0.77), but was statistically significantly lower in the posttreatment period (tamoxifen, 23; placebo, 47; HR = 0.48) [76]. Thus, these results of Royal Marsden trial indicate the long-term breast cancer prevention of ER-negative breast cancer by tamoxifen.

In 1992, The Italian Tamoxifen Study Group initiated a double-blinded randomized trial in women who had no breast cancer and had undergone hysterectomy due to the potential adverse effect of endometrial cancer [77–79]. Between 1992 and 1997, a total of 5,408 women were randomized to take either placebo or tamoxifen (20 mg/day). After a median follow-up of 81.2 months, 79 women had developed breast cancer in which 34 occurred in the tamoxifen arm and 45 in the placebo arm. There was no statistical difference between the two groups. However, tamoxifen significantly reduced the risk of breast cancer in the subgroup of women who also received hormone replacement therapy (17 of 791 in the placebo arm vs 6 of 793 in the tamoxifen arm). In the additional subgroup of women at high risk of ER-positive breast cancer, tamoxifen significantly reduced the incidence of breast cancer by 82% (HR: 0.108, 95% CI = 0.05–0.62). Recently, an updated report after 11 years of follow-up showed similar results, in which tamoxifen only significantly reduced the incidence of breast cancer among women with high risk of developing hormone receptor-positive tumors [80].

Guided by the pilot study of Royal Marsden Hospital trial, the United Kingdom Coordinating Committee for Cancer Research (UKCCCR) at the Royal Marsden Hospital launched the International Breast Cancer Intervention Study (IBIS)-1 trial in UK, Australia, New Zealand, and some European countries [81, 82]. The IBIS-1 trial lasted 5 years and enrolled 7,154 women with high risk of breast cancer. The largest risk group was women who had two or more first-degree or second-degree relatives with breast cancer (62%). Women were randomized to receive either tamoxifen (n = 3,579) or placebo (n = 3,575). A total of 337 breast cancers (invasive and DCIS combined) have been recorded after a median follow-up of 95.6 months. Among them, 195 were from the placebo group and 142 were from the tamoxifen group. The reduction rate was 27% (95% CI = 0.58–0.91). Tamoxifen reduced the risk of both invasive breast cancer (168 vs 124; reduction 26%) and non-invasive breast cancer (27 vs 17; reduction 37%). When ER status was considered in invasive breast cancer, tamoxifen reduced the development of ER-positive breast cancer by 34%, but had no effect in reducing the risk of ER-negative breast cancer. The frequency of endometrial cancer was increased by 1.55-fold (tamoxifen group 17, placebo group 11). Most of the endometrial cancers occurred in women older than 50 years. Venous thromboembolic events were increased by 1.72-fold (95% CI = 1.27–2.36) by tamoxifen. Other side effects that were significantly increased by tamoxifen treatment were vasomotor and gynecological complaints, which include hot flash, vaginal discharge, and abnormal vaginal bleeding. However, these toxicities were observed only in the active treatment phase and not in the subsequent period.

A meta-analysis of the four tamoxifen prevention trials was recently reported [83]. The overall reduction rate of breast cancer by tamoxifen was 38% (95% CI = 0.28–0.46, $p<0.001$). There was no difference in reduction rate between women aged under or over 50 years. Tamoxifen reduced the risk of ER-positive breast cancer by 48%, but had no effect in reducing the risk of ER-negative breast cancer. We performed another meta-analysis based on updated data from these trials (Fig. 4). This analysis shows that tamoxifen still reduced the risk of ER-positive breast cancer by 45% even many years after completing tamoxifen intake. As seen in the previous meta-analysis, the incidence of ER-negative breast cancer was not significantly changed by tamoxifen. Recently, Decansi et al. have found that a reduced dose of tamoxifen ($\leq$ 5 mg/day) can still modulate favorably breast tissue biomarkers in hormone replacement therapy users without increasing endometrial proliferation and menopausal symptoms [84]. These results suggest that it may be possible that low doses of tamoxifen will prevent breast cancer with reduced toxicity.

Raloxifene

Although tamoxifen effectively reduces the risk of ER-positive breast cancer, its tumor-promoting effect on the uterus limits its uses. Raloxifene (Evista) is another SERM that has estrogen agonist effects on bone, but has estrogen antagonist effect on breast and uterus [85]. This agent does not induce endometrial cancer, but retains the favorable activities of tamoxifen on bone [86]. Based on several trials showing that raloxifene prevents bone fractures, this agent was approved for the prevention and treatment of postmenopausal osteoporosis [87]. In the Multiple Outcomes of Raloxifene Evaluation (MORE) trial which aimed to evaluate the effect of raloxifene on bone mineral density and vertebra fracture incidence in postmenopausal women with osteoporosis, the frequency of breast cancer was investigated as a secondary endpoint [88, 89]. The MORE trial had enrolled 7,705 postmenopausal women who were diagnosed with osteoporosis from 1994 to 1998. Women were randomly assigned to receive placebo (n = 2,576), raloxifene 60 mg/day (n = 2,557), or raloxifene 120 mg/day (n = 2,572). After 4 years of follow-up, 77 breast cancers were diagnosed, in which 44 cases occurred in the placebo group, as compared with 33 cases in the two raloxifene groups. The reduction rate was 62%

(raloxifene vs placebo, RR: 0.38, 95% CI = 0.24–0.58). Among the participants who were diagnosed with invasive breast cancer (62), raloxifene reduced the risk by 72% (RR: 0.28, 95% CI = 0.17–0.46). When ER status was considered, raloxifene significantly decreased the incidence of ER-positive breast cancer by 84%, but had no effect to reduce the incidence of ER-negative breast cancer.

As expected, raloxifene significantly reduced vertebral fracture in both 60 mg/day and 120 mg/day groups. Bone mineral density was also increased by 2.1% (60 mg) and 2.4% (120 mg) in the femoral neck and by 2.6% (60 mg) and 2.7% (120 mg) in the spine ($p<0.001$ for all comparisons). The incidence of endometrial cancer had no significant difference among the three groups, but raloxifene significantly increased the risk of venous thromboembolism (RR: 3.1, 95% CI = 1.5–6.2) [88].

The Continuing Outcomes Relevant to Evista (CORE) trial investigated the effect of raloxifene for an additional 4 years on the incidence of invasive breast cancer in women who had participated in the MORE trial [90]. A total of 3,510 women who received raloxifene (either 60 or 120 mg/day) were assigned to continually receive 60 mg/day of raloxifene, and 1,703 of women in the placebo group in MORE trial remained in the placebo group. After 4 years of follow-up, raloxifene reduced the incidence of invasive breast cancer and ER-positive invasive breast cancer by 59% (RR: 0.41, 95% CI = 0.24–0.71) and 66% (RR: 0.34, 95% CI = 0.18–0.66), respectively. Over the 8 years of both trials, the incidence of invasive breast cancer and ER-positive invasive breast cancer was reduced by 66% (RR: 0.34, 95% CI = 0.22–0.50) and 76% (RR: 0.24, 95% CI = 0.15–0.4), respectively.

Both MORE and CORE trials demonstrated that raloxifene is an effective agent to prevent the development of breast cancer in older women with osteoporosis. To directly compare the effectiveness and toxicity profile of raloxifene and tamoxifen, the NSABP launched the Study of Tamoxifen and Raloxifene (STAR) trial [91]. From 1999 to 2005, the STAR trial had recruited 19,747 postmenopausal women who had high risk of breast cancer based on Gail model [49]. Women were randomly assigned to receive either 20 mg/day of tamoxifen or 60 mg/day of raloxifene for a maximum of 5 years. After a mean follow-up of 3.9 years, 4.3 per 1,000 of women in the tamoxifen group developed invasive breast cancer, as compared with 4.41 per 1,000 in the raloxifene group. The preventive effects of these two agents were equivalent. In contrast, there were fewer non-invasive breast cancers in the tamoxifen group (1.51 per 1,000) than in the raloxifene group (2.11 per 1,000; RR: 1.4, 95% CI = 0.98–2.00), although this did not reach statistical significance. As expected, fewer endometrial cancers occurred in the raloxifene group (23 cases vs 36 cases, RR: 0.62, 95% CI = 0.35–1.08), although the difference lacked statistical significance. There was a statistically significant difference between the treatment groups in the incidence of uterine hyperplasia (RR: 0.16, 95% CI = 0.09–0.29), indicating that raloxifene has less effect on uterus than tamoxifen. Overall, raloxifene had a more favorable side effect profile. Women who received raloxifene had less pulmonary emboli and deep venous thromboembolic events than those assigned to tamoxifen. There were fewer complaints of hot flashes and vaginal discharges in women taking raloxifene as compared to those taking tamoxifen. The incidence of cataracts was also less in women taking raloxifene. The risk of other cancers, fractures, ischemic heart disease, and stroke was similar for both agents. There was no difference in the total number of death or in causes of death.

Thus, the results of STAR trial demonstrated that raloxifene had equivalent preventive effect against breast cancer and had less-toxic side effects than those of tamoxifen. However, these results are only relevant to postmenopausal women. Raloxifene has not been tested in premenopausal women and is not approved in this population. Given the strong evidence from the STAR trial, the FDA approved raloxifene for breast cancer risk reduction in postmenopausal women who have osteoporosis or who have a high risk for invasive breast cancer. Thus, two agents (raloxifene and tamoxifen) are available for breast cancer prevention for postmenopausal women.

Other SERMs

The selective effects of SERMs on different tissues have made it possible to develop new SERMs with more favorable selective modulating activity, such as agents with more potent estrogen antagonist effects in the breast, estrogen agonist effects on the bone and on lipid metabolism, and no effect on the uterus. Arzoxifene is a raloxifene derivative that has antiestrogenic effects in breast and uterus while estrogenic effects on bone and lipid metabolism [92]. In structure (Fig. 2), the carbonyl group in raloxifene has been replaced by an ether linkage in arzoxifene, which makes arzoxifene to have higher affinity to the estrogen receptor. The methylated phenolic hydroxyl group gives arzoxifene potent pharmacokinetic activity. It was found to be more potent than raloxifene as an estrogen antagonist on uterus and as an estrogen agonist on bone and lipid metabolism [93]. Therefore, arzoxifene represents a promising SERM for preventing osteoporosis and breast cancer. A phase II clinical trial showed that 20 mg/day of arzoxifene was well tolerated, and was effective for treatment of patients with tamoxifen-sensitive and tamoxifen-resistant breast cancer [94]. Fabian et al. performed two phase I clinical trials to evaluate arzoxifene in women with newly diagnosed DCIS or T1/T2 invasive breast cancer [95]. Both trials demonstrated that arzoxifene decreased in serum insulin-like growth factor I (IGF-I) and serum IGF-I:IGF-binding protein-3 ratio. These data are important because high levels of circulating IGF-I and low levels of IGF-binding protein-3 are clinically associated with increased risk of breast cancer [96, 97]. In addition, a decrease in ER expression was observed with arzoxifene compared with placebo. Given the favorable side effect profile and these biomarker modulations, arzoxifene is a promising agent for breast cancer prevention.

Other SERMs that have favorable selective estrogen modulator profile include lasofoxifene [98], acolbifene [99], and bazedoxifene [100]. All of these novel SERMs have estrogenic effect on bone, antiestrogenic effect on breast, and no undesirable uterotrophic effects of tamoxifen. The ultimate clinical effect and application of these new agents will depend on future clinical trials.

Aromatase Inhibitors

SERMs prevent the development of breast cancer primarily through their estrogen antagonist effect on breast tissue. Aromatase inhibitors (AIs) offer an alternative approach to antagonize the estrogen signaling pathway [101]. Unlike SERMs, AIs work by depleting the availability of estrogen. The estrogen production is determined by the enzyme aromatase and its substrates: testosterone and androstenedione. AIs inhibit the activity of aromatase, a rate-limiting enzyme catalyzing the last step in estrogen synthesis: conversion of androgen to estrogen (Fig. 5) [102]. AIs are effective in reducing circulating estrogen levels in postmenopausal women. However, the premenopausal ovary is relatively resistant to AIs [103]. This is because the ovaries produce large amounts of androstenedione. The feedback increase of LH and FSH hormones when estrogen is low will stimulate ovary to produce more androstenedione and aromatase, which will allow the ovary to continue producing significant amounts of estrogen even during AI treatment. Therefore, AIs are only used in postmenopausal women.

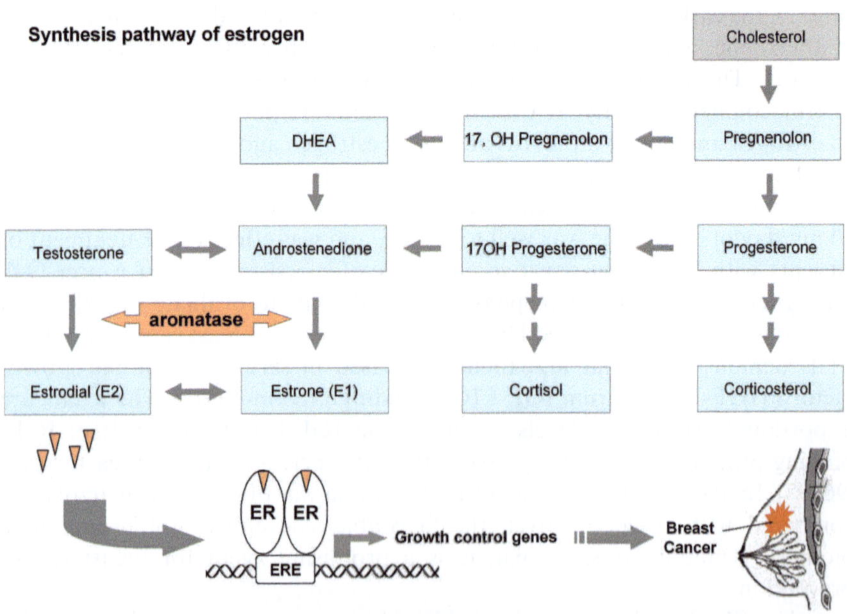

Fig. 5 Biosynthesis of estrogen and the action of aromatase

Compared to SERMs, AIs have some potential advantages. First, some toxicities of SERMs are due to their estrogen agonist effects including increased risk of endometrial cancers seen with tamoxifen and increased risk of thromboembolic events seen with both tamoxifen and raloxifene. AIs have no estrogen agonist activity, and thus do not have these side effects. Second, long-term usage of SERMs may induce drug resistance, which is a common consequence of SERM treatment [104]. Third, SERMs can have partial agonistic activity, and in some cases can stimulate breast cell growth [105]. AIs reduce estrogen levels and thus do not have many of these unfavorable effects of SERMs.

Aminoglutethimide was the first AI introduced and shown to have clinical efficacy in treating ER-positive breast cancer. However, the high toxic profiles had limited its extensive clinical application. It was not until the development of relatively non-toxic third-generation AIs that these drugs were widely used for treatment and prevention of breast cancer. Three third-generation AIs, including non-steroidal AIs, anastrozole and letrozole, and the steroidal AI, exemestane, have been extensively assessed for the treatment of breast cancer. All of these AIs were found to be superior to tamoxifen as first-line treatment for advanced breast cancer. Their chemopreventive effects, like tamoxifen, were first observed in the adjuvant studies.

Results of the Anastrozole, Tamoxifen, Alone or in Combination (ATAC) trial [106] suggests that the aromatase inhibitor anastrozole may be an effective cancer preventive agent. In this trial, 9,366 postmenopausal women with early-stage invasive breast cancer were randomly assigned to receive adjuvant therapy after surgery: anastrozole alone, tamoxifen alone, and the two in combination. Initial analyses of the ATAC trial at 33 and 47 months of median follow-up showed that anastrozole significantly prolonged time-to-recurrence and reduced the incidence of contralateral breast cancer, compared with tamoxifen [106, 107]. After a median follow-up of 68 months, anastrozole significantly prolonged time-to-recurrence (402 vs 498, HR: 0.79, 95% CI = 0.70–0.90, $p = 0.0005$) and greatly reduced contralateral breast cancers by 42% in all patients (59 vs 35, 95% CI = 0.12–0.67, $p = 0.01$) and by 53% in hormone receptor-positive patients (95% CI = 0.25–0.71, $p = 0.001$), as compared with tamoxifen [108]. Thus, while tamoxifen reduces the risk of breast cancer by 50%, the ATAC results suggest that anastrozole reduces this risk even further, possibly as much as by 70–80%.

The occurrence of side effects was similar between the tamoxifen and combination groups. However, in comparison with tamoxifen alone, anastrozole was associated with significantly fewer endometrial cancers, hot flushes, cerebrovascular events, venous thromboembolic events, and less vaginal bleeding and discharge. Not surprisingly, tamoxifen was associated with a significantly reduced rate of musculoskeletal disorders and fractures. Overall, treatment-related adverse events occurred significantly less often with anastrozole than with tamoxifen (61 vs 68%; $p < 0.0001$), as did treatment-related serious adverse events (5 vs 9%; $p < 0.0001$) and adverse events leading to withdrawal (11 vs 14%; $p = 0.0002$) [109]. Thus, in general, anastrozole was better tolerated than tamoxifen and had a more favorable overall risk–benefit profile and lower recurrence rate than tamoxifen.

Results from two additional adjuvant trials also provide evidence that AIs may prevent breast cancer. In the MA-17 trial [110, 111], a total of 5,187 postmenopausal women with breast cancer who completed 5 years of tamoxifen therapy were randomly assigned to receive 5 years more of letrozole (n = 2,593) or placebo (n = 2,594). After a median follow-up of 30 months, women taking letrozole showed a 37.5% relative reduction (HR = 0.63, 95% CI = 0.18–2.21, p = 0.12) in risk of contralateral breast cancer compared with women taking placebo. Moreover, there was a 40% reduction in risk of distant recurrence in the letrozole group as compared with the placebo group (HR = 0.60, 95% CI = 0.43–0.84, p = 0.002). The Intergroup Exemestane Study (IES) trial [112, 113] was a double-blind randomized trial to test whether exemestane was more effective than tamoxifen in breast cancer women who had already received 2–3 years of tamoxifen therapy. About 4,724 participants were randomized to receive either exemestane (n = 2,352) or tamoxifen (n = 2,372) for 5 years. After a median follow-up of 55.7 months, 809 first events (local or metastatic recurrence, contralateral breast cancer, or death) were reported in which 354 were in the exemestane group while 455 were in the tamoxifen group. Exemestane significantly reduced the risk of contralateral breast cancer by 49% (18 in exemestane group vs 35 in tamoxifen group). The results from all the three adjuvant trials suggest that AIs are effective in preventing breast cancer and that AIs have different toxicity profile than SERMs. These promising results have provided a compelling rationale for exploring the use of AIs in breast cancer prevention. A number of AI prevention trials are being conducted in high-risk women (Table 1).

The International Breast Cancer Intervention (IBIS)-2 prevention trial was initiated in 2003 to evaluate the chemopreventive effect of anastrozole in high-risk postmenopausal women [114]. The IBIS-2 trial was split into two parts: the IBIS-2 prevention trial and the IBIS-2 DCIS trial. In the IBIS-2 prevention trial, 6,000 women without breast cancer but who were at increased risk of breast cancer are to be randomized to either anastrozole or placebo for 5 years. In the IBIS-2 DCIS trial, 4,000 women who had a surgery to remove a hormone receptor-positive DCIS will be randomly assigned to receive either anastrozole or tamoxifen for 5 years. The NSABP has initiated a trial similar to the IBIS-2 DCIS trial, the B-35 trial, to compare 5 years treatment of anastrozole and tamoxifen in preventing the recurrence of breast cancer in postmenopausal women with DCIS treated by lumpectomy and radiation therapy [115]. The National Cancer Institute of Canada is also conducting the Mammary Prevention 3 (MAP3) trial to assess the preventive effects of exemestane in postmenopausal women with increased risk of breast cancer. The MAP3 trial was initially designed as a three-arm trial testing placebo, exemestane alone, and exemestane plus celecoxib in breast caner prevention [116]. However, the rare but serious toxicities caused the MAP3 trial to be modified with removal of the exemestane plus celecoxib arm. A total of 4,560 patients (2,280 per treatment arm) are to be

Table 1 Ongoing breast cancer prevention trials using AIs

Trials	Therapy	Planned accrual	1° Endpoint	Eligibility (postmenopausal women)
NSABP B-35 [115]	Anastrozole vs tamoxifen ×5 years	3,000	Ipsilateral/ contralateral breast cancer incidence	ER+/PR+DCIS
IBIS-2 (DCIS) [114]	Anastrozole vs tamoxifen ×5 years	4,000	Ipsilateral/ contralateral breast cancer incidence	ER+/PR+DCIS
IBIS-2 prevention [114]	Anastrozole vs placebo ×5 years	6,000	Breast cancer incidence	Increased risk of breast cancer
APreS [117]	Exemestane vs placebo ×5 years	666	Breast cancer incidence	BRCA 1/2 mutation carriers
NCIC-MAP3 [116]	Exemestane vs placebo ×5 years	4,560	Breast cancer incidence	≥ 35 years of age and increased risk of breast cancer

recruited to receive either exemestane or placebo for 5 years. Italian investigators have initiated the Aromasin Prevention Study (APreS) trial to evaluate the preventive effect of exemestane vs placebo in postmenopausal women who have a BRCA 1 or 2 mutation (and who have not developed breast cancer). The APreS trial accrual goal is 666 such women [117].

Because prevention trials using these third-generation AIs are not yet complete, the American Society of Clinical Oncology (ASCO) has not recommended using AIs for primary prevention of breast cancer outside of research studies.

Novel Agents for the Prevention of ER-Negative Breast Cancer

Despite the promise of SERMs and AIs for breast cancer prevention, these agents are expected to have no effect on the development of ER-negative breast cancer. Mammary tumorigenesis is a diverse and complicated process that involves aberrant regulation of multiple signaling pathways. To effectively prevent and treat breast cancer, especially ER-negative breast cancer, identification of estrogen-independent signaling pathways will be necessary. Recent

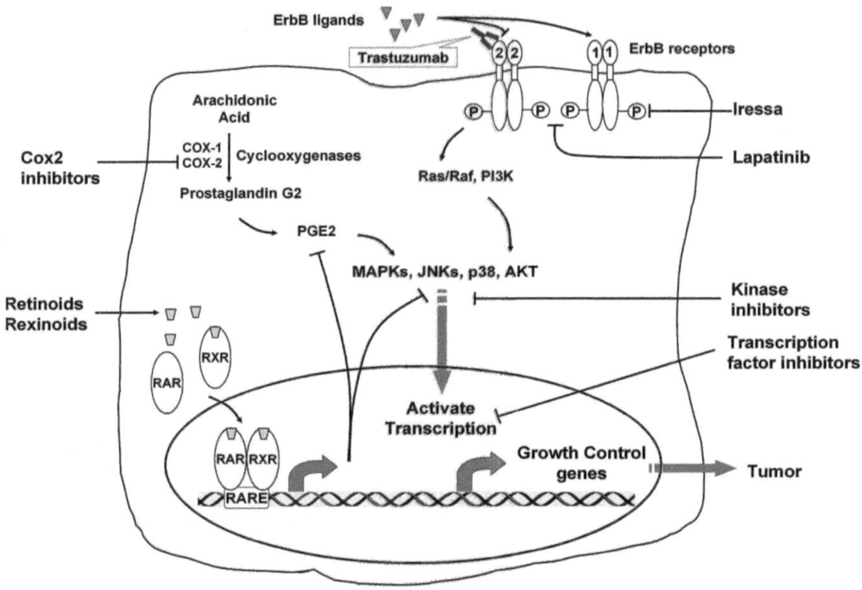

Fig. 6 Novel target for the prevention of ER-negative breast cancer. Novel agents targeting non-endocrine pathways include retinoids, COX-2 inhibitors, EFGR/tyrosine kinase inhibitors, transcription factor inhibitors, and others

research has revealed various signaling pathways that are involved in ER-negative mammary tumorigenesis. Clearly, pharmacologic interventions targeting these pathways represent promising strategies for ER-negative breast cancer prevention. Figure 6 illustrates several estrogen-independent signaling pathways that are important for breast cell growth. Novel agents targeting on these non-endocrine pathways have been shown to prevent ER-negative breast cancer in animal models. Some of these agents are currently being used to treat cancer patients and are well tolerated. Representative agents include tyrosine kinase inhibitors against erbB receptors, selective COX-2 inhibitors, and ligand of nuclear receptor families such as retinoids.

Retinoids are natural and synthetic derivatives of vitamin A (retinol) that have profound effects on development, differentiation, and cell growth [118]. Fenretinide is one of the most extensively studied retinoids due to its favorable toxicological profile in humans. A multicenter phase III chemoprevention trial of fenretinide showed that fenretinide significantly reduced the occurrences of both contralateral and ipsilateral breast cancer incidence in premenopausal women (HR: 0.66, 95% CI = 0.41–1.07 and HR: 0.65, 95% CI = 0.46–0.92, respectively) but not postmenopausal women [119, 120, 121]. We have demonstrated that RXR-selective retinoids, commonly referred as rexinoids, have potent cancer preventive activity, with less toxicity than retinoids in preclinical studies [122]. We also showed that both the rexinoids bexarotene and

LG100268 prevent ER-negative mammary tumorigenesis in multiple mouse models [123–126], suggesting the preventive potential of rexinoids on ER-negative breast cancer.

Besides nuclear receptors, peptide growth factor receptors represent a different group of signaling molecules that are critical for the growth and differentiation of both normal and malignant tissues. Our laboratory has demonstrated that gefitinib (ZD1839 or Iressa), an epidermal growth factor receptor (EGFR; also termed HER-1 or ErbB1) tyrosine kinase inhibitor, suppressed ER-negative mammary tumor formation in MMTV-ErbB2 transgenic mice [127]. In humans, however, gefitinib use is rarely associated with interstitial lung disease (overall incidence at about 1%) [128]. Concerns about this potentially serious side effect caused the FDA to halt clinical cancer preventive trials using gefitinib. We have also shown that lapatinib (GW572016), a dual kinase receptor that targets both EGFR and erbB2 receptors, significantly delays ER-negative breast cancer development in MMTV-erbB2 transgenic mice [129]. Both gefitinib and lapatinib also prevent the development of premalignant mammary lesions in these mice, suggesting that these agents inhibit mammary carcinogenesis at an early step. In addition to lapatinib, a number of novel multitarget inhibitors have been developed [130]. Selection of appropriate candidate agents for prevention studies will depend heavily on the toxicity profiles of these agents.

Accumulating epidemiology data suggest that long-term usage of aspirin or non-steroidal anti-inflammatory drug (NSAIDS) is associated with reduced risk of cancer from various tissues including breast [131, 132]. The main target of NSAID is cyclooxygenase (COX), which consists of two isoforms, COX-1 and COX-2. Aberrant expression of COX-2 is a marker of poor prognosis in human breast cancer and correlates with increased tumor size, negative ER status, HER-2 overexpression, and the presence of metastatic lesions [133–135]. Several preclinical studies have shown that celecoxib, a selective COX-2 inhibitor, reduced the incidence of both ER-positive and ER-negative breast cancers in animal models [136, 137]. Compared to NSAIDs, COX-2 inhibitors have less gastrointestinal toxicity often observed with NSAIDs (believed to occur due to COX-1 inhibition). This promoted extensive clinical testing of the chemopreventive effect of selective COX-2 inhibitors. Unfortunately, increased risk of heart attacks by COX-2 inhibitors was observed in multiple clinical trials [138]. These rare but serious side effects have reduced interest in using COX-2 inhibitors as cancer prevention agents. Researchers are searching for alternative strategies to antagonize the COX-2 pathway. Downstream activation of the COX-2 product, PGE2, is an important mediator for tumorigenesis. Blocking PGE2 activity through targeting prostanoid receptors (EP receptors) is one promising strategy to prevent cancer development [139, 140]. New agents targeting alternative COX-2 pathways are expected to retain the anticancer activity of COX-2 inhibitors, but lack the severe side effect. These new strategies will be the focus of future studies targeting COX-2 pathways.

In addition to the agents summarized above, there is a growing list of molecularly targeted agents that block critical signaling pathways in cancer cells. Promising agents include peroxisome proliferator-activated receptor (PPAR) ligands [141–146], vitamin D analogues [147–150], imatinib mesylate (gleevec) [151], demethylating agents and histone deacetylase inhibitors [152, 153], polyamine synthesis inhibitors [154, 155], metalloprotease inhibitors [156], angiogenesis inhibitors [157], and triterpenoids [158]. Most of these agents have shown anticancer activities in preclinical studies. Future clinical studies are needed to determine the efficacy of these agents in preventing ER-negative breast cancers.

Combination Chemoprevention

It is well accepted that carcinogenesis is a multistep process that involves the activation of multiple signal transduction pathways. Thus, to effectively prevent all forms of breast cancer, multiple drugs that block different pathways may be needed.

Both in vitro and in vivo experiments have shown that combinations of SERMs with retinoids or rexinoids are more effective in preventing breast cancer than the agents alone. In in vitro studies, tamoxifen and all-*trans* retinoic acid (RA) act synergistically to inhibit the growth of MCF-7 human breast cancer cells [159]. In addition to ER-positive breast cancer cells, combination of fenretinide and tamoxifen was found to synergistically inhibit the growth of ER-negative breast cancer cells [160]. In animal studies, fenretinide plus tamoxifen was more effective than either agent alone in preventing chemical-induced mammary tumors [161]. Moreover, the ability of 9cRA against chemical-induced mammary tumorigenesis was enhanced by combination with either tamoxifen or raloxifene [124].

Recently, Michael Sporn's group demonstrated that arzoxifene and the rexinoid LG100268 synergized to prevent the ER-positive breast cancer development in rat models [162–164]. The synergistic effect is primarily through inhibiting proliferation and promoting apoptosis, which result from a combined action of induction of transforming growth factor β by arzoxifene with inhibition of the NFκB and phosphatidylinositol 3$'$ kinase signaling pathways by LG100268. More recently, this group also showed that this combination prevented ER-negative breast cancer in MMTV-erbB2 mice [164]. The synergistic effect was so profound that none of the 12 mice treated with arzoxifene and LG100268 had tumor at the end of the experiment, as compared with 100% of tumor incidence in the control group. Similar preventive effect was also observed by the combination treatment of LG100268 with acolbifene, another SERM. In addition, they developed a new protocol using intermittent high dosing for short periods, followed by more prolonged drug-free rest periods. Such a protocol was highly effective for the prevention of breast cancer in rats. This is clinically important because it maximizes efficacy while minimizing undesirable chronic side effects. It would be interesting to test whether this protocol is applicable to other combination studies.

Combining chemopreventive agents that target non-endocrine signaling pathways represent a promising approach to prevent ER-negative breast cancer. Preclinical studies have found that several combinations had synergistic effect in reducing the mammary tumor growth and development. These combinations include a PPAR-gamma ligand and a retinoid or rexinoid [145, 165] and an EGFR inhibitor with a COX-2 inhibitor [166–168]. Although combination therapy has already been widely used to treat cancer patients, combination of drugs to prevent breast cancer has only recently been tested. In addition to improved effectiveness, a potential advantage of combination chemoprevention is that low doses of each individual agent might decrease the incidence of adverse effects. Such combination chemoprevention is expected to attract more attention in the near future.

Choosing the Right Women for Chemoprevention

Although tamoxifen has shown significant preventive efficacy in multiple clinical trials, most women have not accepted it due to concerns about side effects. When considering preventive therapy, the clinicians should assess the risk of breast cancer in candidates, the risk of adverse effects, and the balance between potential benefits and adverse effects (Fig. 7). Given the fact that BRCA

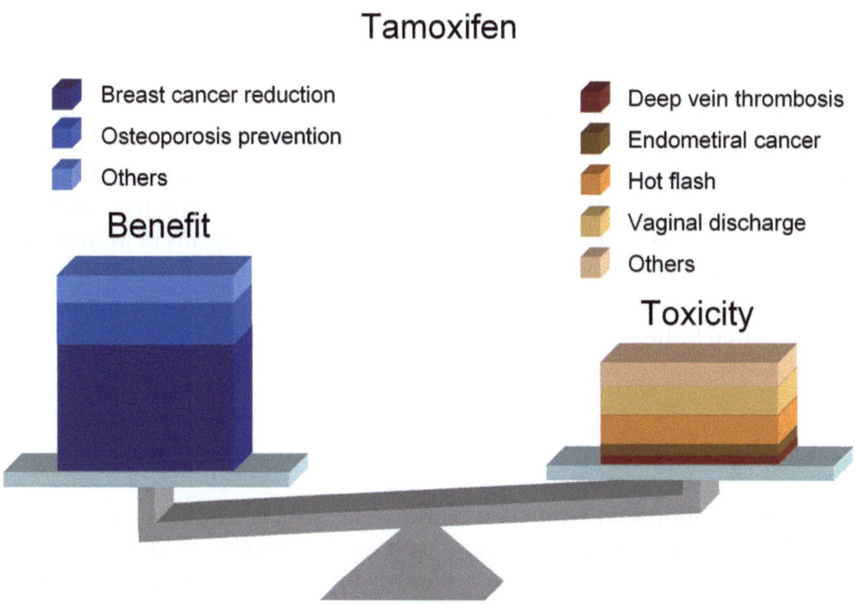

Fig. 7 Balance between benefit and toxicity

mutation carriers have a very high lifetime risk (54–85%) to develop breast cancer, prevention approaches in these patients are highly recommended. Prevention choices for women with BRCA mutations include prophylactic mastectomy, prophylactic oophorectomy, and chemoprevention.

For women who do not have the BRCA mutations, chemoprevention will be primarily used in those who have increased risk of breast cancer. Gail model provides a good assessment for the risk of breast cancer. The US Food and Drug Administration (FDA) has approved the use of tamoxifen to prevent breast cancer in women who are 35 years or older and have a 5-year risk of 1.66% or more as calculated by Gail model. This standard is similar to what has been recommended by ASCO, in which 20 mg/day of tamoxifen for 5 years is recommended to women with a 5-year projected breast cancer risk of 1.66% or higher [169]. In addition to tamoxifen, FDA has recently approved raloxifene for breast cancer risk reduction in postmenopausal women who have osteoporosis or who have high risk for invasive breast cancer.

Consistent with this, USPSTF only recommends the use of tamoxifen or raloxifene for the prevention of breast cancer in women at high risk but not at low or average risk for breast cancer. For example, USPSTF has recommended the usage of tamoxifen only in high-risk women in their 40 s and 50 s due to toxicity consideration [170]. Women younger than 40 years have a low risk of developing breast cancer and will not benefit from chemoprevention. Women older than 60 years will have a higher risk of complications, and thus have a less-favorable balance of benefit and toxicity.

Besides the risk calculated by quantitative risk assessment models, atypia identified in cytological or histological examinations presents a solid evidence of increased risk of developing breast cancer, and women who have it definitely meet the criteria for chemoprevention. Other significant risk factors for breast cancer that confer chemopreventive considerations include personal history of breast cancer or DCIS, breast irradiation prior to age 20 years, presence of LCIS, and combined estrogen–progesterone replacement therapy for more than 10 years [171]. When considering the use of chemopreventive agents in these high-risk women, physicians should avoid using the agents in women who are susceptible to its severe side effects. For example, tamoxifen should not be used in women who have a history of stroke, deep venous thrombosis, or pulmonary embolus.

Conclusions

The demonstration that tamoxifen reduces the incidence of breast cancer has made hormone preventive therapy a standard approach to prevent breast cancer. During the past 20 years, a number of preventive clinical trials have demonstrated significant breast cancer risk reduction using SERMs. However, although SERMs and AIs are promising agents to prevent ER-positive breast cancers, they do not reduce the incidence of ER-negative breast cancers. A growing number of chemopreventive agents have emerged and shown potential values in preventing ER-negative breast cancers in preclinical models. Despite the promising effect of these novel agents, issues of safety and toxicity continually hamper the progression of the field. Clinically observed toxicity has halted the development of several chemoprevention trials including those testing the COX-2 inhibitor celecoxib and the EGFR inhibitor gefitinib. Even tamoxifen or raloxifene, two well-tolerated SERMs that have been shown to be effective in preventing breast cancer, are not recommended for routine use in women at low or average risk of breast cancer due to safety reasons. Therefore, breast cancer risk assessment becomes critical to select the high-risk women who will benefit from chemoprevention. More recently, preclinical studies have shown that combination chemoprevention is a promising strategy that will greatly enhance the efficacy of cancer preventive effect. Thus, to ultimately prevent all forms of breast cancers, it will be necessary to combine both endocrine interventions as well as agents inhibiting critical estrogen-independent pathways.

References

1. Jemal A, Siegel R, Ward E, et al. Cancer statistics, 2007. CA Cancer J Clin. 2007;57(1): 43–66.
2. Ravdin PM, Cronin KA, Howlader N, et al. The decrease in breast-cancer incidence in 2003 in the United States. N Engl J Med. 2007;356(16):1670–4.
3. Beatson G. On the treatment of inoperable cases of carcinoma of the mamma: suggestions for a new method of treatment, with illustrative cases. Lancet 1896;148:101–7.
4. Parkin DM, Bray F, Ferlay J, et al. Global cancer statistics, 2002. CA Cancer J Clin. 2005;55(2):74–108.
5. Ziegler RG, Hoover RN, Pike MC, et al. Migration patterns and breast cancer risk in Asian-American women. J Natl Cancer Inst. 1993;85(22):1819–27.
6. Lambe M, Hsieh CC, Chan HW, et al. Parity, age at first and last birth, and risk of breast cancer: a population-based study in Sweden. Breast Cancer Res Treat. 1996;38(3):305–11.
7. Medina D, Smith GH. Chemical carcinogen-induced tumorigenesis in parous, involuted mouse mammary glands. J Natl Cancer Inst. 1999;91(11):967–9.
8. Rajkumar L, Guzman RC, Yang J, et al. Short-term exposure to pregnancy levels of estrogen prevents mammary carcinogenesis. Proc Natl Acad Sci U S A. 2001;98(20): 11755–9.
9. Russo IH, Koszalka M, Russo J. Comparative study of the influence of pregnancy and hormonal treatment on mammary carcinogenesis. Br J Cancer. 1991;64(3):481–4.
10. Thordarson G, Jin E, Guzman RC, et al. Refractoriness to mammary tumorigenesis in parous rats: is it caused by persistent changes in the hormonal environment or permanent biochemical alterations in the mammary epithelia? Carcinogenesis. 1995; 16(11):2847–53.
11. Sinha DK, Pazik JE, Dao TL. Prevention of mammary carcinogenesis in rats by pregnancy: effect of full-term and interrupted pregnancy. Br J Cancer. 1988;57(4):390–4.
12. Russo J, Moral R, Balogh GA, et al. The protective role of pregnancy in breast cancer. Breast Cancer Res. 2005;7(3):131–42.

13. Trichopoulos D, Lagiou P, Adami HO. Towards an integrated model for breast cancer etiology: the crucial role of the number of mammary tissue-specific stem cells. Breast Cancer Res. 2005;7(1):13–7.
14. Monninkhof EM, Elias SG, Vlems FA, et al. Physical activity and breast cancer: a systematic review. Epidemiology. 2007;18(1):137–57.
15. Lahmann PH, Friedenreich C, Schuit AJ, et al. Physical activity and breast cancer risk: the European Prospective Investigation into Cancer and Nutrition. Cancer Epidemiol Biomarkers Prev. 2007;16(1):36–42.
16. Irwin ML. Randomized controlled trials of physical activity and breast cancer prevention. Exerc Sport Sci Rev. 2006;34(4):182–93.
17. McTiernan A, Tworoger SS, Ulrich CM, et al. Effect of exercise on serum estrogens in postmenopausal women: a 12-month randomized clinical trial. Cancer Res. 2004;64(8):2923–8.
18. Armstrong B, Doll R. Environmental factors and cancer incidence and mortality in different countries, with special reference to dietary practices. Int J Cancer. 1975;15(4): 617–31.
19. Knight DC, Eden JA. A review of the clinical effects of phytoestrogens. Obstet Gynecol. 1996;87(5 Pt 2):897–904.
20. Tham DM, Gardner CD, Haskell WL. Clinical review 97: Potential health benefits of dietary phytoestrogens: a review of the clinical, epidemiological, and mechanistic evidence. J Clin Endocrinol Metab. 1998;83(7):2223–35.
21. Duffy C, Perez K, Partridge A. Implications of phytoestrogen intake for breast cancer. CA Cancer J Clin. 2007;57(5):260–77.
22. Prentice RL, Caan B, Chlebowski RT, et al. Low-fat dietary pattern and risk of invasive breast cancer: the Women's Health Initiative Randomized Controlled Dietary Modification Trial. JAMA. 2006;295(6):629–42.
23. Prentice RL, Thomson CA, Caan B, et al. Low-fat dietary pattern and cancer incidence in the Women's Health Initiative Dietary Modification Randomized Controlled Trial. J Natl Cancer Inst. 2007;99(20):1534–43.
24. Michels KB, Mohllajee AP, Roset-Bahmanyar E, et al. Diet and breast cancer: a review of the prospective observational studies. Cancer. 2007;109(12 Suppl):2712–49.
25. Smith-Warner SA, Spiegelman D, Yaun SS, et al. Alcohol and breast cancer in women: a pooled analysis of cohort studies. JAMA. 1998;279(7):535–40.
26. van den Brandt PA, Spiegelman D, Yaun SS, et al. Pooled analysis of prospective cohort studies on height, weight, and breast cancer risk. Am J Epidemiol. 2000;152(6):514–27.
27. Lynch HT, Lynch J, Conway T, et al. Hereditary breast cancer and family cancer syndromes. World J Surg. 1994;18(1):21–31.
28. Lynch HT, Snyder CL, Lynch JF, et al. Hereditary breast-ovarian cancer at the bedside: role of the medical oncologist. J Clin Oncol. 2003;21(4):740–53.
29. Wirk B. The role of ovarian ablation in the management of breast cancer. Breast J. 2005;11(6):416–24.
30. Struewing JP, Hartge P, Wacholder S, et al. The risk of cancer associated with specific mutations of BRCA1 and BRCA2 among Ashkenazi Jews. N Engl J Med. 1997;336(20):1401–8.
31. Ford D, Easton DF, Bishop DT, et al. Risks of cancer in BRCA1-mutation carriers. Breast Cancer Linkage Consortium. Lancet. 1994;343(8899):692–5.
32. King MC, Marks JH, Mandell JB. Breast and ovarian cancer risks due to inherited mutations in BRCA1 and BRCA2. Science. 2003;302(5645):643–6.
33. Rebbeck TR, Friebel T, Lynch HT, et al. Bilateral prophylactic mastectomy reduces breast cancer risk in BRCA1 and BRCA2 mutation carriers: the PROSE Study Group. J Clin Oncol. 2004;22(6):1055–62.
34. Hartmann LC, Sellers TA, Schaid DJ, et al. Efficacy of bilateral prophylactic mastectomy in BRCA1 and BRCA2 gene mutation carriers. J Natl Cancer Inst. 2001;93(21):1633–7.

35. Pennisi VR, Capozzi A. Subcutaneous mastectomy data: a final statistical analysis of 1500 patients. Aesthetic Plast Surg. 1989;13(1):15–21.
36. Meijers-Heijboer H, van Geel B, van Putten WL, et al. Breast cancer after prophylactic bilateral mastectomy in women with a BRCA1 or BRCA2 mutation. N Engl J Med. 2001;345(3):159–64.
37. Brekelmans CT, Seynaeve C, Bartels CC, et al. Effectiveness of breast cancer surveillance in BRCA1/2 gene mutation carriers and women with high familial risk. J Clin Oncol. 2001;19(4):924–30.
38. Hartmann LC, Schaid DJ, Woods JE, et al. Efficacy of bilateral prophylactic mastectomy in women with a family history of breast cancer. N Engl J Med. 1999;340(2):77–84.
39. Love RR, Philips J. Oophorectomy for breast cancer: history revisited. J Natl Cancer Inst. 2002;94(19):1433–4.
40. Scottish Cancer Trials Breast Group and ICRF Breast Unit. Adjuvant ovarian ablation versus CMF chemotherapy in premenopausal women with pathological stage II breast carcinoma: the Scottish trial. Guy's Hospital, London. Lancet. 1993; 341(8856):1293–8.
41. Love RR, Duc NB, Allred DC, et al. Oophorectomy and tamoxifen adjuvant therapy in premenopausal Vietnamese and Chinese women with operable breast cancer. J Clin Oncol. 2002;20(10):2559–66.
42. Goldhirsch A, Glick JH, Gelber RD, et al. Meeting highlights: International Consensus Panel on the Treatment of Primary Breast Cancer. Seventh International Conference on Adjuvant Therapy of Primary Breast Cancer. J Clin Oncol. 2001;19(18):3817–27.
43. Rebbeck TR, Levin AM, Eisen A, et al. Breast cancer risk after bilateral prophylactic oophorectomy in BRCA1 mutation carriers. J Natl Cancer Inst. 1999;91(17):1475–9.
44. Rebbeck TR, Lynch HT, Neuhausen SL, et al. Prophylactic oophorectomy in carriers of BRCA1 or BRCA2 mutations. N Engl J Med. 2002;346(21):1616–22.
45. Kauff ND, Satagopan JM, Robson ME, et al. Risk-reducing salpingo-oophorectomy in women with a BRCA1 or BRCA2 mutation. N Engl J Med. 2002;346(21):1609–15.
46. Frank TS, Manley SA, Olopade OI, et al. Sequence analysis of BRCA1 and BRCA2: correlation of mutations with family history and ovarian cancer risk. J Clin Oncol. 1998;16(7):2417–25.
47. Schrag D, Kuntz KM, Garber JE, et al. Decision analysis – effects of prophylactic mastectomy and oophorectomy on life expectancy among women with BRCA1 or BRCA2 mutations. N Engl J Med. 1997;336(20):1465–71.
48. Sporn MB, Dunlop NM, Newton DL, et al. Prevention of chemical carcinogenesis by vitamin A and its synthetic analogs (retinoids). Fed Proc. 1976;35(6):1332–8.
49. Gail MH, Brinton LA, Byar DP, et al. Projecting individualized probabilities of developing breast cancer for white females who are being examined annually. J Natl Cancer Inst. 1989;81(24):1879–86.
50. Bondy ML, Lustbader ED, Halabi S, et al. Validation of a breast cancer risk assessment model in women with a positive family history. J Natl Cancer Inst. 1994;86(8):620–5.
51. Rockhill B, Spiegelman D, Byrne C, et al. Validation of the Gail et al. model of breast cancer risk prediction and implications for chemoprevention. J Natl Cancer Inst. 2001;93(5):358–66.
52. Gail MH, Costantino JP, Pee D, et al. Projecting individualized absolute invasive breast cancer risk in African American women. J Natl Cancer Inst. 2007;99(23):1782–92.
53. Claus EB, Risch N, Thompson WD. Autosomal dominant inheritance of early-onset breast cancer. Implications for risk prediction. Cancer. 1994;73(3):643–51.
54. Couch FJ, DeShano ML, Blackwood MA, et al. BRCA1 mutations in women attending clinics that evaluate the risk of breast cancer. N Engl J Med. 1997;336(20):1409–15.
55. Frank TS, Deffenbaugh AM, Hulick M, et al. Hereditary susceptibility to breast cancer: significance of age of onset in family history and contribution of BRCA1 and BRCA2. Dis Markers. 1999;15 (1–3):89–92.

56. Berry DA, Iversen ES, Jr., Gudbjartsson DF, et al. BRCAPRO validation, sensitivity of genetic testing of BRCA1/BRCA2, and prevalence of other breast cancer susceptibility genes. J Clin Oncol. 2002;20(11):2701–12.
57. Tyrer J, Duffy SW, Cuzick J. A breast cancer prediction model incorporating familial and personal risk factors. Stat Med. 2004;23(7):1111–30.
58. Santen RJ, Boyd NF, Chlebowski RT, et al. Critical assessment of new risk factors for breast cancer: considerations for development of an improved risk prediction model. Endocr Relat Cancer. 2007;14(2):169–87.
59. Dupont WD, Parl FF, Hartmann WH, et al. Breast cancer risk associated with proliferative breast disease and atypical hyperplasia. Cancer. 1993;71(4):1258–65.
60. Wrensch MR, Petrakis NL, Miike R, et al. Breast cancer risk in women with abnormal cytology in nipple aspirates of breast fluid. J Natl Cancer Inst. 2001;93(23):1791–8.
61. Dupont WD, Page DL. Risk factors for breast cancer in women with proliferative breast disease. N Engl J Med. 1985;312(3):146–51.
62. Hartmann LC, Sellers TA, Frost MH, et al. Benign breast disease and the risk of breast cancer. N Engl J Med. 2005;353(3):229–37.
63. Fabian CJ, Kimler BF, Zalles CM, et al. Short-term breast cancer prediction by random periareolar fine-needle aspiration cytology and the Gail risk model. J Natl Cancer Inst. 2000;92(15):1217–27.
64. Fisher B, Costantino JP, Wickerham DL, et al. Tamoxifen for prevention of breast cancer: report of the National Surgical Adjuvant Breast and Bowel Project P-1 Study. J Natl Cancer Inst. 1998;90(18):1371–88.
65. Dooley WC, Ljung BM, Veronesi U, et al. Ductal lavage for detection of cellular atypia in women at high risk for breast cancer. J Natl Cancer Inst. 2001;93(21):1624–32.
66. Ozanne EM, Esserman LJ. Evaluation of breast cancer risk assessment techniques: a cost-effectiveness analysis. Cancer Epidemiol Biomarkers Prev. 2004;13(12):2043–52.
67. Lerner LJ, Holthaus FJ, Jr., Thompson CR. A non-steroidal estrogen antiagonist 1-(p-2-diethylaminoethoxyphenyl)-1-phenyl-2-p-methoxyphenyl ethanol. Endocrinology. 1958;63(3):295–318.
68. Riggs BL, Hartmann LC. Selective estrogen-receptor modulators – mechanisms of action and application to clinical practice. N Engl J Med. 2003;348(7):618–29.
69. Osborne CK, Zhao H, Fuqua SA. Selective estrogen receptor modulators: structure, function, and clinical use. J Clin Oncol. 2000;18(17):3172–86.
70. Honig SF. Tamoxifen for the reduction in the incidence of breast cancer in women at high risk for breast cancer. Ann N Y Acad Sci. 2001;949:345–8.
71. Fisher B, Costantino J, Redmond C, et al. A randomized clinical trial evaluating tamoxifen in the treatment of patients with node-negative breast cancer who have estrogen-receptor-positive tumors. N Engl J Med. 1989;320(8):479–84.
72. Cuzick J, Baum M. Tamoxifen and contralateral breast cancer. Lancet. 1985;2(8449):282.
73. Early Breast Cancer Trialists' Collaborative Group. Tamoxifen for early breast cancer: an overview of the randomised trials. Lancet. 1998;351(9114):1451–67.
74. Fisher B, Costantino JP, Wickerham DL, et al. Tamoxifen for the prevention of breast cancer: current status of the National Surgical Adjuvant Breast and Bowel Project P-1 study. J Natl Cancer Inst. 2005;97(22):1652–62.
75. Powles T, Eeles R, Ashley S, et al. Interim analysis of the incidence of breast cancer in the Royal Marsden Hospital tamoxifen randomised chemoprevention trial. Lancet. 1998;352(9122):98–101.
76. Powles TJ, Ashley S, Tidy A, et al. Twenty-year follow-up of the Royal Marsden randomized, double-blinded tamoxifen breast cancer prevention trial. J Natl Cancer Inst. 2007;99(4):283–90.
77. Veronesi U, Maisonneuve P, Costa A, et al. Prevention of breast cancer with tamoxifen: preliminary findings from the Italian randomised trial among hysterectomised women. Italian Tamoxifen Prevention Study. Lancet. 1998;352(9122):93–7.

78. Veronesi U, Maisonneuve P, Rotmensz N, et al. Italian randomized trial among women with hysterectomy: tamoxifen and hormone-dependent breast cancer in high-risk women. J Natl Cancer Inst. 2003;95(2):160–5.
79. Veronesi U, Maisonneuve P, Sacchini V, et al. Tamoxifen for breast cancer among hysterectomised women. Lancet. 2002;359(9312):1122–4.
80. Veronesi U, Maisonneuve P, Rotmensz N, et al. Tamoxifen for the prevention of breast cancer: late results of the Italian Randomized Tamoxifen Prevention Trial among women with hysterectomy. J Natl Cancer Inst. 2007;99(9):727–37.
81. Cuzick J, Forbes J, Edwards R, et al. First results from the International Breast Cancer Intervention Study (IBIS-I): a randomised prevention trial. Lancet. 2002;360(9336): 817–24.
82. Cuzick J, Forbes JF, Sestak I, et al. Long-term results of tamoxifen prophylaxis for breast cancer – 96-month follow-up of the randomized IBIS-I trial. J Natl Cancer Inst. 2007;99(4):272–82.
83. Cuzick J, Powles T, Veronesi U, et al. Overview of the main outcomes in breast-cancer prevention trials. Lancet. 2003;361(9354):296–300.
84. Decensi A, Gandini S, Serrano D, et al. Randomized dose-ranging trial of tamoxifen at low doses in hormone replacement therapy users. J Clin Oncol. 2007;25(27):4201–9.
85. Grese TA, Sluka JP, Bryant HU, et al. Molecular determinants of tissue selectivity in estrogen receptor modulators. Proc Natl Acad Sci U S A. 1997;94(25): 14105–10.
86. Delmas PD, Bjarnason NH, Mitlak BH, et al. Effects of raloxifene on bone mineral density, serum cholesterol concentrations, and uterine endometrium in postmenopausal women. N Engl J Med. 1997;337(23):1641–7.
87. Ettinger B, Black DM, Mitlak BH, et al. Reduction of vertebral fracture risk in post-menopausal women with osteoporosis treated with raloxifene: results from a 3-year randomized clinical trial. Multiple Outcomes of Raloxifene Evaluation (MORE) Investigators. JAMA. 1999;282(7):637–45.
88. Cummings SR, Eckert S, Krueger KA, et al. The effect of raloxifene on risk of breast cancer in postmenopausal women: results from the MORE randomized trial. Multiple Outcomes of Raloxifene Evaluation. JAMA. 1999;281(23):2189–97.
89. Cauley JA, Norton L, Lippman ME, et al. Continued breast cancer risk reduction in postmenopausal women treated with raloxifene: 4-year results from the MORE trial. Multiple outcomes of raloxifene evaluation. Breast Cancer Res Treat. 2001;65(2):125–34.
90. Martino S, Cauley JA, Barrett-Connor E, et al. Continuing outcomes relevant to Evista: breast cancer incidence in postmenopausal osteoporotic women in a randomized trial of raloxifene. J Natl Cancer Inst. 2004;96(23):1751–61.
91. Vogel VG, Costantino JP, Wickerham DL, et al. Effects of tamoxifen vs raloxifene on the risk of developing invasive breast cancer and other disease outcomes: the NSABP Study of Tamoxifen and Raloxifene (STAR) P-2 trial. JAMA. 2006;295(23):2727–41.
92. Sato M, Turner CH, Wang T, et al. LY353381.HCl: a novel raloxifene analog with improved SERM potency and efficacy in vivo. J Pharmacol Exp Ther. 1998;287(1):1–7.
93. Munster PN, Buzdar A, Dhingra K, et al. Phase I study of a third-generation selective estrogen receptor modulator, LY353381.HCL, in metastatic breast cancer. J Clin Oncol. 2001;19(7):2002–9.
94. Buzdar A, O'Shaughnessy JA, Booser DJ, et al. Phase II, randomized, double-blind study of two dose levels of arzoxifene in patients with locally advanced or metastatic breast cancer. J Clin Oncol. 2003;21(6):1007–14.
95. Fabian CJ, Kimler BF, Anderson J, et al. Breast cancer chemoprevention phase I evaluation of biomarker modulation by arzoxifene, a third generation selective estrogen receptor modulator. Clin Cancer Res. 2004;10(16):5403–17.
96. Renehan AG, Zwahlen M, Minder C, et al. Insulin-like growth factor (IGF)-I, IGF binding protein-3, and cancer risk: systematic review and meta-regression analysis. Lancet. 2004;363(9418):1346–53.

97. Pollak MN, Schernhammer ES, Hankinson SE. Insulin-like growth factors and neoplasia. Nat Rev Cancer. 2004;4(7):505–18.
98. Ke HZ, Foley GL, Simmons HA, et al. Long-term treatment of lasofoxifene preserves bone mass and bone strength and does not adversely affect the uterus in ovariectomized rats. Endocrinology. 2004;145(4):1996–2005.
99. Labrie F, Champagne P, Labrie C, et al. Activity and safety of the antiestrogen EM-800, the orally active precursor of acolbifene, in tamoxifen-resistant breast cancer. J Clin Oncol. 2004;22(5):864–71.
100. Komm BS, Kharode YP, Bodine PV, et al. Bazedoxifene acetate: a selective estrogen receptor modulator with improved selectivity. Endocrinology. 2005;146(9):3999–4008.
101. Cuzick J. Aromatase inhibitors for breast cancer prevention. J Clin Oncol. 2005;23(8):1636–43.
102. Smith IE, Dowsett M. Aromatase inhibitors in breast cancer. N Engl J Med. 2003;348(24):2431–42.
103. Santen RJ, Samojlik E, Wells SA. Resistance of the ovary to blockade of aromatization with aminoglutethimide. J Clin Endocrinol Metab. 1980;51(3):473–7.
104. Osborne CK, Fuqua SA. Mechanisms of tamoxifen resistance. Breast Cancer Res Treat. 1994;32(1):49–55.
105. Levenson AS, Jordan VC. The key to the antiestrogenic mechanism of raloxifene is amino acid 351 (aspartate) in the estrogen receptor. Cancer Res. 1998;58(9):1872–5.
106. Baum M, Budzar AU, Cuzick J, et al. Anastrozole alone or in combination with tamoxifen versus tamoxifen alone for adjuvant treatment of postmenopausal women with early breast cancer: first results of the ATAC randomised trial. Lancet. 2002;359(9324):2131–9.
107. Baum M, Buzdar A, Cuzick J, et al. Anastrozole alone or in combination with tamoxifen versus tamoxifen alone for adjuvant treatment of postmenopausal women with early-stage breast cancer: results of the ATAC (Arimidex, Tamoxifen Alone or in Combination) trial efficacy and safety update analyses. Cancer. 2003;98(9):1802–10.
108. Howell A, Cuzick J, Baum M, et al. Results of the ATAC (Arimidex, Tamoxifen, Alone or in Combination) trial after completion of 5 years' adjuvant treatment for breast cancer. Lancet. 2005;365(9453):60–2.
109. Buzdar A, Howell A, Cuzick J, et al. Comprehensive side-effect profile of anastrozole and tamoxifen as adjuvant treatment for early-stage breast cancer: long-term safety analysis of the ATAC trial. Lancet Oncol. 2006;7(8):633–43.
110. Goss PE, Ingle JN, Martino S, et al. Randomized trial of letrozole following tamoxifen as extended adjuvant therapy in receptor-positive breast cancer: updated findings from NCIC CTG MA.17. J Natl Cancer Inst. 2005;97(17):1262–71.
111. Goss PE, Ingle JN, Martino S, et al. A randomized trial of letrozole in postmenopausal women after five years of tamoxifen therapy for early-stage breast cancer. N Engl J Med. 2003;349(19):1793–802.
112. Coombes RC, Hall E, Gibson LJ, et al. A randomized trial of exemestane after two to three years of tamoxifen therapy in postmenopausal women with primary breast cancer. N Engl J Med. 2004;350(11):1081–92.
113. Coombes RC, Kilburn LS, Snowdon CF, et al. Survival and safety of exemestane versus tamoxifen after 2–3 years' tamoxifen treatment (Intergroup Exemestane Study): a randomised controlled trial. Lancet. 2007;369(9561):559–70.
114. Cuzick J. Aromatase inhibitors in prevention – data from the ATAC (arimidex, tamoxifen alone or in combination) trial and the design of IBIS-II (the second International Breast Cancer Intervention Study). Recent Results Cancer Res. 2003;163:96–103; discussion 264–6.
115. Vogel VG, Costantino JP, Wickerham DL, et al. National surgical adjuvant breast and bowel project update: prevention trials and endocrine therapy of ductal carcinoma in situ. Clin Cancer Res. 2003;9(1 Pt 2):495S–501S.

116. Richardson H, Johnston D, Pater J, et al. The National Cancer Institute of Canada Clinical Trials Group MAP.3 trial: an international breast cancer prevention trial. Curr Oncol. 2007;14(3):89–96.
117. Bevilacqua G, Silingardi V, Marchetti P. Exemestane for the prevention of breast cancer in postmenopausal unaffected carriers of BRCA1/2 mutations – Aromasin Prevention Study (Apres). In: 24th Annual San Antonio Breast Cancer Symposium; 2001; San Antonio: Breast Cancer Research and Treatment; 2001. p. S226.
118. Aranda A, Pascual A. Nuclear hormone receptors and gene expression. Physiol Rev. 2001;81(3):1269–304.
119. Veronesi U, De Palo G, Marubini E, et al. Randomized trial of fenretinide to prevent second breast malignancy in women with early breast cancer. J Natl Cancer Inst. 1999;91(21):1847–56.
120. Decensi A, Serrano D, Bonanni B, et al. Breast cancer prevention trials using retinoids. J Mammary Gland Biol Neoplasia. 2003;8(1):19–30.
121. Veronesi U, Mariani L, Decensi A, et al. Fifteen-year results of a randomized phase III trial of fenretinide to prevent second breast cancer. Ann Oncol. 2006;17(7):1065–71.
122. Wu K, Kim HT, Rodriquez JL, et al. Suppression of mammary tumorigenesis in transgenic mice by the RXR-selective retinoid, LGD1069. Cancer Epidemiol Biomarkers Prev. 2002;11(5):467–74.
123. Wu K, Kim HT, Rodriquez JL, et al. 9-cis-Retinoic acid suppresses mammary tumorigenesis in C3 (1)-simian virus 40 T antigen-transgenic mice. Clin Cancer Res. 2000;6(9):3696–704.
124. Anzano MA, Byers SW, Smith JM, et al. Prevention of breast cancer in the rat with 9-cis-retinoic acid as a single agent and in combination with tamoxifen. Cancer Res. 1994;54(17):4614–7.
125. Wu K, Zhang Y, Xu XC, et al. The retinoid X receptor-selective retinoid, LGD1069, prevents the development of estrogen receptor-negative mammary tumors in transgenic mice. Cancer Res. 2002;62(22):6376–80.
126. Li Y, Zhang Y, Hill J, et al. The Rexinoid LG100268 Prevents the Development of Preinvasive and Invasive Estrogen Receptor Negative Tumors in MMTV-erbB2 Mice. Clin Cancer Res. 2007;13(20):6224–31.
127. Lu C, Speers C, Zhang Y, et al. Effect of epidermal growth factor receptor inhibitor on development of estrogen receptor-negative mammary tumors. J Natl Cancer Inst. 2003;95(24):1825–33.
128. Nagaria NC, Cogswell J, Choe JK, et al. Side effects and good effects from new chemotherapeutic agents. Case 1. Gefitinib-induced interstitial fibrosis. J Clin Oncol. 2005;23(10):2423–4.
129. Strecker TE, Brown PH. Lapatinib, in preparation.
130. McNeil C. Two targets, one drug for new EGFR inhibitors. J Natl Cancer Inst. 2006;98(16):1102–3.
131. Khuder SA, Mutgi AB. Breast cancer and NSAID use: a meta-analysis. Br J Cancer. 2001;84(9):1188–92.
132. Johnson TW, Anderson KE, Lazovich D, et al. Association of aspirin and nonsteroidal anti-inflammatory drug use with breast cancer. Cancer Epidemiol Biomarkers Prev. 2002;11(12):1586–91.
133. Zerkowski MP, Camp RL, Burtness BA, et al. Quantitative analysis of breast cancer tissue microarrays shows high cox-2 expression is associated with poor outcome. Cancer Invest. 2007;25(1):19–26.
134. Liu CH, Chang SH, Narko K, et al. Overexpression of cyclooxygenase-2 is sufficient to induce tumorigenesis in transgenic mice. J Biol Chem. 2001;276(21):18563–9.
135. Ristimaki A, Sivula A, Lundin J, et al. Prognostic significance of elevated cyclooxygenase-2 expression in breast cancer. Cancer Res. 2002;62(3):632–5.

136. Harris RE, Alshafie GA, Abou-Issa H, et al. Chemoprevention of breast cancer in rats by celecoxib, a cyclooxygenase 2 inhibitor. Cancer Res. 2000;60(8):2101–3.
137. Howe LR, Subbaramaiah K, Patel J, et al. Celecoxib, a selective cyclooxygenase 2 inhibitor, protects against human epidermal growth factor receptor 2 (HER-2)/neu-induced breast cancer. Cancer Res. 2002;62(19):5405–7.
138. Lenzer J. FDA advisers warn: COX 2 inhibitors increase risk of heart attack and stroke. BMJ. 2005; 330(7489):440.
139. Thorat MA, Morimiya A, Mehrotra S, et al. Prostanoid receptor EP1 expression in breast cancer. Mod Pathol. 2008;21(1):15–21.
140. Ma X, Kundu N, Rifat S, et al. Prostaglandin E receptor EP4 antagonism inhibits breast cancer metastasis. Cancer Res. 2006;66(6):2923–7.
141. Elstner E, Muller C, Koshizuka K, et al. Ligands for peroxisome proliferator-activated receptorgamma and retinoic acid receptor inhibit growth and induce apoptosis of human breast cancer cells in vitro and in BNX mice. Proc Natl Acad Sci U S A. 1998;95(15):8806–11.
142. Clay CE, Namen AM, Atsumi G, et al. Influence of J series prostaglandins on apoptosis and tumorigenesis of breast cancer cells. Carcinogenesis. 1999;20(10):1905–11.
143. Suh N, Wang Y, Williams CR, et al. A new ligand for the peroxisome proliferator-activated receptor-gamma (PPAR-gamma), GW7845, inhibits rat mammary carcinogenesis. Cancer Res. 1999;59(22):5671–3.
144. Yin F, Bruemmer D, Blaschke F, et al. Signaling pathways involved in induction of GADD45 gene expression and apoptosis by troglitazone in human MCF-7 breast carcinoma cells. Oncogene. 2004;23(26):4614–23.
145. Mehta RG, Williamson E, Patel MK, et al. A ligand of peroxisome proliferator-activated receptor gamma, retinoids, and prevention of preneoplastic mammary lesions. J Natl Cancer Inst. 2000;92(5):418–23.
146. Larsson SC, Kumlin M, Ingelman-Sundberg M, et al. Dietary long-chain n-3 fatty acids for the prevention of cancer: a review of potential mechanisms. Am J Clin Nutr. 2004;79(6):935–45.
147. Mehta RG, Hussain EA, Mehta RR, et al. Chemoprevention of mammary carcinogenesis by 1alpha-hydroxyvitamin D5, a synthetic analog of Vitamin D. Mutat Res. 2003; 523–524:253–64.
148. Matsumoto H, Iino Y, Koibuchi Y, et al. Antitumor effect of 22-oxacalcitriol on estrogen receptor-negative MDA-MB-231 tumors in athymic mice. Oncol Rep. 1999;6(2):349–52.
149. Hussain EA, Mehta RR, Ray R, et al. Efficacy and mechanism of action of 1alpha-hydroxy-24-ethyl-cholecalciferol (1alpha[OH]D5) in breast cancer prevention and therapy. Recent Results Cancer Res. 2003;164:393–411.
150. Abe J, Nakano T, Nishii Y, et al. A novel vitamin D3 analog, 22-oxa-1,25-dihydroxyvitamin D3, inhibits the growth of human breast cancer in vitro and in vivo without causing hypercalcemia. Endocrinology. 1991;129(2):832–7.
151. Lev DC, Kim SJ, Onn A, et al. Inhibition of platelet-derived growth factor receptor signaling restricts the growth of human breast cancer in the bone of nude mice. Clin Cancer Res. 2005;11(1):306–14.
152. Davis T, Kennedy C, Chiew YE, et al. Histone deacetylase inhibitors decrease proliferation and modulate cell cycle gene expression in normal mammary epithelial cells. Clin Cancer Res. 2000;6(11):4334–42.
153. Margueron R, Duong V, Castet A, et al. Histone deacetylase inhibition and estrogen signalling in human breast cancer cells. Biochem Pharmacol. 2004;68(6):1239–46.
154. Davidson NE, Hahm HA, McCloskey DE, et al. Clinical aspects of cell death in breast cancer: the polyamine pathway as a new target for treatment. Endocr Relat Cancer. 1999;6(1):69–73.

155. Fabian CJ, Kimler BF, Brady DA, et al. A phase II breast cancer chemoprevention trial of oral alpha-difluoromethylornithine: breast tissue, imaging, and serum and urine biomarkers. Clin Cancer Res. 2002;8(10):3105–17.
156. Winding B, NicAmhlaoibh R, Misander H, et al. Synthetic matrix metalloproteinase inhibitors inhibit growth of established breast cancer osteolytic lesions and prolong survival in mice. Clin Cancer Res. 2002;8(6):1932–9.
157. Schneider BP, Miller KD. Angiogenesis of breast cancer. J Clin Oncol. 2005;23(8):1782–90.
158. Liby KT, Yore MM, Sporn MB. Triterpenoids and rexinoids as multifunctional agents for the prevention and treatment of cancer. Nat Rev Cancer. 2007;7(5):357–69.
159. Wang Y, He QY, Chen H, et al. Synergistic effects of retinoic acid and tamoxifen on human breast cancer cells: proteomic characterization. Exp Cell Res. 2007;313(2): 357–68.
160. Aoyama Y. Experimental studies on the effects of the combined use of *N*-(4-hydroxyphenyl)retinamide (4-HPR) and tamoxifen (TAM) for estrogen receptor (ER)-negative breast cancer. Kurume Med J. 2002;49(1–2):27–33.
161. Moon RC, Kelloff GJ, Detrisac CJ, et al. Chemoprevention of MNU-induced mammary tumors in the mature rat by 4-HPR and tamoxifen. Anticancer Res. 1992;12(4): 1147–53.
162. Suh N, Lamph WW, Glasebrook AL, et al. Prevention and treatment of experimental breast cancer with the combination of a new selective estrogen receptor modulator, arzoxifene, and a new rexinoid, LG 100268. Clin Cancer Res. 2002;8(10):3270–5.
163. Rendi MH, Suh N, Lamph WW, et al. The selective estrogen receptor modulator arzoxifene and the rexinoid LG100268 cooperate to promote transforming growth factor beta-dependent apoptosis in breast cancer. Cancer Res. 2004;64(10): 3566–71.
164. Liby K, Rendi M, Suh N, et al. The combination of the rexinoid, LG100268, and a selective estrogen receptor modulator, either arzoxifene or acolbifene, synergizes in the prevention and treatment of mammary tumors in an estrogen receptor-negative model of breast cancer. Clin Cancer Res. 2006;12(19):5902–9.
165. Elstner E, Williamson EA, Zang C, et al. Novel therapeutic approach: ligands for PPARgamma and retinoid receptors induce apoptosis in bcl-2-positive human breast cancer cells. Breast Cancer Res Treat. 2002;74(2):155–65.
166. Dannenberg AJ, Lippman SM, Mann JR, et al. Cyclooxygenase-2 and epidermal growth factor receptor: pharmacologic targets for chemoprevention. J Clin Oncol. 2005;23(2):254–66.
167. Buchanan FG, Wang D, Bargiacchi F, et al. Prostaglandin E2 regulates cell migration via the intracellular activation of the epidermal growth factor receptor. J Biol Chem. 2003;278(37):35451–7.
168. Tortora G, Caputo R, Damiano V, et al. Combination of a selective cyclooxygenase-2 inhibitor with epidermal growth factor receptor tyrosine kinase inhibitor ZD1839 and protein kinase A antisense causes cooperative antitumor and antiangiogenic effect. Clin Cancer Res. 2003;9(4):1566–72.
169. Chlebowski RT, Col N, Winer EP, et al. American Society of Clinical Oncology technology assessment of pharmacologic interventions for breast cancer risk reduction including tamoxifen, raloxifene, and aromatase inhibition. J Clin Oncol. 2002;20(15):3328–43.
170. Chemoprevention of breast cancer: recommendations and rationale. Ann Intern Med. 2002;137(1):56–8.
171. Hollingsworth AB, Singletary SE, Morrow M, et al. Current comprehensive assessment and management of women at increased risk for breast cancer. Am J Surg. 2004;187(3):349–62.

Estrogen Receptor Phenotypes Defined by Gene Expression Profiling

Marleen Kok, Sabine Linn, and Marc van de Vijver

Introduction

Breast cancer is a heterogeneous disease and existing clinicopathological classifications do not fully capture the diversity in clinical disease course. Since the estrogen receptor (ER) α plays a central role in the cross-talk between different signaling pathways in breast cancer, the expression of this receptor is important for the behavior of breast cancer cells and is reflected in gene expression patterns of breast tumors.

High throughput analysis of gene expression of breast cancer has increased the insights in ER signaling, including its relation with disease outcome and therapy response.

Expression of ER and its numerous downstream targets are driving patterns of gene expression and dominate unsupervised analyses in breast cancer specimens studied to date, regardless of microarray platform or statistical approach.

This chapter reviews gene expression studies either attempting to unravel the functional effect of ER or describing the gene expression profiles driven by ER in breast tumors. In addition, the development of molecular signatures predicting response to endocrine treatment will be discussed.

Gene Expression Profiling Technology

Gene expression is a general term used to describe the transcription of information encoded within the DNA into messenger RNA (mRNA). It is assumed that for many genes there is a linear relation between the number of mRNA transcripts and functional proteins expressed in a cell. Gene expression profiling, in turn, is defined as the simultaneous measurement of the expression of a

M.van deVijver (✉)
Academic Medical Center, Amsterdam, The Netherlands
e-mail: mj.vandevijver@amc.uva.nl

S.A.W. Fuqua (ed.), *Hormone Receptors in Breast Cancer*,
Cancer Treatment and Research 312, DOI 10.1007/978-0-387-09463-2_11,

large number of genes. With gene expression profiling it has been possible to group gene transcripts of human tumors to create 'molecular signatures' that give more insight in the biology of cancer and consequently may predict clinical outcome.

Table 1 summarizes the current applications of gene expression profiling. There are three techniques commonly used for gene expression profiling in clinical specimens [1]. These include gene expression profiling using two different microarray platforms (complementary DNA (cDNA) and oligonucleotide arrays) and multiplex quantitative reverse transcriptase polymerase chain reactions (qRT-PCR).

On the cDNA microarray, double-stranded PCR products amplified from expressed sequences tag (EST) clones (length 300–1000 nucleotides) are spotted. Several ten thousands of different cDNA clones can be spotted onto the surface of a glass slide to produce a high-density cDNA array. The affixed DNA segments are known as probes. The drawback of studying gene expression using cDNA arrays is the frequent cross-hybridization amongst homologous genes, alternative splice variants and antisense RNA.

These problems have been overcome by oligonucleotide arrays, which use shorter probes of uniform length, usually 20–80 nucleotides. By constructing oligonucleotide arrays, complete control of the sequence is guaranteed, several different probes per gene can be spotted and many control spots provide information on contamination and hybridization kinetics. Currently, there are three approaches for the production of oligonucleotide arrays. First, the oligonucleotides can be synthesized, purified and then printed by a robot or inkjet process onto glass slides (Agilent). Second, microarrays can be produced by in situ synthesis of oligonucleotides directly onto a solid surface using photolithographic technology (Affymetrix). Recently, a third technology was introduced [2] based on bead-based arrays where the oligonucleotides are attached to microbeads which are then put onto microarrays (Illumina).

Finally, the third technique to measure gene expression in a high throughput fashion is real-time qRT-PCR, which is based on the quantification of mRNA after each round of amplification by PCR using a fluorescent reporter [3]. Current qRT-PCR assays can determine the expression of up to a few hundred genes simultaneously and may have an increased sensitivity compared to the array-based technology.

For the analysis and interpretation of microarray data, a range of computational tools are available. The two basic approaches are unsupervised hierarchical clustering analysis, which orders both samples and genes on the basis of their similarity of gene expression, and supervised methods, which identify gene expression patterns that discriminate samples on the basis of predefined clinical information [4, 5].

Statistical analysis of expression data is complex and prone to false discoveries, e.g., identifying genes of interest just by chance. Therefore, it is crucial to validate molecular signatures in large independent series of patients before clinical application.

Table 1 Gene expression profiling technologies

	cDNA arrays		Oligoarrays		Multiplex RT-PCR
Manufacture	Academic microarray facility, Clontech	Agilent, academic microarray facility	Affymetrix	Illumina	Taqman, Molecular Beacons, Scorpions
Probe	300–1000 nucleotide cDNA clones	60 mer oligonucleotides	20 mer oligonucleotides	50 mer oligonucleotide	~20b PCR primers
Probes per array	up to 20,000	44,000	500,000	48,000	up to 400
General information	Use is decreasing	Dual-channel system: expression values relative to reference	Single-channel system: absolute expression values	Oligo's attached to beads	Most sensitive detection of mRNA levels

Genome-Wide Analyses of Estrogen Receptor Function

Estrogens are known to regulate the proliferation of breast cancer cells and to alter phenotypical properties. However, the mechanisms and pathways by which estrogens regulate these events are only partially understood. With the sequencing of the human genome as well as the advent of microarray technology, it is now possible to investigate the complexities of ER-mediated gene transcription on a more global scale rather than studying one estrogen-responsive target at a time.

Using gene expression profiling, Frasor and colleagues identified patterns of genes that are either stimulated or inhibited by estradiol (E2) in ER-positive MCF-7 human breast cancer cells [6]. Their findings reveal that almost 70% of the genes regulated by E2 are, in fact, downregulated. In addition they show that numerous cell cycle-associated genes as well as expression of novel transcription factors, receptors and signaling pathways are modulated by E2, many of which could play roles in mediating the effects of E2 on breast cancer proliferation.

Subsequently, to better understand the actions of endocrine treatment, microarray analysis was performed after exposure of breast cancer cells to different estrogen receptor-targeted drugs [7, 8]. The gene expression changes induced as a response to selective estrogen receptor modulators (SERMs) such as tamoxifen and raloxifene or the anti-estrogen fulvestrant indicated the agonistic and/or antagonistic actions on a large set of estrogen-regulated genes. Although the regulation of the majority of E2-regulated genes is either partially or fully reversed by SERMs and fulvestrant, differences can be observed among these ligands in their balance of agonistic, partial antagonistic or fully antagonistic activities on E2-regulated genes.

In addition, in 2006 Oh and colleagues used this strategy to classify ER or progesterone receptor (PR)-positive breast carcinomas [9], applying supervised analysis (significant analysis of microarray data 'SAM,' software for expression data mining) on gene expression data of ER-positive MCF-7 cells treated with E2 [10]. Using this approach, they identified 822 genes that were shown to be estrogen regulated. These genes were used to develop an outcome predictor, which was then validated on independent published breast cancer datasets.

Translational research performed at the Netherlands Cancer Institute, the Netherlands, showed that combining *in vitro* experiments with gene expression analyses of clinical breast cancer samples can improve the understanding of ER function in cancer patients. Using fluorescence resonance energy transfer (FRET) that detects changes in the conformation of ER, the efficacy of anti-estrogens to inactivate ER was studied [11, 12]. Phosphorylation of serine 305 in the hinge region of ER by protein kinase A (PKA) induced resistance to tamoxifen. In clinical samples, the downregulation of a negative regulator of PKA, PKA-RIα, was associated with tamoxifen resistance. Activation of PKA by downregulation of PKA-RIα converted tamoxifen from an ER inhibitor into a growth stimulator.

ER-mediated transcription has been intensively studied on a small number of endogenous target promoters [13, 14]. Recently, ER-binding sites were mapped in a less-biased way that did not depend on preexisting concepts of classic promoter domains and subsequently several new features of ER-Mediated transcription were identified, such as the facilitation of ER binding to chromatin leading to gene transcription [15]. Subsequently, all ER and RNA polymerase II binding sites were mapped on a genome-wide scale in breast cancer cells stimulated by E2, identifying a broad range of *cis*-binding sites and target genes [16]. Since the *cis*-regulatory elements can be located in the promoter region 5′ to the gene it controls, as well as in the intron, or in the 3′ region, this study found a more complete set of ER-binding sites across the genome. Combining this unique resource with gene expression data from breast cancer patients, it correctly predicted that the genes co-expressed with the ER and thereby identified important and previously unexplored regions of the genome that could be the critical regulators of the estrogen dependence of breast cancer.

Gene Expression Profiles Driven by Estrogen Receptor

The first large-scale study of gene expression profiling in breast cancer was performed by Perou and colleagues who showed that based on overall gene expression profiles, breast carcinomas can be subdivided into five molecular subtypes (Fig. 1) [17]. Three biologically distinct subgroups of ER-negative breast tumors have been identified: the 'basal-like' group, which expresses cytokeratin-5 and cytokeratin-17; the 'HER2-positive' group, expressing several genes located in the HER2 amplicon including HER2 and the gene encoding for growth factor receptor-bound protein 7 (GRB7); and the 'normal-breast-like' group, which expresses genes usually expressed in normal breast. The ER-positive tumors that were originally found to be a single group have in subsequent studies been separated into at least two distinct groups: the 'luminal A' subtype, which expresses high levels of cytokeratin-8 and cytokeratin-18 and other breast luminal genes, and the 'luminal B' subtype, expressing low levels of these genes [18]. Importantly, these five subtypes also represent clinically distinct subgroups of patients. For example, the ER-negative 'basal-like' and 'HER2-positive' subtypes are associated with a shorter overall and disease-free survival, whereas the ER-positive 'luminal A' tumors have the best outcome. These findings have been confirmed in independent datasets [19, 20].

It has to be realized that classifications generated by hierarchical clustering may be unstable. For example, adding more breast cancer samples resulted in a changed dendrogram, as demonstrated by the disappearance of the luminal C subtype [19]. Furthermore, it can be argued that these analyses do not provide more information than currently given by histological grade and immunohistochemistry (IHC) for ER and HER2 of the tumor. When interpreting these

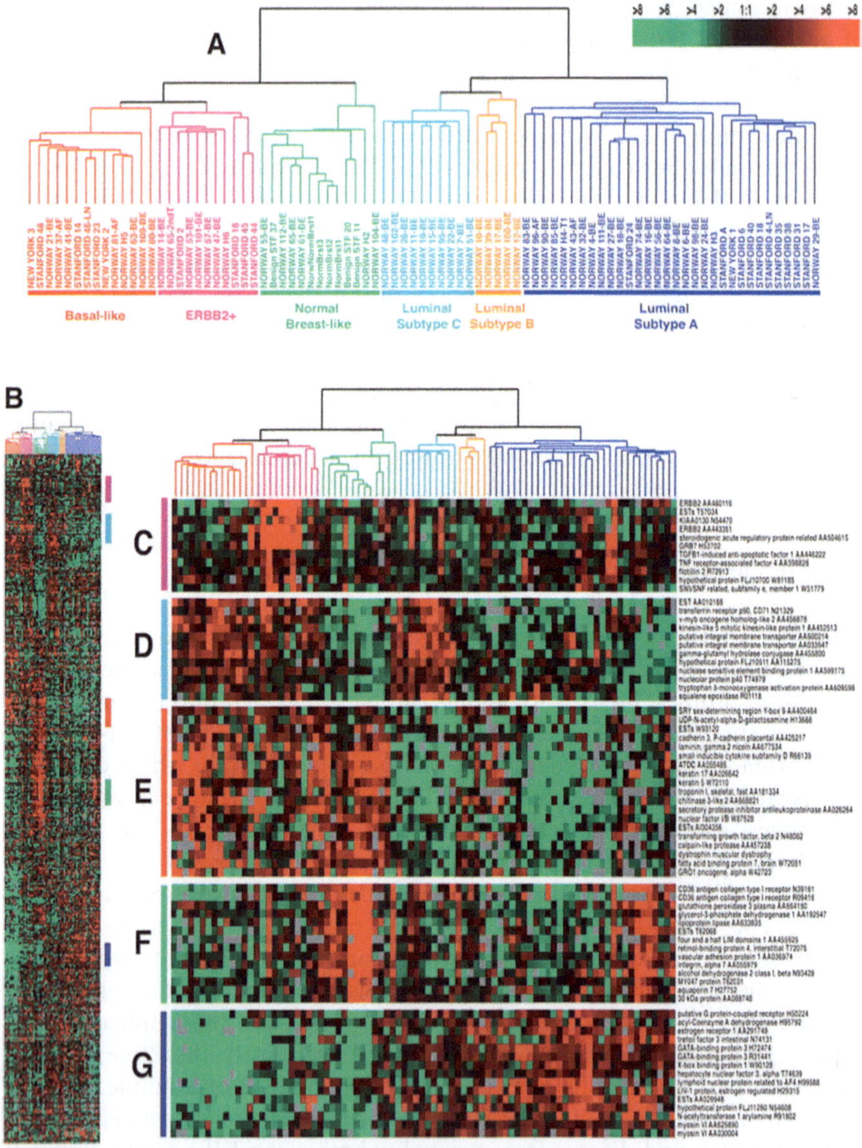

Fig. 1 Molecular subtypes of breast cancer. Gene expression patterns of 85 experimental samples representing 78 carcinomas, 3 benign tumors and 4 normal tissues analyzed by hierarchical clustering of cDNA clones. **a** Tumor specimens were divided into five (or six) subtypes based on differences in gene expression: *dark blue*: luminal A, *yellow*: luminal B, *light blue*: luminal C, *green*: normal breast like, *red*: basal like and *pink*: HER2+. **b** Full cluster diagram scaled down, colored bars on the right represent the inserts present in **c**–**g**. **c** HER2 amplicon. **d** Unknown cluster. **e** Basal epithelial cell-enriched cluster. **f** Normal breast-like cluster. **g** Luminal epithelial gene cluster containing ER. Copyright © 2001 by The National Academy of Science of the United States of America, all rights reserved [18]

observations, it is important to keep in mind that many of these correlations are expected because of the strong association between molecular class and conventional histopathological variables.

The gene expression grade index (GGI), which defines histological grade based on gene expression profiles [21], could also define two ER-positive molecular subgroups (high and low genomic grade) [22]. Despite tracking a single biological pathway, these subgroups were highly concordant with the previously described luminal A and B classifications.

Subsequent studies confirmed that there are large-scale gene expression differences between ER-positive (most 'luminal-like') and ER-negative (most 'basal-like') cancers. Table 2 summarizes different studies describing the dominant gene expression pattern in breast carcinomas driven by ER. To study the characteristics of ER-positive and ER-negative breast tumors in more detail, Gruvberger and colleagues profiled a homogeneous group of lymph node-negative breast cancers [23]. They reported that ER-positive and ER-negative tumors display remarkably different molecular phenotypes. To gain insight into the genes of this dominant expression signature, van't Veer et al. associated gene expression data with ER expression as determined by IHC [24]. Out of 39 tumors stained negative for ER by IHC, 34 clustered together. By this unsupervised approach, known ER target genes formed a cluster with the ER-α gene (ESR1). Supervised classification showed that 550 genes optimally reported the dominant pattern associated with ER status; reporter genes included cytokeratin-18, bcl-2, HER3 and HER4 (see Fig. 2). Twenty-one out of the 50 ER reporter genes as determined by Gruvberger et al. were also present in the 550 gene list [23].

Since the introduction of high throughput analysis of gene expression, several molecular signatures predicting prognosis in breast cancer patients have been developed [25–28]. All classifiers have been developed using different microarray platforms and approaches to select genes. Consequently a direct comparison between the various gene lists generated is difficult. However, these different gene sets show significant agreement in the outcome predictions for individual patients and are probably tracking a common set of biological phenotypes [20]. In addition to the degree of proliferation and histological grading, information on ER signaling is present in all prognostic signatures. Wang and colleagues included this information in the development of their prognostic test [28]. Tumors used for their discovery study were allocated to one of two subgroups stratified by ER status. Each subgroup was analyzed separately for selection of genes. Markers selected from each subgroup (60 genes for ER-positive tumors and 16 for ER-negative tumors) were combined to form a single signature to predict tumor metastasis in a subsequent independent validation consisting of both ER-positive and ER-negative tumors. This result supports the idea that the extent of heterogeneity and the underlying mechanisms for disease progression could differ for the two ER-based subgroups of breast cancer patients.

Tabel 2 Gene expression profiling to identify genes related to ER

Microarray type	Samples	ER related genes	Identified by	Prediction results	Reference
Oligonucleotide 25 k, Agilent	98 breast tumors	550	Unsupervised clustering	95% of ER status (IHC) predicted correctly (training only)	[24]
cDNA array 10 k ESTs	38 breast tumors	105	Supervised analysis	16/20 ER status (IHC) predicted correctly (validation)	[30]
cDNA array 4.5 k ESTs	38 breast tumors	98	Median difference per gene in ER + vs ER – tumors	46 genes more expressed in ER + 52 genes more expressed in ER –	[53]
cDNA array 6.728 clones	58 breast tumors	Top 100	Artificial neural networks models	100% of ER status (LBA) predicted correctly (validation)	[23]
cDNA array 8.102 clones	85 breast tumors and normal tissues	427	Differentially expressed between subtypes of breast tumors (17)	Discrimination of ER + (luminal) vs ER – tumors (basal, HER2 +, normal-like subtypes)	[17, 18]
Oligonucleotide Hu6800, Affymetrix	49 breast tumors	Top 100	Correlation coefficient per gene with ER + vs ER – tumors	8/9 ER status (IHC) predicted correctly (validation)	[52]
Oligonucleotide 44 k, Agilent	65 breast tumors and MCF-7 cell line	822	Stimulation of MCF-7 cells with estradiol	Good discrimination of relapse-free survival	[9]

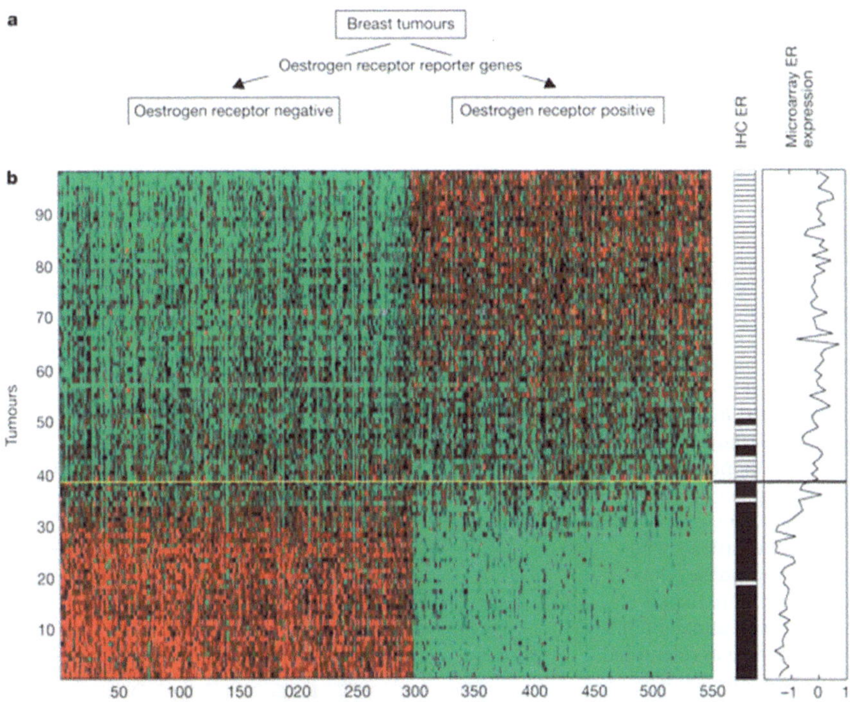

Fig. 2 Supervised classification by ER status. **a** Outline of classification system: 98 breast tumors are classified into an ER-positive and ER-negative group. **b** Expression data matrix across 550 optimal ER reporter genes. The contrasting patterns discriminate between tumors with an ER-negative signature (*below solid line*) and an ER-positive signature (*above solid line*). The reporter genes were ordered on the basis of their level of contribution to the classifier. Tumors are arranged according to the leave-one-out correlation coefficients to the average signatures of the classifier. The ER status, as determined by IHC and microarray, are indicated in the two right panels. Adapted by permission from Macmillan Publishers Ltd: Nature (van't Veer et al. copyright 2002 [24])

In addition, Dai et al. showed within a subset of young patients (<55 years) characterized by relatively high ER expression for their age (i.e., the ER/age high group) that the occurrence of metastases is strongly predicted by a homogeneous gene expression pattern almost entirely consisting of cell cycle genes [29]. By combining information on expression of ER with clinical variables such as age at diagnosis, a subgroup of patients was identified in which expression of proliferation-associated genes is a very strong predictor of outcome.

All the above findings describe the marked influence of ER and its numerous targets on gene expression in breast cancer. Expression of ER drives patterns of gene expression and dominates unsupervised analyses in breast cancer specimens studied to date, regardless of microarray platform or statistical approach.

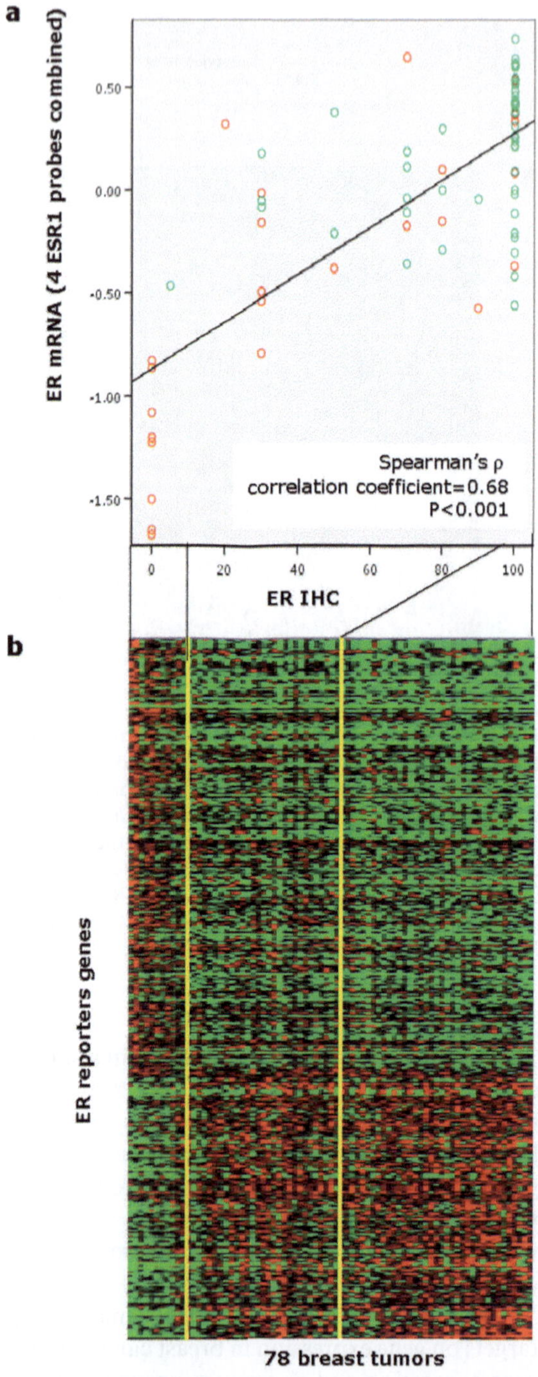

Fig. 3 Relation of ER protein expression, ER mRNA levels and the corresponding expression of ER-related genes with tamoxifen response. **a** Scatter plot depicting ER as determined by IHC (*x*-axis, % of tumor cells positive) and mRNA level (*y*-axis, calculated using four probes for ESR1 on 44 k Agilent array) expressed in log-ratio relative to reference consisting of pool of breast tumors. *Red circles* indicate patients resistant to tamoxifen in metastatic disease setting (≤6 months benefit), *green circles* indicate the patients who showed a response (clinical benefit for more than 6 months). **b** Heatmap of 385 ER-related genes (identified by mapping the 550 ER reporter gene described by van't Veer et al. to the 44 k Agilent array). Tumors ranked based on ER determined by IHC. Genes ranked based upon correlation coefficient with ESR1 as determined in dataset of van't Veer et al. *Yellow lines* group tumors in ER negative (*left*), ER low (*middle*) and ER high (*right*) (Kok et al. unpublished data; [24])

mRNA levels of ER (gene name ESR1) show strong correlation with protein expression as depicted in Fig. 3 (Kok et al. unpublished data; [17, 24, 30]). Although there is preliminary evidence that quantitative mRNA levels of ESR1 and gene lists containing ER target genes could be predictive for outcome after endocrine treatment [27], clinical application of these tests requires further investigation.

While most gene expression studies have focused on the presence or absence of ER, Creighton et al. examined RNA expression of ER+ breast cancers in relation to the presence of PR [31]. ER+/PR– breast cancer defined by gene expression profiling (i.e., tumors neither truly ER+/PR+ nor ER–/PR– but sharing expression patterns with both) tended to have poor outcome and this was not observed when using the IHC assays to determine ER and PR status. This shows that gene expression profiles may provide a clinically relevant tool to assess PR levels for diagnostic or therapeutic purposes.

Molecular Signatures Predicting Response to Endocrine Treatment

Adjuvant tamoxifen treatment reduces the breast cancer death rate with 31% in patients with ER-positive disease [32]. However, a substantial proportion of patients develop metastases despite tamoxifen treatment. Moreover, only half of the recurrences in ER-positive breast tumors respond to tamoxifen while the other half is resistant [33]. Gene expression studies have consistently confirmed the heterogeneity of ER-positive breast cancer and may provide insights into the mechanisms of response to endocrine treatment.

Current research efforts are focusing on the discovery of molecular signatures that might identify those patients most responsive to tamoxifen. The expression of ER does not guarantee functional activity and other molecular events unrelated to ER signaling can also influence sensitivity to endocrine treatment regimens. A multigene assay calculating a recurrence score (Onco*type* DX^{TM}) represents an important conceptual evolvement in the diagnosis of ER-positive breast cancer [26]. This RT-PCR-based assay was derived from 250 candidate genes selected by a literature search of the most important microarray studies in breast cancer. For the recurrence score, out of these 250, 16 genes were selected as well as 5 control genes. This assay measures ER mRNA levels in a quantitative and reproducible manner and also measures expression of several downstream ER-regulated genes (PR, bcl2 and SCUBE2) that probably contain information on functionality of ER. The same assay also quantifies HER2 expression and proliferation-associated genes (Ki67, cyclin B1 and survivin). This RT-PCR-based test has been optimized for paraffin-embedded material and has been shown to accurately identify a group of patients with excellent prognosis when treated with adjuvant tamoxifen [26, 34]. Notably, the predictive power was independent of age and tumor grade or size. A disadvantage included the preselection of genes and a subsequent algorithm that may not encompass more than quantitative ER and PR levels, proliferation and HER2 expression, all currently easy to test and hence may provide no new biological insights into tamoxifen response.

Another study, conducted in 60 ER-positive breast carcinomas treated with adjuvant tamoxifen, suggested the utility of a two-gene-index of HOXB13 and IL17BR in identifying a subset of patients who are at risk for relapse of disease [27]. In an independent dataset of patients receiving tamoxifen, Reid et al. reported that the two-gene-index failed to detect differences in outcome [35]. Taking into account that Fan and colleagues calculated the two-gene-index using microarray data, again no association with outcome was seen [20]. However, in three other large cohorts the two-gene-index showed a relation with tumor aggressiveness and response to first-line tamoxifen monotherapy for relapse of disease [36–38]. In studies of relatively small sample size, a model based on analysis of only two genes is much more likely to be sensitive to technical differences or patient selection. Further, in a substantial proportion of ER-positive tumors HOXB13 expression was below the detection level [38]. Rodriguez et al. showed by functional experiments that HOXB13 is an ER target gene and that its repression is mediated by DNA methylation in ER-positive tumors [39]. The observation by Wang et al. that HOXB13 and IL17BR expression strongly correlates with the expression of ER, PgR and HER2 as determined by the routinely used immunohistochemistry supports this regulation mechanism [40]. Independent studies will reveal whether HOXB13 and IL17BR might be useful predictive markers when used instead of immunohistochemistry or add information to the standard markers.

In addition, using Affymetrix Gene Chip arrays, investigators from the Jules Bordet Institute, Belgium, selected 62 genes by Cox proportional regression analysis to predict patients having an early relapse after adjuvant tamoxifen treatment [41]. In a large validation set, they were able to identify patients who will probably have more benefit from other endocrine approaches such as upfront treatment with aromatase inhibitors.

While the recurrence score and two-gene-index might be very helpful in predicting the likelihood of relapse of disease, a major limitation of these tests is that tamoxifen is prescribed as adjuvant treatment. A disadvantage of assessing response in the adjuvant setting is that both response of tumor cells to tamoxifen as well as intrinsic aggressiveness of the malignancy are measured. Furthermore, some resistant tumors will not recur because they were already cured by surgery and radiation. The proportion of this group of patients is unknown.

In contrast, Jansen and colleagues discovered, using cDNA microarrays, an 81-gene signature in tumors of breast cancer patients treated with tamoxifen for their metastases [42]. In this palliative setting, tumor response can be visualized. The 81 genes were found – by supervised hierarchical clustering – to be differentially expressed between tamoxifen-sensitive and tamoxifen-resistant, ER-positive breast tumors (n = 46, heatmap of genes shown in Fig. 4).

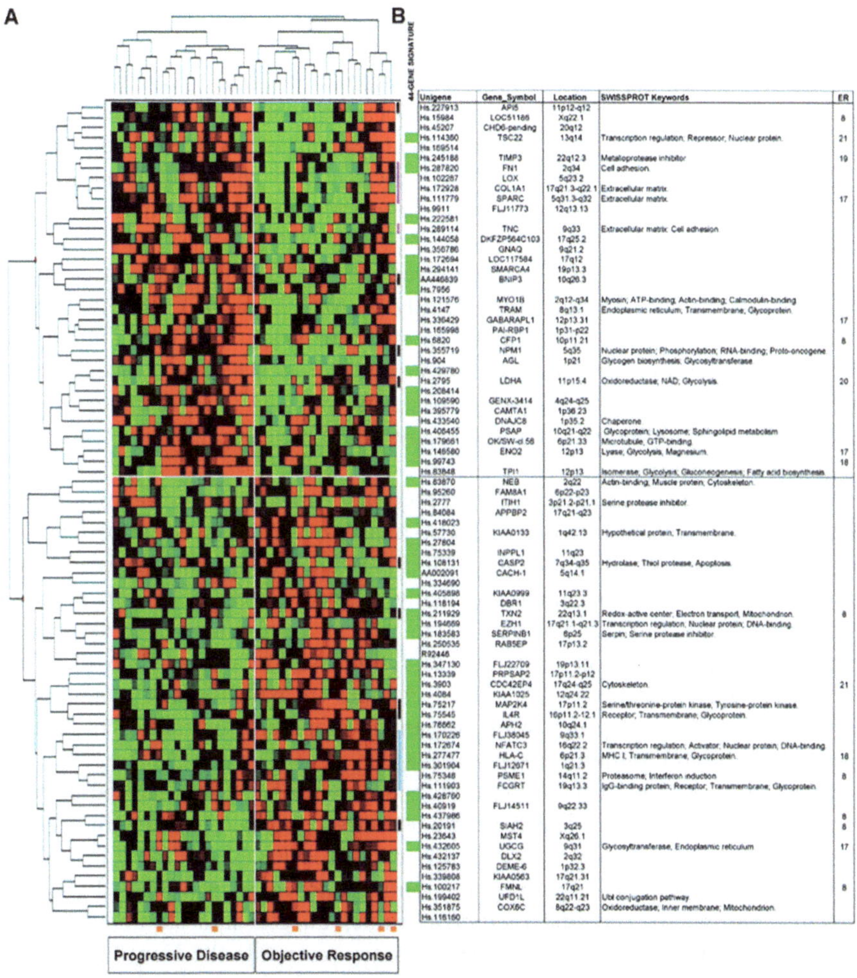

Fig. 4 Supervised clustering of tamoxifen-resistant and -sensitive breast carcinomas (n = 46) using the 81-gene signature. **a** Expression plot showing clusters of tumors with progressive disease and objective response. *Orange* bars below indicate misclassified tumors. *Red* indicates upregulated genes and *green* indicates downregulated genes. **b** Bars next to plot indicate genes of predictive signature (*green*), apoptosis (*black*), extracellular matrix (*purple*) and immune system (*blue*). Information includes cytoband location and references of estrogen function. Reprinted with permission from the American Society of Clinical Oncology: Jansen et al. [42]

Subsequently, this response profile was tested on 66 independent cases and could select patients who had a short time to tumor progression (TTP). The genes were involved in estrogen action, apoptosis, extracellular matrix formation and immune response.

Recently, these 81 genes were validated in tumor samples from another hospital using a more advanced microarray platform [43]. Combining this tamoxifen response profile with PR determined by IHC, patients with an excellent TTP could be identified. It is provocative to speculate on the predictive value of this tool if used for adjuvant treatment decisions. Identification of a subset of patients who might have more chance to be cured by tamoxifen instead of an aromatase inhibitor may open the door to more individualized medicine.

While adjuvant tamoxifen treatment reduces the risk of breast cancer death by 31% [32], aromatase inhibitors slightly prolong disease-free survival compared to tamoxifen [44], In addition, a survival benefit has been shown for sequential tamoxifen and an aromatase inhibitor [45, 46]. A molecular test helping clinicians to make a choice between starting with tamoxifen, an aromatase inhibitor or rather with chemotherapy would have enormous potential for tailoring treatment.

Mackay et al. conducted gene expression profiling on pretreatment and posttreatment biopsies of breast cancer patients who received an aromatase inhibitor for 2 weeks before surgery [47]. Profound changes in gene expression were seen after treatment, including many classical estrogen-dependent genes (TFF1, CCND1, PDZK1 and AGR2) as well as a prominent decrease in the expression of proliferation-related genes. Using a similar approach, Miller and colleagues identified letrozole-induced changes in expression in genes associated with cell cycle progression, organ development, extracellular matrix regulation and inflammatory response [48].

Since most of the aromatase inhibitors are prescribed for advanced disease after adjuvant tamoxifen, Lin et al. retrospectively studied primary tumors of this group of patients and subsequently measured levels of E2-related genes using RT-PCR [49]. An algorithm combining mRNA levels of ER, PgR and BRCA1 resulted in the best predictive value. Larger datasets and samples derived from a randomized trial are necessary to enable the identification of markers or gene signatures specifically associated with aromatase inhibitor response.

Currently, the use of microarray technology in clinical practice is being tested (EORTC trial: http://www.eortc.be/services/unit/mindact/) and we speculate that a gene expression profile predicting treatment response might provide additional information on top of measurement of nuclear receptors. Thereby, endocrine treatment decisions can be tailored, e.g., starting tamoxifen, an aromatase inhibitor or rather focus on disease control by chemotherapy. Nevertheless, most algorithms developed to predict outcome after tamoxifen are based on adjuvant treatment [26, 27, 41]. Further investigations are needed to elucidate whether these gene profiles truly predict drug response or solely prognosis. In the absence of frozen material obtained in a randomized controlled trial addressing whether a drug is effective in the adjuvant setting including a control arm with untreated patients, response to treatment can only be visualized in neoadjuvant treatment settings [50, 51] or in patients with measurable disease in metastatic disease setting [42, 43].

Perspectives

In a short period of time, analysis of gene expression in breast cancer has increased the understanding of ER signaling and the diversity of ER-positive and -negative breast cancer subtypes. However, there are still many questions remaining which could be answered by continuing research using gene expression profiling of human tumor samples.

The advantage of microarray technology is that thousands of genes can be studied at the same time instead of focusing on a single gene of interest. Regarding the genes responding to activation of ER, several lists of either putative ER targets or genes correlating with ER expression have been published [9, 16, 23, 24, 52, 53]. However, currently there is no consensus on the comprehensiveness of these gene sets. A complete overview of genes also including processes in which ER is influencing gene expressing by functioning as a transcriptional co-factor or driving other co-factors is still lacking. Furthermore, gene expression profiling is not suitable to pinpoint posttranslational modifications of ER or epigenetic regulation by ER by binding to chromatin.

While the description of breast cancer phenotypes in distinct molecular subtypes, as first portrayed by Perou and colleagues, has been exciting, further refinement of subdivision of ER-positive breast cancer is needed [17]. How to define the group of patients with a very good outcome for which systemic treatment can be safely omitted? And since some ER-positive tumors show a moderate response to chemotherapy, it will be very interesting to screen this subgroup for specific drug targets. If these can be identified, clinicians can offer endocrine treatment combined with targeted therapy.

Although the high throughput analysis of gene expression of breast cancer cells has increased the insights in the behavior of the disease, the relation with outcome and therapy response, accurate and robust validation of the candidate response profiles is necessary before clinical application. Standardization of technology and properly designed clinical trials performed at large scale will be essential. Moreover, the discrimination of the prognostic value of a set of genes, e.g., aggressiveness of tumor cells regardless of systemic treatment, versus the capacity to predict response to a specific drug needs more detailed investigation. In ideal clinical practice, a single platform will be used that is able to provide prognostic (who to treat?) as well as predictive information (how to treat?).

The perspective for the coming years is that the normal function of the ER and its downstream targets will continue to be unraveled and that combining this knowledge with gene expression profiling of breast cancers of patients in defined clinical settings will lead to diagnostic tests that can guide endocrine treatment, and finally to more insight in mechanisms underlying resistance to endocrine therapy that can help in developing novel treatment strategies.

References

1. Tan P, Downey T, Spitznagel E, Xu P, Fu D, Dimitrov D, et al. Evaluation of gene expression measurements from commercial microarray platforms. Nucl Acids Res. 2003;31:5676–84.
2. Fan JB, Gunderson KL, Bibikova M, Yeakly JM, Chen J, Wickham Garcia E, et al. Illumina universal bead arrays. Methods Enzymol. 2006;410:57–75.
3. Walker SJ, Worst TJ, Vrana KE. Semiquantitative real-time PCR for analysis of mRNA levels. Methods Mol Med. 2003;79:211–27.
4. Golub TR, Slonim DK, Tamayo P, Huard C, Gaasenbeek M, Mesirov JP, et al. Molecular classification of cancer: class discovery and class prediction by gene expression monitoring. Science. 1999;286:531–7.
5. Quackenbush J. Computational analysis of microarray data. Nat Rev Genet. 2001;2: 418–27.
6. Frasor J, Danes J, Komm B, Chang K, Lyttle CR, Katzenellenbogen B. Profiling of estrogen up- and down-regulated gene expression in human breast cancer cells: insights into gene networks and pathways underlying estrogenic control of proliferation and cell phenotype. Endocrinology. 2003;144:4562–74.
7. Frasor J, Stossi F, Danes J, Komm B, Lyttle CR, Katzenellenbogen B. Selective estrogen receptor modulators: discrimination of agonistic versus antagonistic activities by gene expression profiling in breast cancer cells. Cancer Res. 2004;64:1522–33.
8. Fan M, Yan P, Hartman-Frey C, Chen L, Paik H, Oyer S, et al. Diverse gene expression and DNA methylation profiles correlate with differential adaptation of breast cancer cells to the antiestrogens tamoxifen and fulvestrant. Cancer Res. 2006;66: 11954–66.
9. Oh D, Troester M, Usary J, Hu Z, He X, Fan C, et al. Estrogen-regulated genes predict survival in hormone receptor-positive breast cancers. J Clin Oncol. 2006;24:1656–64.
10. Tusher V, Tibshirani R, Chu G. Significance analysis of microarrays applied to the ionizing radiation response. PNAS. 2001;98:5116–21.
11. Michalides R, Griekspoor A, Balkenende A, Verwoerd D, Janssen L, Jalink K, et al. Tamoxifen resistance by a conformational arrest of the estrogen receptor [alpha] after PKA activation in breast cancer. Cancer Cell. 2004;5:597–605.
12. Zhang J, Campbell R, Ting A, Tsien R. Creating new fluorescent probes for cell biology. Nat Rev Mol Cell Biol. 2002;3:906–18.
13. Shang Y, Hu X, DiRenzo J, Lazar M, Brown M. Cofactor dynamics and sufficiency in estrogen receptor-regulated transcription. Cell. 2000;103:843–52.
14. Metivier R, Penot G, Hubner M, Reid G, Brand H, Kos M, et al. Estrogen receptor-[alpha] directs ordered, cyclical, and combinatorial recruitment of cofactors on a natural target promoter. Cell. 2003;115:751–63.
15. Carroll J, Liu XS, Brodsky A, Li W, Meyer C, Szary A, et al. Chromosome-wide mapping of estrogen receptor binding reveals long-range regulation requiring the forkhead protein FoxA1. Cell. 2005;122:33–43.
16. Carroll J, Meyer C, Song J, Li W, Geistlinger T, Eeckhoute J, et al. Genome-wide analysis of estrogen receptor binding sites. Nat Genet. 2006;38:1289–97.
17. Perou C, Sorlie T, Eisen M, van de Rijn M, Jeffrey S, Rees C, et al. Molecular portraits of human breast tumours. Nature. 2000;406:747–52.
18. Sorlie T, Perou C, Tibshirani R, Aas T, Geisler S, Johnsen H, et al. Gene expression patterns of breast carcinomas distinguish tumor subclasses with clinical implications. PNAS. 2001;98:10869–74.
19. Sorlie T, Tibshirani R, Parker J, Hastie T, Marron JS, Nobel A, et al. Repeated observation of breast tumor subtypes in independent gene expression data sets. PNAS. 2003;100:8418–23.
20. Fan C, Oh D, Wessels L, Weigelt B, Nuyten D, Nobel A, et al. Concordance among gene-expression-based predictors for breast cancer. N Engl J Med. 2006;355:560–9.

21. Sotiriou C, Wirapati P, Loi S, Harris A, Fox S, Smeds J, et al. Gene expression profiling in breast cancer: understanding the molecular basis of histologic grade to improve prognosis. J Natl Cancer Inst. 2006;98:262–72.
22. Loi S, Haibe-Kains B, Desmedt C, Lallemand F, Tutt A, Gillet C, et al. Definition of clinically distinct molecular subtypes in estrogen receptor-positive breast carcinomas through genomic grade. J Clin Oncol. 2007;25:1239–46.
23. Gruvberger S, Ringner M, Chen Y, Panavally S, Saal L, Borg A, et al. Estrogen receptor status in breast cancer is associated with remarkably distinct gene expression patterns. Cancer Res. 2001;61:5979–84.
24. van't Veer L, Dai H, van de Vijver M, He Y, Hart A, Mao M, et al. Gene expression profiling predicts clinical outcome of breast cancer. Nature. 2002;415:530–6.
25. van de Vijver M, He Y, van't Veer L, Dai H, Hart A, Voskuil D, et al. A gene-expression signature as a predictor of survival in breast cancer. N Engl J Med. 2002;347:1999–2009.
26. Paik S, Shak S, Tang G, Kim C, Baker J, Cronin M, et al. A multigene assay to predict recurrence of tamoxifen-treated, node-negative breast cancer. N Engl J Med. 2004;351: 2817–26.
27. Ma X, Wang Z, Ryan P, Isakoff S, Barmettler A, Fuller A, et al. A two-gene expression ratio predicts clinical outcome in breast cancer patients treated with tamoxifen. Cancer Cell. 2004;5:607–16.
28. Wang Y, Klijn J, Zhang Y, Sieuwerts A, Look M, Yang F, et al. Gene-expression profiles to predict distant metastasis of lymph-node-negative primary breast cancer. Lancet. 2005;365:671–9.
29. Dai H, van't Veer L, Lamb J, He Y, Mao M, Fine B, et al. A cell proliferation signature is a marker of extremely poor outcome in a subpopulation of breast cancer patients. Cancer Res. 2005;65:4059–66.
30. Pusztai L, Ayers M, Stec J, Clark E, Hess K, Stivers D, et al. Gene expression profiles obtained from fine-needle aspirations of breast cancer reliably identify routine prognostic markers and reveal large-scale molecular differences between estrogen-negative and estrogen-positive tumors. Clin Cancer Res. 2003;9:2406–15.
31. Creighton CJ, Osborne CK, van de Vijver M, Foekens J, Wang Y, et al. Gene expression profiles of ER+/PR– breast cancer are associated with genomic instability and Akt/mTOR signaling, and predict poor patient outcome better than clinically assigned PR status. Breast Cancer Res Treat. 2007;106:S10.
32. Effects of chemotherapy and hormonal therapy for early breast cancer on recurrence and 15-year survival: an overview of the randomised trials. Early breast cancer trialists' group. Lancet. 2005;365:1687–717.
33. Pritchard K. Endocrine therapy of advanced disease: analysis and implications of the existing data. Clin Cancer Res. 2003;9:460S–7S.
34. Paik S, Shak S, Tang G, Kim C, Joo H, Baker J, et al. Expression of the 21 genes in the Recurrence Score assay and prediction of clinical benefit from tamoxifen in NSABP study B-14 and chemotherapy in NSABP study B-20. J Clin Oncol. 2005;23:16S.
35. Reid J, Lusa L, De Cecco L, Coradini D, Veneroni S, Daidone M, et al. Limits of predictive models using microarray data for breast cancer clinical treatment outcome. J Natl Cancer Inst. 2005;97:927–30.
36. Ma X, Hilsenbeck S, Wang W, Ding L, Sgroi D, Bender R, et al. The HOXB13:IL17BR expression index is a prognostic factor in early-stage breast cancer. J Clin Oncol. 2006;24:4611–9.
37. Goetz M, Suman V, Ingle J, Nibbe A, Visscher D, Reynolds C, et al. A two-gene expression ratio of homeobox 13 and interleukin-17B receptor for prediction of recurrence and survival in women receiving adjuvant tamoxifen. Clin Cancer Res. 2006;12: 2080–7.

38. Jansen MP, Sieuwerts AM, Look MP, Ritstier K, Meijer-van Gelder ME, van Staveren IL, et al. HOXB13-to-IL17BR expression ratio is related with tumor aggressiveness and response to tamoxifen of recurrent breast cancer: a retrospective study. J Clin Oncol. 2007;25:662–8.
39. Rodriguez B, Jin V, Cheng A, Davuluri R, Gray J, Huang T. HOXB13 is an estrogen receptor responsive gene preferentially methylated in ER-positive breast cancer. AACR Meeting Abstracts. 2006;2006:377.
40. Wang Z, Dahiya S, Provencher H, Muir B, Carney E, Coser K, et al. The prognostic biomarkers HOXB13, IL17BR, and CHDH are regulated by estrogen in breast cancer. Clin Cancer Res. 2007;13:6327–34.
41. Loi S, Piccart MJ, Desmedt C. Prediction of early distant relapses on tamoxifen in early-breast cancer (BC): a potential tool for adjuvant aromatase inhibitors (AI) tailoring. Proc Am Soc Clin Oncol. 2005;23.
42. Jansen M, Foekens J, van Staveren I, Dirkzwager-Kiel M, Ritstier K, Look M, et al. Molecular classification of tamoxifen-resistant breast carcinomas by gene expression profiling. J Clin Oncol. 2005;23:732–40.
43. Kok M, Linn S, Wessels L, Jansen M, Van den Berg TM, Delahaye L, et al. Robust independent validation of the 81-gene breast cancer tamoxifen response profile. Breast Cancer Res Treat. 2006;100.
44. Results of the ATAC (Arimidex, Tamoxifen, Alone or in Combination) trial after completion of 5 years' adjuvant treatment for breast cancer. ATAC trialists' group. Lancet. 2005;365:60–2.
45. Jonat W, Gnant M, Boccardo F, Kaufmann M, Rubagotti A, Zuna I, et al. Effectiveness of switching from adjuvant tamoxifen to anastrozole in postmenopausal women with hormone-sensitive early-stage breast cancer: a meta-analysis. Lancet Oncol. 2006;7: 991–6.
46. Coombes RC, Kilburn LS, Snowdon CF, Paridaens R, Coleman RE, Jones SE, et al. Survival and safety of exemestane versus tamoxifen after 2–3 years' tamoxifen treatment (Intergroup Exemestane Study): a randomised controlled trial. Lancet. 369:559–70.
47. Mackay A, Urruticoechea A, Dixon JM, Dexter T, Fenwick K, Ashworth A, et al. Molecular response to aromatase inhibitor treatment in primary breast cancer. Breast Cancer Res. 2007;9:R37.
48. Miller W, Larionov A, Renshaw L, Anderson T, White S, Murray J, et al. Changes in breast cancer transcriptional profiles after treatment with the aromatase inhibitor, letrozole. Pharmacogenet Genomics. 2007;17:813–26.
49. Lin Z, Reierstad S, Cotteril H, Rademaker A, Khan S, Haynes B, et al. Messenger RNA levels of estrogen-related genes in malignant breast tumor tissue predict responsiveness to aromatase inhibitors. Breast Cancer Res Treat. 2006;100:S9.
50. Chang J, Wooten E, Tsimelzon A, Hilsenbeck S, Gutierrez MC, Elledge R, et al. Gene expression profiling for the prediction of therapeutic response to docetaxel in patients with breast cancer. Lancet. 2003;362:362–9.
51. Hannemann J, Oosterkamp H, Bosch C, Velds A, Wessels L, Loo C, et al. Changes in gene expression associated with response to neoadjuvant chemotherapy in breast cancer. J Clin Oncol. 2005;23:3331–42.
52. West M, Blanchette C, Dressman H, Huang E, Ishida S, Spang R, et al. Predicting the clinical status of human breast cancer by using gene expression profiles. PNAS. 2001;98:11462–7.
53. Nagai MA, Da Ros N, Neto MM. Gene expression profiles in breast tumors regarding the presence or absence of estrogen and progesterone receptors. Int J Cancer. 2004;111: 892–9.

Index

Q

R

X

MIX
Papier aus verantwortungsvollen Quellen
Paper from responsible sources
FSC® C105338

If you have any concerns about our products,
you can contact us on
ProductSafety@springernature.com

In case Publisher is established outside the EU,
the EU authorized representative is:
Springer Nature Customer Service Center GmbH
Europaplatz 3, 69115 Heidelberg, Germany

Printed by Libri Plureos GmbH
in Hamburg, Germany